Advance Praise for *In the FLO*

"When I first heard Alisa explain the Cycle Syncing Method, I was floored. As someone who has struggled with hormones, I couldn't believe what we don't know about our bodies. I didn't realize how my everyday routine was affecting my mood, my weight, and my energy. Working with Alisa has shown me how to take care of my biological rhythms so I stay in a peak flow state. It's given me back my energy, made me a happier mom, and made me passionate about sharing this information with other women—it's about time for us to get *In the FLO*."

> —Gabrielle Union-Wade, actor, activist, and *New York Times* bestselling author of *We're Going to Need More Wine*

"Living in alignment with our cycle is the next frontier for women's health. Alisa's book provides a tool for reconnecting with your unique female biorhythms—a powerful offering toward helping women reclaim hormone health and much-needed life balance."

> —Aviva Romm, MD, author of *The Adrenal Thyroid Revolution*

"This book teaches you how to use your biology to tune in to your inner guidance and to create optimal flow in every area of your life. It offers a path toward your highest power and potential."

> —Gabrielle Bernstein, #1 *New York Times* bestselling author of *The Universe Has Your Back*

"*In the FLO* is Whole30 meets Bulletproof meets 4-Hour Workweek—but designed exclusively for a woman's body. This book will change the way you eat, work out, manage your time, and do your work—all in harmony with your body! It's the next wave in women's health and, best of all, there aren't any complicated rules to follow—it's liberating and logical. Alisa will help you achieve your optimal health and live your best life."

> —JJ Virgin, nutrition expert and *New York Times* bestselling author of *The Virgin Diet*

"Alisa is a true pioneer in biohacking for women, and the Cycle Syncing Method is an effective way for women to align with their biological rhythms to optimize not only their health but every other aspect of their lives from career to relationships to motherhood. Every woman should read this book!"

> —Mark Hyman, MD, *New York Times* bestselling author of *The Blood Sugar Solution*

"Trying to operate on a 24-hour clock can leave moms exhausted. Alisa's revolutionary cyclical time management method will liberate you from the stress and exhaustion of trying to 'do it all' and instead adopt a more sustainable approach. Finally you'll replace guilt over all the things you aren't doing with guidance on the best ways to bond with your child and care for yourself week by week."

—**Shefali Tsabary, PhD, psychologist, educator, speaker, and** *New York Times* **bestselling author of** *The Conscious Parent*

"In this must-read hormonal guidebook, Alisa Vitti takes readers on a fascinating voyage inside the female body and brain to demystify the science of hormones. And she lays out a one-of-a-kind nutrition and lifestyle plan to balance hormones so you can think smarter, feel better, and stress less. Your body and brain will thank you for it."

—**Daniel Amen, MD, psychiatrist, neuroscientist, and** *New York Times* **bestselling author of** *Unleash the Power of the Female Brain*

"Alisa walks you through the miraculous wonder that is your female body and how to connect your health, career, and even sex and relationships with your cycle to achieve amazing results *with less effort*—better orgasms included."

—**Regena Thomashauer,** *New York Times* **bestselling author of** *Pussy: A Reclamation*

IN THE FLO

ALSO BY ALISA VITTI

WomanCode

IN THE FLO

UNLOCK YOUR HORMONAL ADVANTAGE
AND REVOLUTIONIZE YOUR LIFE

ALISA VITTI

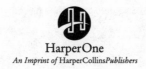

HarperOne
An Imprint of HarperCollins*Publishers*

HarperOne

This book contains advice and information relating to health care. It should be used to supplement rather than replace the advice of your doctor or another trained health professional. If you know or suspect you have a health problem, it is recommended that you seek your physician's advice before embarking on any medical program or treatment. All efforts have been made to ensure the accuracy of the information contained in this book as of the date of publication. This publisher and the author disclaim liability for any medical outcomes that may occur as a result of applying the methods suggested in this book.

FIRST EDITION

Designed by Terry McGrath

Library of Congress Cataloging-in-Publication Data has been applied for.

ISBN 978-0-06-287048-3

20 21 22 23 24   LSC   10 9 8 7 6 5 4 3 2 1

"Those who flow as life flows know they need no other force."
LAO TZU

This book is dedicated to my daughter, Ariana.
May you always know the gifts of nature that you contain
and the force of nature that you are.

CONTENTS

Part 3 Getting Your Life in the FLO

FEEL BETTER AND LIVE SMARTER WITH *IN THE FLO*

I've created a special bundle of resources to help you put into action what you learn in this book, including a **quick-start program** to help you get started, a **bonus self-care guide,** a **community** where you can connect with other readers, special **downloads,** and more! You can access everything for free at www.IntheFLObook.com/bonus.

Introduction

What's the greatest lesson a woman should learn? That
since day one, she's already had everything she needs within
herself. It's the world that convinced her she did not.
—RUPI KAUR

I remember from a young age hearing from multiple sources that to succeed as a woman you have to work hard—twice as hard as a man, in fact. Early on, I felt a drive to do as much as I could and to push myself. In school, I took all of the hardest classes, worked for top grades, and was involved in activities to develop my creative talents and practice leading teams. These are all admirable pursuits—but I noticed that my drive came with a cost. In high school I was regularly up past midnight trying to complete homework. I was spread as thin as I could be, and now, looking back, I can see the toll it was taking on my body. The pressure I felt to perform, create, achieve, and work only grew, however, as I continued on through college and into my career. All the while, my health issues became more problematic. My anxiety went from occasional to constant, my insomnia became a nightly problem, I was gaining weight despite being active daily, my skin was breaking out, my periods were missing, and I felt more and more overwhelmed by all that I had to do. Instead of being invigorated by the things I wanted to do, I felt unable to tackle them and drained. I criticized myself for procrastination, for inefficient time management, and for not having my body and my life perfectly together. I tried diets, workouts, and planners, and I bought every inspirational book I thought might help me figure out how to do it all. I see my struggles reflected all the time in the lives of other women—and the fact is we're working long hours but struggling to get everything done, caretaking children and friends with little time left over to rest, exercising constantly but not seeing results, trying to eat well but still feeling blah—and we find we have less and less energy left to create our best work, nurture our relationships, and access our joy for life in general. We're all looking for a way to make everything more doable, but doing everything still leaves us feeling like somehow we've failed.

Our culture forces us to keep pushing, pushing, pushing. We overstretch ourselves, our expectations, our bodies, and our time. We race breathlessly to keep up with never-ending to-do lists, put everybody else's needs first, and juggle career and family. We look outside ourselves—relying on magazine articles or male-centered health research—for healthy living strategies rather than listening to the inner wisdom of our biochemistry.

As a result, our physical health is deteriorating. Fibroids, endometriosis, polycystic ovary syndrome (PCOS), infertility, low sex drive, premature ovarian failure (POF), and challenging perimenopause are all on the rise. Chronic stress takes a toll on our bodies, our abilities to pursue our dreams, and our bonds with the people we love. At our deepest levels, we feel we're not good enough, not smart enough, not organized enough to achieve what we desire in our lives.

What if I told you that there was a secret blueprint you've had available to you for years—a simple way to be more powerful and more effective in all areas of your life? Not only have you been ignoring it, you've viewed it as a liability. You've even tried to override this powerful tool, unintentionally dampening its force and causing it to work against you. As a result, it's sapping your energy, making you sick, and holding you back from getting everything you want—and deserve—in life.

The secret isn't really a secret—it's been within you all along. I'll cut right to the chase: your female biochemistry, and more specifically, your hormonal cycle—the one you probably lament on a monthly basis—is an incredible asset. Think of it as our unique and miraculous female advantage. It's a game-changing tool we can use to empower every aspect of our lives—if we will only leverage it.

The problem is, we've been taught the opposite about our hormonal cycle. From the moment women get our first periods, we're told about the cramps, the premenstrual syndrome (PMS), the burden our bodies must now take on. From a young age, we're taught to feel ashamed rather than empowered by our bodies. Something that is so fundamental to us—our biochemistry, our reproductive system, our menstrual cycle—is twisted into "the curse" that we must hide or "deal with" rather than celebrate and use. We've been conditioned to ignore our hormonal cycle until something goes wrong with it. Then we treat it like an adversary that needs to be tamed with medication or other interventions so we can go back to ignoring it. This treatment has created a dysfunctional relationship with our hormones, our bodies, and ourselves—obliterating the power of our hormones and rendering them ineffective at best and a stumbling block at worst.

The good news is, with some simple lifestyle tweaks you can tap into this natural power source to biohack your way to better health and fitness, enhance your productivity, master time management, and enjoy greater success in every area of your life. Best of all, it's really easy (compared with exhausting yourself trying to cram as much as possible into your day, striving to accomplish impossible to-do lists, and ignoring your most basic physical needs). By living, eating, and working in synchrony with your cyclical nature rather than fighting against it, you can unleash your creativity, fire up your energy, strengthen your relationships, and even be a better mom (if you're a mom). You'll use time strategically instead of being a slave to your calendar, increasing your energy and ultimately getting more done with fewer struggles. You'll tap into that elusive sensation of "flow"—that incredible feeling you have when everything just clicks. You'll be able to reframe your concept of success to feel great about yourself rather than tear yourself down. You'll intuitively understand how to manage stress, increase self-satisfaction, quiet your inner critical voice, improve your health, and empower yourself to become productive and efficient in ways that are sustainable for you.

All this is achievable, but we can't access our full potential when we're living by someone else's rules and not listening to the wisdom within. Simply put, we are round pegs trying to fit ourselves into square holes—no wonder we're exhausted. We live out of sync with our unique female brain and body chemistry; we don't eat in a pro-hormonal way that gives our endocrine system the building blocks it needs to keep our hormones balanced, and too often we're prescribed medications like synthetic hormones that further prevent us from accessing the inherent gifts inside our bodies that could help us live our best lives. Our non-female-centric diet and lifestyle put a strain on a system that is perfectly equipped by nature to keep our hormones balanced and health optimized. Being out of sync with our female chemistry weakens our thyroid, our ovaries, our livers, our adrenals, our immunity, and our digestion. In fact, being out of sync weakens everything about our physical health, makes our thinking foggy, and takes us out of our creative zone.

The truth is, all the cultural myths about women's bodies—that we are inherently weaker, more vulnerable to aging, less worthy of study—are BS. We've been sold a lie—harmful propaganda that says our body and biochemistry are a disadvantage. It's time to flip the script. I've pioneered the groundbreaking Cycle Syncing Method™ to empower women, finally, to use their hormones in ways that are nothing short of revolutionary.

Syncing with your cycle is all about knowing where you are in your menstrual cycle and using that knowledge to understand yourself better and support yourself as hormone levels change. In my first best-selling book, *WomanCode*, I shared the eye-opening message that you could put your hormonal problems—think PMS, PCOS, fibroids, and endometriosis—into remission naturally with food and diet changes. I knew this message would create an "aha moment" for many women, but I was absolutely blown away by the response. What I learned from the hundreds of thousands of women who have reached out to me since then—at our center, at wellness conferences where I speak, via social media, and through the MyFLO app—was even more important. Listening to their stories, I realized there was a much bigger message to share—that the false notions about our female biochemistry have robbed us of far more than just our hormonal health. They've stolen our confidence, our vitality, and the very opportunity to live our best lives.

Enough!

The time to reclaim your female biochemistry is now. You just need to learn how to start tapping into its power. This book will help you do it. Drawing on leading-edge research in the fields of neuroendocrinology, functional medicine, nutritional genomics, chronobiology, integrative nutrition, and behavioral psychology, this book will explore the intersection of hormones, neurochemistry, and productivity—all in an effort to allow you to reconnect with the feminine advantage that resides within you. The book will also give you a new female-centered paradigm to manage your time and productivity more effortlessly, in ways specifically tailored to your female needs.

Once you have the foundational, perspective-shifting knowledge needed to reverse the cultural conditioning that's been holding us back, I'll break down the four phases of your hormonal cycle and how they affect your brain, moods, energy, and behaviors. You'll learn how to care for yourself in each unique phase and harness strengths around your creativity, energy, emotions, and sexuality. I'll also introduce you to a female-centered form of time management that works with your hormonal phases to help you get more done with less stress and get more enjoyment out of everything you do. In other words, we'll throw out living exclusively by the standard 24-hour clock (which—no surprise—happens to be in alignment with the male hormonal cycle) and shift to a more sustainable 28-day approach. This book provides a clear plan to biohack your health and fitness in ways that are specifically tailored to your unique biochemistry, and offers tips to help you bring these insights beyond self-care and personal time management, into your interactions with the larger world around you. Believe me, we get into the nitty-gritty. You'll know on what day to ask for that promotion, the best time to do yoga or cardio, when to double up on leafy greens, the best week to spend time being introspective and gentle with yourself, and when to unleash your social butterfly.

The book also provides a planner and evaluation tool to help you engage this superpower, and teaches you how to heal the root causes of your hormone imbalances to create a lifestyle that keeps you from being vulnerable to new imbalances, and lets you harness your body's innate patterns as a tool for peak productivity, flow, and happiness. Even if you aren't suffering from hormonal imbalance, you can benefit from tuning in to your female biochemistry to help you achieve more with less stress.

I teach women of all ages all across the world how to use the Cycle Syncing Method™ every day—and their hormonal health and lives are transforming in ways they never dreamed possible. (Take note: you can engage this cycle even if you're postmenopausal or are no longer bleeding.) Whether you're coming to this book to relieve health issues, decrease stress, or just to figure out how to live your best life, there's something here for you.

This is the right book for you if any of these statements rings true:

- You feel like you are always trying to do it all, but there's never enough time.
- You strive to give 100 percent in every area of your life, but it's hard to keep up with your own expectations.
- You want to be more creative, more enterprising, more consistent, but you feel like you start and then don't follow through.
- You have tried every kind of planner to be more organized.
- You've tried every diet and fitness program and don't get the results you want.
- You're interested in biohacking, but not sure where to start.
- You feel continually drained and overwhelmed by all the commitments in your life.
- You want to be having more fun and pleasure in your life, but you struggle to stay up with your to-do list and often feel like you haven't earned enjoyment.
- You have PMS, PCOS, fibroids, endometriosis, ovarian cysts, infertility, or any other period problems.
- You've already seen functional medicine doctors *and* your regular ob-gyn and tried everything—acupuncture, in vitro fertilization (IVF), birth control, other medications, antidepressants, skincare treatments, diuretics for bloating, ibuprofen for cramps—and you're still not getting the results you want.

- You're eating a healthy diet but you're still having symptoms.
- You're a mom with a tween or teen struggling with her period, skin, weight, or moods.
- You are in the first half of perimenopause and are experiencing symptoms.
- You're not enjoying your relationship or sex life as much as you'd like to be.
- You feel disconnected from your body or feminine energy.
- You think being a woman means you're destined to suffer.
- You want to live your best life, but need a sustainable way to do it.

IS THIS BOOK FOR YOU?

This book is written for women, but some people who identify as women may not have the biochemical or physical makeup being explored here. What if you're trans, nonbinary, or taking estrogen or testosterone as you undergo gender transition? You may not fit into a traditional gender box. However you self-identify or wherever you are in your gender journey, understand that working with your unique reality is a gift that is available to everyone. How should you approach using the Cycle Syncing Method™ if you're transgender, for example? For people transitioning to female, following this program may help you feel more connected to your feminine energy even if you're not menstruating. For those who are transitioning to male but still menstruating, you may prefer to get in tune with the more linear, 24-hour male pattern. In that case, you may not want to follow a cyclical program. The bottom line is that it's entirely up to you.

In these pages, you'll meet some of the amazing real-life women who have adopted this program and not only have found solutions to their hormonal problems, but also have unlocked their potential—gaining the confidence to do the things they'd always dreamed of doing. You can gain this confidence, too.

Once you understand the concept, it's all very simple. You just need to cut through the misinformation and turn on the power of your body and the time it keeps. After reading this book, you will take with you the scientific understanding, the tactical plan, and the inspiration to change your life immediately.

In addition to these practical benefits for your health and productivity, you'll gain the opportunity to come home to yourself—to heal the wounds of feminine disconnection. We have tried to survive in a noninclusive culture for too long by compromising too much of ourselves. We don't have to squeeze ourselves into this paradigm. What women are in desperate need of now is a female-centered framework for how to live. That's where this book comes in.

This book:

- will give you the freedom and permission to do what's right for you more of the time.
- will end the confusion about how your hormones work and how they affect more than your period and fertility so you'll know what to expect and what your hormonal advantages are.
- will teach you to biohack so hormonal issues never sideline you again.
- will give you a blueprint to use your hormonal advantages to create a life of more ease, joy, and flow.

In chapter 1, you'll discover the truth about the amazing female body and unlearn some of the misinformation that's been keeping us confused, ashamed, and struggling with an array of health issues. You'll hear about my own hormonal saga and understand why we're so often misunderstood and misdiagnosed.

Chapter 2 will describe the differences between the 24-hour circadian clock and the 28-day infradian clock (yes, there are two!), offering you a new approach to time management, productivity, and success that will help you step off the proverbial treadmill and start living in sync with your natural rhythms.

Chapter 3 will explore the workings of the female system and show you how your hormones affect your moods, brain chemistry, immune system, energy, and more. The chapter will remind you that whenever negative voices pipe up to deny the power of your female system, it's just cultural conditioning—*not* fact—that leads you to doubt the workings of your body. Science proves nature intended you to be in sync with your cycle, so you can be confident in embracing this new female-centered way of living.

In chapters 4, 5, and 6, you'll discover how to apply the simple, female-centered Cycle Syncing Method™ around diet, fitness, and time management. This is where biohacking meets self-care. You'll learn how to use food to support your hormones during each phase of your cycle, reveal the secrets to getting better results with less sweat, and introduce you to planning tools that will help you achieve more with less effort.

A Biohacking Tool Kit following chapter 6 introduces you to approachable steps to balance your uniquely female hormones and neurochemistry to troubleshoot period, fertility, and other hormonal problems to transform your cycle into a source of empowerment and wisdom rather than pain. I want to help you solve your period issues, so you can start accessing the amazing benefits of living in sync with your cycle!

Chapter 7 shows you how to navigate your work life and reenvision productivity and success through the lens of cyclical living and your four-part creative cycle, so you can work in a more sustainable way—whether you're an entry-level employee trying to chart your career path, an entrepreneur in the trenches of the start-up phase, a corporate exec leading a team of hundreds, or a volunteer in the nonprofit sector trying to make a difference in the world.

Chapter 8 debunks the myths we've all learned about love and sex and delivers the ultimate guide to communication, connection, intimacy, orgasm, and foreplay—all based on your hormonal cycle.

In Chapter 9, you'll find out how to let go of the pressure to be the perfect mom at all times and discover how to embrace the different emotional realities of all four phases of your cycle.

Chapter 10 encourages you to embrace your feminine energy and tap into your power, because your health, success, relationships, and daughters are counting on you.

The Cyclical Promise

This is more than a book. It's a language and a model for female-centered living. It's a reclamation and a positive galvanizing force for women today to truly embrace ourselves, making our point of view and our bodies the center point of our self-reference. This book will be the catalyst for an entirely new lifestyle for you regardless of your background, age, or stage in life. We're not meant to be in perpetual productivity mode, pushing all the time for results. Nothing in nature works that way. We simply need to get back into sync with the four-part blueprint that our female body maps out for us. Then and only then will we be able to pursue the life we're meant to live as women—liberated and free.

Once you discover this blueprint for yourself, you might wonder why we aren't taught this as young women. Wouldn't it be amazing to know all this from puberty onward? How much more strategically could you design your life with your best interests at the center? As frustrating as these revelations might be, they motivate us to work toward a better future for ourselves and for women and girls to come.

Now is a pivotal moment to seize this opportunity. Times are changing—we're in the midst of a long overdue, much-needed shift in our perceptions of our bodies and in our expectations regarding our health care. In the past few years, in large part thanks to millennials taking to social media, we're realizing some key things:

1. The taboos and myths surrounding menstrual periods are outdated, false, and a tool of patriarchal oppression that holds us back.
2. Hormones affect everything beyond our periods—our moods, creativity, energy, and more.
3. Our menstrual needs are not being effectively addressed by conventional health care services.
4. Our hormonal cycle is not being adequately factored into emerging conversations in functional medicine and biohacking, or medical research.

As we work to reduce gender disparity in the workplace and in society in general, this desire for adequate care for our hormonal needs might be the final frontier of smashing the patriarchy. After menstrual mainstreaming, women deserve more: more transparency in information about birth control side effects, more health care options for menstrual problems, more gender-tailored biohacking suggestions and research.

We deserve better.

We deserve to live on our own terms and on our own time.

PART I

OUR BODIES, OUR TIME

It takes years as a woman to unlearn
what you have been taught to be sorry for.

—AMY POEHLER

CHAPTER 1

Ending Your Mys-education

Girls are taught to view their bodies as unending projects
to work on, whereas boys from a young age are taught to
view their bodies as tools to master the environment.
—GLORIA STEINEM

I remember it vividly—the day we were finally getting to the human reproduction section of our textbook in eighth-grade biology class. I loved my
teacher, Mr. Bing. I loved school. And I loved biology most of all. For me, it
represented the intersection of philosophy, art, and nature—I was perfectly
suited to its study. I was expecting a banner day in class. We began as we always did, with Mr. Bing giving a brief introduction to the subject, followed
by a fifteen-minute period to read the related section in the textbook, then
discussion, questions, and a project assignment. In the past, these assignments included replicating a DNA model, making a cross-section of a cell,
and dissecting cow eyeballs and frogs. One of my favorite projects involved
selecting a tree to observe from winter to spring bloom and collecting sam-
ples of the development from bud to flower, pressing them, and sketching
the components of the plants. The project taught me a lot about the natural
rhythm of life—waiting for a tiny seed to grow, then watching it bloom and
finally wither away. That lesson stuck with me, but as much as I liked that
one, this day's subject was on a whole other level. I sat at my desk, barely
able to control my excitement as Mr. Bing introduced the topic—human

reproduction. Then I got down to reading. It just so happened that, sequentially, we read about sperm production first. The language was potent—it
read something like:

> The testes are powerhouses of efficient production. They produce two to
> three hundred million spermatozoa daily. Each sperm itself is a perfect deliv-
> ery system for genetic material to the egg—the shape, the tail, the nutrients
> that give the sperm its mobility and motility—all in perfect concert for its
> ultimate goal—getting to the egg first to share genes.

"Wow! Nature is brilliant by design, and if I had balls, I'd be proud," I
thought.

I moved on to the section about women's reproduction. I couldn't wait
to read about the incredible inner workings of my own body. But what I got
was something like this:

> After the development and release of one egg from the ovary, the female re-
> productive process is twofold. In the case of conception, the lining thickens,
> the uterus grows, the placenta forms, and the miracle of life begins in the safe
> confines of the womb. If not, then the lining sheds and is lost and the cycle
> begins again.

"That's it?" I thought.

I was struck by the change in tone, the light treatment of the process, and
the glossing over of the major things we do—you know, bleed and not die,
and—oh yeah—3-D print tiny humans. No biggie! The textbook hinted at
disappointment if we didn't conceive. It painted our hormonal process as
belonging in value only to those outside of us—men for procreation, and
babies for the 3-D printing. Sure, I was only fourteen—what did I know?
But I was the girl who was so fascinated and excited about this phase of
my life that I had started the "Period Club" with my three best friends a
few years earlier after our very first sex ed class in sixth grade. The Period
Club had two main functions: (1) to share guesses about which member
would get her period first, and (2) to justify frequent trips to the bathroom
during lunch and recess to see whether any of us had started bleeding. I was
years into being awestruck by the thought of my approaching womanhood.

I took the sex ed textbook's lackluster description of the female system personally. I found it hurtful.

And the disconnect didn't stop there. I would encounter this same weird tone and deeply disturbing oversight of the obvious power of our bodies in every context describing our biological process as my studies progressed over the years—from Mr. Bing's biology class to the hallowed halls of Johns Hopkins University, where I went to college for my undergraduate degree. From the mechanical descriptions of how long a "normal" cycle should be, to the time frame given for dilation of the cervix during labor—all was presented in a dry, clinical way that was definitely not empowering for women. The insidious implication, of course, was that if we deviated from that standard performance, we were abnormal disappointments of nature and needed medical intervention.

What I read didn't just make me feel hurt. I was pissed. Where was the description matching the positive view of sperm production? I wanted to see a description that read like this:

The female reproductive system is the crowning achievement of human evolution and reproduction. Efficient and highly adaptable, seven hormones work in symphonic relationship to cause four highly refined processes to take place in a given monthly cycle: the development of multiple follicles, ovulation, the building of the lining of the uterus (to prepare for possible conception), and the release of that lining when conception does not occur. When conception does occur, the process of gestation is absolutely breathtaking. The rate of growth of the fetus made possible by changes in the woman's hormones, immune function, and metabolism is astonishing. And the fact that this process is also beneficial to the mother is remarkable as well. The process of labor and delivery—one that seems to pose extreme physical danger—is the peak example of how women's bodies transform into a channel of power to safely deliver the baby and preserve themselves. The female body, biologically potent, supports this menstrual and reproductive process by being the more efficient extractor of micronutrients from food, by having the more developed immune system, by having a slightly slower metabolic system to retain nutrients for as long as possible before the elimi-

nation system gets to them, and by having more connections of nerve fibers between the two hemispheres of the brain. This biological precision ensures that a woman is sensitive to herself, her body, her community, and her environment, so she can make the best decisions for her well-being, as she is the one privileged by nature's design to carry the intense responsibility of creating the next generation of humans. And when not creating a human, all of these same systems support her in being a strong and attuned leader in her community and in the world.

The fact that this isn't what young people—both girls and boys—are taught is tragic and JUST. SO. WRONG. As someone who has spent her life studying the female hormonal symphony and who has dedicated her career to helping women get in sync with their cycles, I can tell you that any less awe-inspiring description does not capture the truth—not even close.

Many years passed before I stumbled upon the reason that the female reproductive process wasn't described in all its glory, the way it should be. What I discovered floored me. Quite simply, acknowledging the power of the female reproductive process would shift the power dynamics in our global culture. If we all agreed that, biologically, women are not the weaker sex, then pretty much everything about our societal norms would have to change to make space for women to have equal footing. And it seems the patriarchy hasn't been interested in this happening. You don't need me to tell you about the thousands of years of female oppression across every culture. But it's eye-opening to realize that even the education we receive about our bodies—from how it's described in textbooks to how it's handled (or pejoratively represented) in the medical community—not only supports and deepens that oppression, but worse, also makes women complicit as self-oppressors. If we believe that we're destined to suffer and that we shouldn't expect our bodies to function symptom-free, we won't believe that we have any power to improve our hormonal functioning.

When we do not know what is really going on with our bodies—when our biology is our blind spot—we don't have our own legs to stand on. We don't know who we are. We don't grow up believing we are gifted by nature's design to be fully equipped to lead. And because of that, we give away our power in a thousand ways every day—from denying our own nature by trying to fit into our male-dominated culture, to suffering needlessly due to rampant hormonal dysfunction, to holding back our potent life force because we've never been taught how to care properly for our beautifully complex system.

Let's be real. Your sex ed class sucked. Media and advertising messages hammered it into your head that your period was something dirty you needed to hide. This mythology and lack of education keeps you from appropriate self-care. Our culture convinced us our bodies are projects to endlessly work on, while boys' bodies are power tools that help them master their lives. Is it any surprise we're out of sync with our bodies? Because of this faulty introduction to womanhood, *we seek to suppress our biology because we believe it will help us be more successful.* And it isn't working. Everything you've tried to get rid of—your unwanted weight, PMS, and breakouts—is a bust. Your efforts to move up the corporate ladder or launch your own business compromise your health more than you'd like. In addition to being overextended with invisible work, actual work, and motherhood, we add our drive to be perfect to our wellness activities, too. What you don't realize is that we struggle needlessly, drained of the energy we need to create, because we look for help from diets, healing protocols, and time management tools that leave the female cycle *out* of the equation. Most of the advice you're following is intended for men with the assumption—*and it's a big one*—that the same advice will translate to women. I've got news for you—it doesn't.

Our mys-education runs deep. And it has to end *now*!

The Truth Behind the Most Common (and Harmful) Period Myths

Our mys-education is responsible for some very common myths about menstruation that make us feel bad about our hormonal cycles, our bodies, and about womanhood in general. It's time to set the record straight.

Myth 1: PMS is just part of having a period

Mood swings. Bloating. Breakouts. We're told these premenstrual symptoms are normal. News flash: They're not. This myth about PMS is very harmful because it forces you to suffer unnecessarily. When you're conditioned to believe that pain and problems are par for the course, you're prevented from looking for solutions. The PMS myth does further damage, as it is used against women to dismiss our feelings, opinions, and judgments. People put us in the box of "being hormonal" (as if men don't have hormones too!) as a way to devalue women.

The truth: Science shows us that PMS symptoms arise only when there is an imbalance of estrogen and progesterone during the luteal phase. This imbalance can be triggered by diet choices—such as coffee, sugar, dairy, dieting, juice fasts, and low-fat fads—or by the more insidious suppression of feminine energy—the energy of change. According to the National Institutes of Health's BioCycle Study, the longer PMS goes unchecked and untreated, the greater the risk for cancer, heart disease, diabetes, and dementia postmenopausally. When women live in tune with their cycle, eating the right foods and nurturing their feminine energy, PMS symptoms disappear. The premenstrual phase can actually be a time of insight, clarity, and direction. It can fill you with a can-do, get-it-done attitude and a desire to clean house—literally and metaphorically. I have renamed PMS "prioritizing my self," and if more women did the same, we would have far fewer premenstrual symptoms.

Myth 2: Cramps are unavoidable

More than half of all women of reproductive age say they have some period pain for one to two days each month. Have you ever caught yourself thinking you're *supposed* to have cramps, or that as a woman you were destined to be cursed with painful periods? When you've been told your whole life that period pain is just a reality to "deal with" or "get over," you accept it and don't expect it to be any better. It's time for a reality check—you don't have to suffer from cramps.

The truth: Yes, your body produces one type of prostaglandin—PgE2—that causes uterine contractions and in excess can lead to cramps. But did you know that your body also pumps out two additional types of prostaglandin—PgE1 and PgE3—that are antispasmodic in nature and counteract those contractions? Thanks to these natural painkillers, your body effectively has twice the capacity to relieve pain than to cause cramps. The good news is that when you consume the right foods for your cycle, you provide the building blocks your body needs to promote the production of the good prostaglandins that ease period pain.

Myth 3: Being on the pill helps you regulate your period

If you're like most of the women I talk with, you probably believe that you still menstruate when you're taking synthetic birth control pills. After all, many women on the pill bleed each month.

The truth: What you experience when you're on the pill is not a real period. It's actually a "withdrawal bleed" that bears no physiological resemblance to the natural period that comes at the end of your monthly hormonal cycle. You may be surprised to discover that the placebo week found in most birth control packs was created as a marketing ploy. In the early days of the pill, manufacturers thought women would be so disturbed by the idea of not bleeding at all that they wouldn't want to use it. That's how the placebo week was born. For real menstruation to occur, you need to be ovulating; but the pill prevents this critical phase of your cycle. Without ovulation, your gorgeous hormonal cycle gets stuck in a static low-hormone phase and can't create a period. Furthermore, synthetic birth control does not correct hormonal imbalances; it merely suppresses your own hormonal function and allows you to go years or decades without addressing the root causes of symptoms, which makes your overall health worsen. And then there are all the nasty side effects to consider—and I don't mean just the ones listed in the little pamphlet that comes with your synthetic birth control packet. In the upcoming Biohacking Tool Kit section, you'll learn that there are many more downsides your gynecologist probably never informed you about—

for example, that the pill depletes nutrients, disrupts your microbiome, and increases depression.

Myth 4: You don't *need* to have a period

Every few years, an article will come out claiming that there's no reason for modern-day women to have a period and that we would actually be better off and healthier if we didn't bleed on a monthly basis. Some ob-gyns give their patients the green light to toss the placebos and take the active birth control pills continuously to skip bleeding indefinitely.

The truth: Yes, it's amazing that as a species we've discovered how to outsmart our bodies by suppressing our cycle, but that doesn't mean we should. Nature is infinitely more intelligent than we are and gave us the gift of the cycle as a way to protect our long-term health. Tampering with that system by intentionally skipping your period comes with real side effects and health dangers. Ovulation, and therefore menstruation, plays an important role in safeguarding our health for decades to come and protecting us from osteoporosis, heart disease, breast disease, and dementia. Every ovulation and cycle puts protective benefits into your health "bank account" for the years when you stop having a cycle. Our menstrual cycle is so critical to our overall health and well-being that the American College of Obstetricians and Gynecologists has decreed that menstruation is the fifth vital sign, just as important as pulse, temperature, breathing rate, and blood pressure. If your period has gone MIA, it is considered a sign of a health issue such as low estrogen levels, which have been linked to heart issues and bone weakness. If you're missing periods due to polycystic ovary syndrome (PCOS), or if you have irregular cycles, it's a sign your hormonal system is off-kilter and will likely be accompanied by symptoms like acne, mood swings, or weight gain. A period that arrives like clockwork each month is just as important as having healthy blood pressure levels at your annual checkup. I recommend monitoring your period—tracking the color and consistency, duration, and intensity—to stay on top of your hormonal health. In the Biohacking Tool Kit section, we'll take a deeper dive into menstruation to help you interpret the color of your monthly bleed, fix your specific period problems, and have a happier cycle.

Myth 5: If you have a bad period, there's not much you can do

When you get a cold, do you just let it run its course, or do you take action to promote faster healing? Of course it makes sense to pop vitamin C, get more rest, and take better care of ourselves. It's odd that when we're having period-related symptoms—cramps, heavy bleeding, or spotting—we tend to ignore our problems. We believe it's our lot in life to have painful periods, so we don't do anything about it.

The truth: This way of thinking is the direct result of the paltry education we receive about our hormones and what kind of support they need, because the reality is you can do something. You can take action, change your hormonal reality, and have a better period. Just as you wouldn't let your cold linger unnecessarily, you don't have to put up with problem periods. With some simple cyclical lifestyle hacks—think food, exercise, supplements, and the way you manage your time—you could see results as soon as your next cycle.

YOU ARE A BIOLOGICAL POWERHOUSE

Women are inherently abundant by design. We can make multiple babies, we bleed every month, we produce milk—heck, we even secrete vaginal bacteria that's vital for a baby's optimal gut health. Nearly every function of our body replenishes life. For example, check out the life-giving power of your reproductive fluids.

- **Menstrual blood:** Researchers have discovered that stem cells found in menstrual blood may have the potential to be used in treatments for stroke, liver damage, and other conditions. *Period blood doesn't seem so "dirty" anymore, does it?*

- **Breast milk:** New science suggests that nipples absorb a baby's saliva, which may program the mammary glands to pump out made-to-order germ fighters the baby needs. One study in 2013 showed that immune factors in a mother's milk change quickly in response to a baby's infection. *It's Mommy, MD, to the rescue!*

- **Vaginal secretions:** Bacteria in the birth canal seeds a baby's gut microbiome for optimal health. Babies born by cesarean section, who miss out on this bacterial bath, have a much higher risk of developing chronic immune disorders, such as asthma, allergies, juvenile arthritis, inflammatory bowel disease, and even leukemia, according to a study published in 2014 that included two million children over a span of 35 years. The medical community is finally tuning in to this critical process; a 2016 pilot study that involved swabbing C-section babies' mouths and bodies with their mothers' vaginal bacteria showed promise for restoring the babies' gut microbiome. *Now that's pussy power!*

Meanwhile, more research is being done on fecal transfers—which involve transplanting fecal matter from a healthy donor into the gastrointestinal tract of another—to treat conditions like Crohn's disease and ulcerative colitis. Why not look to the female body's treasures instead? Our much-maligned fluids have so much untapped potential. Who knows what could be possible if researchers devoted as much interest to women's fluids as they do to, well, poop?

Life in the Boys' Club

There's no denying it: we have been living in a man's world—although, thankfully, with more women in leadership positions in the private and public sectors, this reality is bound to change, and soon. Our cultural values prioritize masculine energy of individuality and linear progression at the expense of all else, which is reflected in the breakdown of our communities and the disregard for the health of our planet. In addition, our foundational beliefs about our own health are largely informed by research done by men, on male subjects. Even our daily routines are all based on the 24-hour male cycle. Yes, men have a hormonal cycle too! We just never talk about their cycle, because we cater to it every day. We'll learn more about our own hormonal symphony soon, but for now, let's look at a day in the life of male hormones.

Male 24-Hour Hormonal Cycle

- **Morning:** Testosterone and cortisol levels are at their highest when he wakes up, making him energetic, communicative, laser-focused, ready for sex (cue the morning erection), and super-efficient at getting stuff done.

- **Afternoon:** Declining testosterone puts him in the mood to socialize and connect with people. This is when he wants to pitch ideas to clients, network with colleagues, and meet up for a date.

- **Evening:** Testosterone levels wane, making him more sensitive to his estrogen, and generally more interested in cocooning on the couch or finding other ways to quiet his mind.

Notice anything? This schedule lines up almost perfectly with the way a typical day in a typical life—male or female—plays out. We wake up early and immediately start fielding email. We spend the early part of the workday tearing through our agenda. Then in the afternoon we continue to work through our to-do list, though our productivity has already peaked. After work, it's happy hour—time to commiserate and blow off steam! Finally, we collapse in front of the TV, ready to relax after a day full of ups and downs.

Just hit repeat on this cycle day after day, 365 days a year. It's that simple. Or is it? Women's 28-day cycle bears no resemblance to this 24-hour schedule, but we have been forced to live according to the male hormonal rhythm for so long we don't even question it. Have we ever stepped back to ask if it makes sense to operate our lives this way? Hormonally, each day is a new start for men, so we structure our workdays and social lives thinking only about the day of the week or the time of day. But women's bodies don't work that way. Our energy is not static day to day and week to week. Our productivity could be completely different depending on where we are in our 28-day cycle. The time we feel most social isn't dictated by the time happy hour starts. And while men tend to recharge in the evening, our cocooning period is tied to a certain time of the month.

We're overlooking a crucial component that governs the moods and emotions of half the population—it's no wonder women don't feel that they are thriving as much as they would like to be. The lack of knowledge about women's biochemistry and cyclical nature extends to the medical community too. As far back as 1995, a paper in *Epidemiological Review* noted that medical research basically ignores women's hormonal cycles. This ignorance plays out in the care and treatment we receive.

All too often when we visit the doctor for our symptoms, we are told, "it's all in your head," and are sent home to suffer in silence. This treatment is especially common for menstrual issues like fibroids, endometriosis, and dysmenorrhea. As a result, women often are not properly evaluated or diagnosed until years after their symptoms begin. I know. For me, this process took seven years, and I had to bring the diagnosis myself to my doctor to confirm my PCOS, because she never considered it! Sometimes, we're labeled "chronic complainers," as evidenced in a study by the American Autoimmune Related Diseases Association, which found that nearly half of people who were eventually diagnosed with an autoimmune disease (remember, 75 percent of people with autoimmune diseases are women) were initially told they were "too concerned about their health." Think about that phrase for a minute. A 2010 analysis on chronic pain in women found that health care professionals were more likely to dismiss women's complaints of pain as "emotional, psychogenic, hysterical, or oversensitive."

Instead of your health issues being taken seriously, you're told that you're "hormonal," that you were dealt the short end of the biological stick, that your treatment options are limited to taking the pill or possibly having surgery, and that ultimately you should just accept that suffering and feeling crappy is your genetic destiny. Can you imagine men being told to be passive, do nothing, and just learn to live with their symptoms? It's unacceptable that women are relegated to suffering. In her book, *Doing Harm: The Truth About How Bad Medicine and Lazy Science Leave Women Dismissed, Misdiagnosed, and Sick,* author Maya Dusenbery summed it up succinctly: "Women's symptoms are not taken seriously because medicine doesn't know as much about their bodies and health problems. And medicine doesn't know as much about their bodies and health problems because it doesn't take their symptoms seriously."

On the flip side, some physicians are quick to dole out prescriptions—synthetic birth control that hijacks your natural hormonal cycle, antidepressants that alter your neurochemistry, and the list goes on. More than half of all US women are taking at least one prescription medication, and about twenty-six million are taking five or more doctor-ordered meds. And that's not taking into account the billions and billions of over-the-counter pills, tablets, caplets, gels, and other remedies we take to try to heal the side effects of neglecting our cycles—acne, headaches, exhaustion, weight gain, insomnia, bloating, and more.

Even the new trend toward biohacking—using food, supplements, and more to optimize our well-being—falls short because it doesn't take our cyclical nature into consideration. Just look at the diet and fitness industry. Can you show me one trendy, well-known diet or workout that's based on women's hormonal cycle? That's because most diet and exercise research has been conducted on men, not women. Check out these sad statistics:

• Women account for only 39 percent of participants in exercise
  studies.
• When the XX-chromosome crowd does make the cut in sports
  and exercise research, we are often studied only during the first half
  of our cycle, when hormone levels are low, or only if we're taking
  hormonal birth control.

In fact, women have been historically underrepresented in all health, drug, and biological research. Here's a quick timeline of some of the most foundational health research and the shocking absence of women.

- **The year 1958:** A trial on the physical and cognitive changes and chronic diseases that come with natural aging called the Baltimore Longitudinal Study of Aging was launched; for its first twenty years, it included more than one thousand men and exactly zero women. It wasn't until 1978 that women were added to the roster of participants.
- **The year 1973:** The first study looking into the effects of estrogen on the prevention of heart disease included 8,341 men and—*you guessed it!*—no women.
- **The year 1982:** The landmark Physician's Health Study reported the now widely held belief that taking low-dose aspirin can lower the risk for heart disease. The only problem? The study tracked 22,071 men and not a single woman.
- **The year 1985:** By this date, the Public Health Service Task Force on Women's Health Issues concluded that "the historical lack of research focus on women's health concerns has compromised the quality of health information available to women as well as the health care they receive."

Today, we're still trying to catch up. Why did women get left out of scientific research while men became the standard human representative in clinical trials? There are many reasons, but here are a couple of biggies:

- **Men are preferred research subjects.** Men have only one biological clock—that simple, rhythmic 24-hour hormonal circadian pattern—while women also have the more complex 28-day cycle. Researchers have argued that it's easier and less expensive to facilitate for experiments for the male pattern than for women's hormonal fluctuations.
- **A major drug trial on women went tragically wrong.** Another factor that played into our exclusion was a sense of needing to protect women's reproductive processes. Birth defects from the drug thalidomide in the 1960s resulted in the FDA adopting guidelines in 1977 essentially banning women of "childbearing age" from

participating in clinical research. These guidelines effectively cut women who weren't postmenopausal out of the research game.

It wasn't until 1993 when the National Institutes of Health Revitalization Act attempted to change things by requiring researchers to include women in human studies and to note any results that differed in women compared with men. We've made inroads since then, but "progress has been painfully slow—stalling for long periods or sometimes reversing direction—and, consequently, not nearly enough progress has been made," according to a 2015 review in *BMC Women's Health*.

When you realize that our culture's foundational health research has largely excluded women, it's easy to grasp why our health issues are sometimes misunderstood and misdiagnosed. The fact that many of the diseases that affect women in greater numbers receive less funding for research compounds the problem. Trying to fit into the boys' club actually prevents you from being oriented to your own body and from doing self-care in a way that supports your biochemical needs.

The lack of understanding of women's health issues can feel isolating. In our sessions, when we talk about the issues my clients are having, women often start by saying, "I must be one in a million, because I have this symptom." And it's a symptom that I know is actually very common. I let them know they're not one *in* a million with their period problem, they're one *of* millions struggling alone and unnecessarily confused. The fact is that your problems are not the result of a deficiency in synthetic hormones. The problem is twofold: (1) we don't talk enough about the epidemic of women's chronic hormonal problems, and (2) the one-size-fits-all health care, fitness, and life management advice we're getting *doesn't* fit all—it's designed primarily for the male hormonal ecosystem. The solution is to redefine women's health care, time management, and our concept of success from a totally female-centered standpoint. That's the only way you're going to live your best life. Even if you don't suffer from any hormonal health issues, honoring your cyclical nature is the only way to take advantage of all the gifts your body inherently offers.

My Hormone Story

I know firsthand how stressful hormonal problems can be. I struggled with them for a decade, and my journey with a debilitating hormonal condition changed my career and my life. My issues started in junior high school. I was a very late bloomer in the puberty department. Even though I was the president and founder of the Period Club, I was the last one in the club to actually start my period. I was almost sixteen when I got my first bleed, although it was brown and not healthy. I went to my gynecologist annually but was offered no diagnosis or explanation for the laundry list of issues I was having. Meanwhile, my symptoms worsened throughout high school and in college. At one point, I tipped the scales at 205 pounds; my face, chest, and back were covered in severe, painful cystic acne; and I hadn't had my period more than a handful of times in a decade. Things got so bad for me, I couldn't sleep, I binged on food to deal with fatigue and anxiety, I felt depressed, and I struggled to do basic things like be on time for appointments and stick with plans to go out with friends. I was a mess and felt trapped in my own body. One night when I was suffering with my usual insomnia, I headed to the library at Johns Hopkins, where I was a student, and I came across a brief article in an obstetrics journal about Stein-Leventhal disease, which is now called polycystic ovary syndrome (PCOS). As I scanned the symptoms associated with this condition, I recognized myself immediately. "This is it," I thought!

In my book *WomanCode*, I described in detail how that discovery prompted me to demand that my gynecologist give me a test to diagnose PCOS—a transvaginal ultrasound along with bloodwork. When the test revealed the telltale signs of PCOS—multiple cysts on both of my ovaries—I finally knew what was causing all of my issues. It suddenly made sense to me that all the diets, exercise, and skin care treatments hadn't worked for me. My symptoms weren't caused by my not trying hard enough; my hormonal system was so severely out of tune that no ordinary diet or skin cream was going to help. My prognosis was grim—a lifetime of cystic acne and an increased risk for obesity, diabetes, infertility, heart disease, and cancer. As I sat in stunned silence, the doc dispassionately informed me there was no cure, only a litany of prescriptions—birth control pills to artificially regulate my period, Accutane for acne, Glucophage for insulin problems, Aldactone for hirsutism issues, blood pressure medicine, Clomid when it came time to conceive, and on and on—that I would likely have to take for the rest of my life. The message was clear: go home and suffer quietly.

As I was reeling from the notion of a lifetime of pills and problems, a voice welled up from deep inside, calmly reassuring me: "That's not your path." My body was sending me a strong message that there had to be a better way. I didn't realize it in that moment, but looking back, my body was letting me know I had the power to do something, to change my hormonal situation and create a better future for myself. In that moment, I made the switch from having a passive relationship with my body to becoming a champion for my health and well-being. I was in a fight for my quality of life, literally, and if traditional medicine was going to leave me unsupported, I'd look elsewhere for a remedy. For the next two years, I embarked on an exploratory journey to learn as much as I could from experts in a variety of health specialties, including naturopaths, herbalists, and acupuncturists. I tried elimination diets, candida diets, herbs, and supplements, and nothing worked for me. Although these therapies can provide relief for many conditions, they didn't heal my hormonal problems. In fact, my condition continued to worsen.

Out of desperation, I went on the pill, but after just ten days I temporarily lost vision in one eye from an ocular migraine and suffered a cardiac episode of low blood pressure and heart palpitations. After medical evaluation, I was told to avoid synthetic birth control. Finally, after exhausting all of the existing treatments, I tapped into my inner strength as a researcher (I had studied biology and wanted to become an ob-gyn) and began looking into the endocrine system, epigenetics, circadian patterns of the body and hormones (chronobiology), and the five-phase theory from Chinese medicine. My findings encouraged me to experiment and create a revolutionary new way of eating that ultimately put my symptoms and condition into remission naturally. This is the basis of the FLO protocol I described in *WomanCode*, which includes using food to stabilize your blood sugar levels and insulin, reduce cortisol levels, restore microbial balance in the gut, and improve the breakdown of estrogen in the liver.

Within nine months of following this protocol, my period came back, I lost sixty pounds, my skin cleared up, and my mood and life were transformed. I was beyond thrilled with this transformation, but my journey wasn't over. I needed to find a way to maintain the changes I had made, and I wanted to get in touch with my cyclical nature by reclaiming a female-centered way of living. The Cycle Syncing Method™ was born from these two fundamental needs. The method is based on the extraordinary blueprint for self-care, biohacking, and optimization on every level provided by our cyclical hormonal patterns. The method allows us to stay connected to our feminine energy despite the cultural conditioning that dictates a linear, repetitive way of living. I certainly wish somebody had taught me about my cyclical nature when I was a little girl. Where was the textbook that had this description of our female process?

> *On the day when you start your first period, you'll be entering a wondrous, cyclical phase of your life. Your second biological clock becomes activated. Your body's cyclical nature empowers you with an abundance of gifts and offers a clear road map to take advantage of each of them at the most opportune time. Syncing with your cycle is the simplest, most effective way to enhance your hormonal health and create sustainable success in all areas of your life—career, relationships, sex, and motherhood.*

Can you imagine reading something like this when you were a preteen, and the influence it might have had on your self-esteem and sense of how you could thrive in our society? How might information about syncing with your cycle have shaped the way you think about your body, your period, and your hormonal patterns? How might that information have impacted the way you approach every aspect of your life? I'm convinced that living in tune with our cyclical nature is the key to optimal living for women. Honoring yourself as a cyclical being isn't just about achieving better hormonal health; it can boost every area of your life. I've seen this transformation happen to thousands of women around the world. This book is based on the work I've been doing for the past two decades at the FLO Living Hormone Center, a first-of-its-kind company dedicated to modernizing menstrual health care. The FLO Living Hormone Center gives women around the world virtual access to products and programs like the MyFLO app that help them evaluate their hormonal problems, track their symptoms, and naturally address their hormone imbalances. And women can talk at length with a hormone coach about their issues and learn about the benefits of getting in sync with their cyclical nature.

SIDE EFFECTS OF SYNCING WITH YOUR CYCLE

- Finding yourself building energy, not draining it
- Finding yourself in the right place at the right time more often
- Feeling really good about who you are
- Feeling good in your body all month
- Feeling powerful and confident
- Having time work for you, rather than twisting yourself around for time
- Feeling less stress, but getting more done
- Effortlessly maintaining a healthy weight
- Deriving more enjoyment from your work
- Feeling aligned with the process of creation
- Not feeling so much pressure to be perfect
- Feeling like your body is a clear channel for your passion and purpose to come through

---

Living in harmony with your nature makes you healthier, happier, and symptom-free, and allows you to pursue your creative and career passions more successfully and sustainably. Syncing with your cycle is *the* ultimate biohack for women's health and success. Like your cycle, this biohack is efficient, elegant, and direct. All you have to do is access what's already inside you.

Biohacking, Functional Medicine, and the Cycle Syncing Method™—What's the Difference?

Most women I connect with all have a similar adverse reaction to the term *biohacking*. There is something about the word that feels invasive, and I think that our collective unconscious wounding around our physical safety has us balk at this term on an emotional level. We don't want to be hacked into or hack into ourselves. It feels intrusive and violent, acting against the body's propensities and—possibly—its permission. However, *biohacking* really is a term that can be used to describe a proactive relationship with your body, its systems, and your health. Let's reclaim this term, which has tremendous positive advantages, and understand the different types of biohacking available.

Biohacking, in the wellness community, is using devices, supplements, food, and lifestyle modifications to change the performance of an already normally functioning body system with the aim of enhancing physical performance and achievement in other areas of your life. Its goal is to push the limits of what can be achieved in the 24-hour window. On the positive side, biohacking is about trying to increase the performance of the body beyond its points of natural limitation or to respond better to its environment—for example, using caffeine to increase energy or concentration, or using adaptogens to improve its stress response. It can go as far as genetic modification and device implantation in the body. Some of these are necessary, like artificial valve replacements in the heart or robotic limbs, but I'm talking more about the nonessential versions of these, like chips implanted in the body to track your activity. I think it is part of our nature and our culture to continue to figure out how we can outsmart nature's processes and succeed in spite of our body's limitations.

Functional medicine involves a variety of testing followed by food and supplement modification to heal a body system that is in crisis, restoring homeostasis so that the body can perform normally. For example, if you have a diagnosis of PCOS or fibroids, there is an imbalance in the endocrine system that needs support. Initial healing work is essential to get your body back to normal endocrine performance. This is a form of biohacking to restore homeostasis and health.

The Cycle Syncing Method™ is about working with your body's natural processes to both optimize your health and your life *without* adding anything to the body system. Because you have a second clock, you have an internal code, or "preferred performance pattern," in your body. All you have to do to feel the best possible way and to live the life you want for yourself is to align with this pattern and support it as much as you can. You don't have to try to extend your energy in a 24-hour pattern, because you have the expanse of 28 days to play with. When you run out of energy today, you can stop and rest, knowing that you have a whole variety of energy and creativity to play with over the whole month. This form of biohacking is about aligning with your body's biological rhythms, and it's much more collaborative, grounding, anxiety-reducing, and embracing of your feminine energy.

Free Your Feminine Energy for Change

Today's patriarchal society doesn't really offer a clear space for this powerful female energy that creates continuous change. But you can make space in your own life the way I did—carefully, thoughtfully, intentionally. I let the truth of science guide me. And science shows me that I am designed to be strong, emotionally attuned, analytical, insightful, creative, playful, nurturing, spontaneous, dynamic, and reliable. Only when we learn how to leverage our natural patterns are we able to thrive in our bodies, our careers, and our relationships, so we can live our optimal lives.

When enough women tap into this personal power, we can collaborate and begin to drive change in our culture to reflect our needs and values of sustainability and well-being—increasingly critical issues for a society moving toward increased dependence on technology and increased damage to our environment. As we head into a future in which more women are rising to positions of power, it is more important than ever to make sure our education about how we self-reference and perform self-care matches the truth of our biology and empowers us. We need to give ourselves permission to lead like women and embrace our dynamic energy to help us champion the changes our world so clearly needs.

I'm constantly surprised that every women's event or conference—whether focused on business or wellness—does not always include panels, segments, or presentations about hormones and mental health, hormones and energy, or hormones and wellness. I'm always so happy when the people in charge of the conference realize this topic has been left out inadvertently and create some space for it. As we include this in our conversations, we shift how we feel about our female biochemistry.

In fact, we live in an amazing time for periods! Millennials and celebrities are opening up on social media and other platforms about their experiences riding the "crimson wave" and are truly breaking down all the bloody barriers that hold us back from knowing how our bodies work and what's possible for them. But it's also a fascinating time as next-generation advances in technology—think artificial intelligence (AI), artificial simulation of the menstrual cycle, and "BioBags" to grow babies outside the uterus—seem to be paving the way for a future where life can be created artificially in response to the decline in everyone's hormonal health. It's up to us to protect our hormones and our cycles now and for the seven future generations genetically affected by the self-care choices we make today.

This is the conversation we need to have, not the one we got in our severely inadequate sex ed class, not the one about the "curse." I actually count myself lucky that as a preteen I never got "the talk" from my mom. She never mentioned one word about menstruation to me. But because I didn't get the talk, I had no preconceived notions about menstruation being dirty or something to be ashamed of. So when I heard about this mysterious monthly visitor for the first time in my sixth-grade class (a few years before Mr. Bing's biology class), I was absolutely enchanted. "Ah-mazing!" I thought. I couldn't wait to start having a cycle. My organic reaction to the idea of having a period was utter joy and enthusiasm. I thought of it as a gift, not a curse. That's the experience I want for you and for all women—to find the joy in our cycles and to use it to heal our symptoms and help us live our best lives.

CHAPTER 2

Break Free from the 24-Hour Clock

The psyches and souls of women also have their own cycles
and seasons of doing and solitude, running and staying, being
involved and being removed, questing and resting, creating
and incubating, being of the world and returning.
—CLARISSA PINKOLA ESTÉS

think we're all wired to try to figure out how to be happy. I remember that in my quest for happiness, I stumbled across an important concept: most of us are going about being happy the wrong way. It's the "have-do-be" concept. Essentially, we believe, as I sure did, that once I *had* acquired a goal (like the perfect weight, or the right job, or quality friends), then I'd *do* all the things I wanted to do (like wear a bikini to the beach, have lots of money to spend, go out and do fun things), and then finally I'd *be* happy! The truth is, however, that the process works in the opposite direction. While I understood this concept intellectually, it was a whole other thing to actually live it. I'm from New England—maybe there is something in the water up there that makes a person want very practical solutions to esoteric questions. I wanted to know how to generate feelings of well-being and enjoyment consistently. It turns out that the answer was waiting for me all along in my biochemistry.

In the previous chapter I revealed how misinformation about our biochemistry is preventing us from taking advantage of the natural competitive edge women possess. In this chapter I'll unpack a fundamental truth about female biology that most women are ignoring: while children, men, and postmenopausal women are operating on a single biological clock, women of reproductive age are blessed to have two powerful inner clocks that create an organic framework for optimizing our energy, nurturing our creativity, maintaining our health, and making sustainable our productivity. Just as we now appreciate taking serious care of our circadian clock, it is equally critical to take care of your monthly hormonal clock, as you'll see in this chapter. Honoring both these clocks can help you access the gifts of your cyclical nature so you can optimize your performance and achieve more with less effort and less stress. On the other hand, continuing to ignore your second clock can ravage your health and make it harder for you to experience more flow and ease in your life.

Chronobiology and You

I've always been fascinated by chronobiology. It's the field within biology that seeks to understand the cyclical phenomena in organisms and their adaptation to physiological rhythms. The term comes from the ancient Greek words *chronos*, the word for time, and *bios logia*, the study of life. These cycles are known as *biological rhythms* and they impact anatomy, physiology, genetics, molecular biology, behavior, epigenetics, reproduction, and even our planet's ecology. Basically, *everything* is affected by this action of cycles and timing, and yet we don't get exposed to this perspective when we are learning about basic biology as we're growing up. Timing is essential for many key biological processes: from sleeping to cellular regeneration and even bacterial activity, its impact on your well-being is enormous. We should all have a basic understanding of the timing of our bodies' functions.

In addition to most of us not having a strong understanding about this field of study, we usually only hear about one of the timing cycles: the circadian rhythm and its connection to the solar rhythm. *Circadian* is from the Latin words *circa* (around) and *diem* (day), describing the solar cycle of one day. Of course, there are some cultural reasons behind this cycle being so well-known compared to others: the sun, from Greek mythology to modern religion, has always been associated with male power. Unfortunately, due to this patriarchal agenda and the association between the menstrual cycle and lunar rhythms, the menstrual biological rhythm has become culturally devalued to the point where we're not even taught its proper name.

Well, here it is. Your menstrual cycle is an *infradian* rhythm, a cycle longer than a day. There are also *ultradian* rhythms that refer to cycles shorter than a day, like REM cycles and growth hormone cycles. Lunar rhythms are actually a separate cycle, and, from a chronobiological standpoint, they typically refer to tidal activity. The facts that our bodies are 80 percent water and women observe a correlation between their infradian rhythm and their lunar cycle mean that there might be more connection there than we have research for currently. However, because they have been associated together historically and they don't fit well with religious and patriarchal values, we don't know much about our biological rhythms, and we ourselves don't believe they have much value.

But science transcends cultural narratives: what you're about to learn is a real and missing piece of your understanding of your biology, and as such you can feel confident in reclaiming your hormonal advantage and revolutionizing your life accordingly. We've all learned how to orient ourselves around a day and to connect with the timing of the world outside. We need to learn to leverage our infradian rhythm for our success and well-being—we need to learn to connect with our inner timing.

Meet Your 24-Hour Clock—the Circadian Rhythm

Let's look at your 24-hour clock first. Inside all of us—women and men—we have a circadian rhythm that regulates our daily bodily processes, including digestion, body temperature, metabolism, sleep, elimination, and the production of certain hormones. This circadian clock kicks into action the day you're born, and continues ticking day in and day out throughout your entire life. Michael Breus, in his book *The Power of When*, explores how the circadian rhythm reigns over your body's processes—cuing cortisol to spike in the morning to rev you up, boosting alertness in late morning, and secreting melatonin around 9 p.m. to help you wind down for sleep. Here's a breakdown of how your 24-hour clock primes your body for a variety of processes throughout the day:

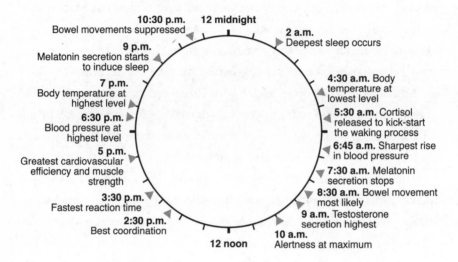

In traditional Chinese medicine, the organs also have peak activity times during the day, and practitioners use this clock to understand which organs need extra support:

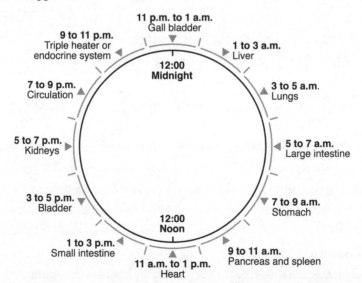

A master timekeeper, which is composed of a cluster of about 20,000 neurons, is found in the brain's hypothalamus and keeps all of these internal processes in sync. For science geeks, this structure is called the suprachiasmatic nucleus, or SCN. Throughout human history, this circadian clock has dictated our daily lives—prompting us to wake when the sun rises and sleep when nighttime falls.

Our modern-day lifestyle, however, is increasingly at odds with our inner clock. Ever since Thomas Edison patented the light bulb in 1879, we've lived in a world of never-ending bright light. Want to go dancing until 2 a.m.? Write your screenplay at midnight? Eat dinner at 10 p.m.? No problem. But when our lifestyle doesn't sync with our circadian clock, it can impact our well-being and has been associated with a litany of physical, mental, and cognitive issues, according to numerous studies. For example, a 2014 paper in *International Review of Psychiatry* linked circadian misalignment with an increased risk for cardiovascular disease, diabetes, obesity, cancer, depression, bipolar disorder, schizophrenia, and ADHD, and research in the *Annals of the New York Academy of Sciences* found that any disregulation of our circadian clock could potentially trigger metabolic, autoimmune, or mood disorders.

CONDITIONS LINKED TO A CIRCADIAN DISRUPTION INCLUDE THE FOLLOWING:

- Cancer
- Cardiovascular disease
- Diabetes
- Obesity
- Irritable bowel syndrome (IBS)
- Inflammatory bowel disease
- Gastroesophageal reflux disease (GERD)
- Ulcers
- Gut dysbiosis
- Small intestine bacterial overgrowth
- Depression
- Bipolar disorder
- Attention deficit disorder (ADD)
- Attention deficit hyperactivity disorder (ADHD)
- Schizophrenia
- Lack of alertness
- Reduced cognitive function

Our daily timekeeper has been deemed so critical to our health and well-being that three scientists were awarded the 2017 Nobel Prize, the world's highest scientific honor, for pinpointing the gene that keeps this daily timekeeper ticking. Now that the rest of us understand how important it is to sync with our circadian rhythms, we're taking action to avoid anything that disrupts our 24-hour clock. We've inadvertently deregulated our circadian clock and have gotten to a point where we have to biohack our lives to reverse the damage. Just look at how popular those glasses that filter the blue light from our tech gadgets have become. It's common knowledge now that the blue light from all our devices is messing with our sleep. But many of us don't know that blue light diminishes the pineal gland's ability to make melatonin, which can disrupt ovulation and decrease fertility.

Becoming more aware of how critical it is to live in tune with our circadian clock is great, but women need to understand that we have a second clock that is equally important. Unfortunately, this clock hasn't received nearly the same amount of attention from the scientific community or the media. In fact, this second clock has been largely ignored, and we've been left in the dark about its inner workings and its profound impact on our health, moods, and performance. It's time to change that.

Say Hello to Your Second Clock—the 28-Day Infradian Rhythm

As a woman, you're blessed with a second clock, starting at puberty and continuing until you reach menopause at about age fifty. It deeply impacts your experience of life for approximately forty years. This infradian rhythm is tied to your monthly menstrual cycle, which includes four distinct phases—follicular, ovulatory, luteal, and menstrual. The same way your circadian clock plays a role in your daily bodily functions, your 28-day infradian clock influences your brain chemistry and physiology, providing you with unique gifts and strengths at different times of the month.

28-Day Infradian Rhythm (aka Your Monthly Cycle)			
Phase 1	Phase 2	Phase 3	Phase 4
Follicular	Ovulatory	Luteal	Menstrual
7–10 days	3–4 days	10–14 days	3–7 days

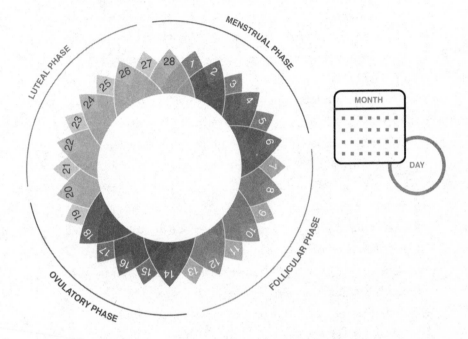

Your two clocks are tightly linked. The four phases of your cycle influence your 24-hour circadian rhythms, and vice versa. For example, did you know that hormonal fluctuations affect your body temperature, sleep patterns, and heart rate throughout your cycle? On the flip side, your 24-hour clock plays a role in how well your 28-day clock functions. Any disturbance in your 24-hour clock can disrupt your 28-day cycle, leading to problems such as irregular periods and longer menstrual cycles.

As we've seen, mountains of research show that living out of sync with your circadian clock can damage your physical and mental health. The same is true if you ignore your monthly cycle. Neglecting this vital inner infradian clock exacts a heavy price from your hormonal, physical, and mental well-being. In addition to the influence of endocrine-disruptive chemical exposure, trying to fit into a 24-hour pattern by ignoring our own hormonal needs is taking a dramatic toll on our bodies. Just look at the numbers:

- Five million women suffer from polycystic ovary syndrome (PCOS).
- Seventy to 80 percent of women will develop fibroids by age fifty.
- One in ten of women will suffer from endometriosis during the reproductive years.
- Nine to fourteen out of one hundred women have heavy periods.
- Ten percent of women experience period pain so intense they can't perform everyday routines.
- Twelve percent of women of reproductive age have difficulty getting pregnant or carrying a pregnancy to term.
- About 600,000 women undergo a hysterectomy every year.
- Women are five to eight times more likely to have thyroid problems.
- More than 75 percent of all people diagnosed with autoimmune diseases are women.
- As many as 50 million women suffer from one or more neglected chronic pain conditions.
- Women are twice as likely as men to have chronic fatigue syndrome.
- Women account for up to 90 percent of all people with fibromyalgia.
- Eighty-five percent of chronic migraine sufferers are women.
- About two-thirds of Alzheimer's disease patients are women.
- Women in their childbearing years are more than twice as likely as men to develop an anxiety disorder.
- One in eight women experience depression in their lifetime, twice the rate as men.

For optimal health and performance, you need to learn as much as you can about your second clock and then nurture it with phase-specific self-care. Syncing with your monthly clock is the key to taking full advantage of your cyclical nature for the three to four decades when it forms the foundation of your life. Before puberty and after menopause, it's your circadian clock and static hormonal pattern that guide the rhythm of your life and allow you to engage in more gender-neutral biohacking. During your reproductive years, however, you need to biohack like a woman.

A Better Way to Think About Time

When you have two biological clocks, you also need to rethink your relationship with time and time management. Are you struggling to balance career, family, friends, volunteer work, workouts, and self-care? Are you constantly stressed trying to wade through your to-do list? Do you feel like there aren't enough hours in the day to get it all done? Want to stop worrying about time, get more done, and actually enjoy what you're doing? The secret lies in timing your life with your second clock in mind rather than simply adhering to the 24-hour clock.

I know what you're thinking. Sounds too good to be true. We're all tired of the media telling us we can "have it all," when we're just trying to get through each day intact. I understand. I've got a lot on my plate: I'm a mom, a wife, a daughter, a business owner, an author, and a speaker. I have a vital self-care practice. I love to cook. I love to read. I can easily get overwhelmed by my to-do list. The fact is that the "you can have it all" credo is steeped in the conditioning that women must "do it all" to earn love, acceptance, and security in our patriarchal society. In a culture that ignores the wisdom of our second clock, what else could we expect? However, when you yourself insist in your own life that you orient everything you do around your 28-day clock, the pressure to do it all and have it all simply drops away. Rushing in to fill the place of that pressure are discernment, desire, and an increased quality of life. Before I incorporated my second clock in my life, if I had a major deadline or project due, I would just push myself to the point of misery and exhaustion to get it done and deal with the health consequences afterward. After I started orienting my life around my second clock, I changed my approach; for example, when I came back on the speaking circuit following the birth of my daughter, I'd schedule those talks only during my ovulatory phases to make sure I didn't burn myself out too quickly.

This change is not some big thing—it's a million little moments when you include your female reality in the choices you make, reclaim your sovereignty, and increase your enjoyment and well-being. I know for a fact that I couldn't perform at a high level, or attempt to accomplish all that I do, if

I weren't managing my time and energy in a cyclical fashion. Before I realized I had to honor my second clock, my hormonal problems had drained my energy to the point where I was barely able to accomplish the basics of daily living. Just getting off the couch to go to a doctor's appointment required a monumental effort. After years of syncing with my cycle, I've learned how to plan ahead to stay in a peak flow state as much as possible. I prime my body with cycle-specific self-care and schedule my days, weeks, months, and year with the four phases of my cycle in mind. I hold brainstorming meetings on the days when my creative energy is highest. I slot my speaking engagements for the dates when communication skills are on point. I tackle detail-oriented tasks during those times when awareness and attention are locked in. I take stock of how I'm doing and where I'm heading in the phase when changes in my neurochemistry encourage self-analysis. Most important, this practice demands that I make choices continually about what works for me and what doesn't. Making these choices is a huge departure from what I had been conditioned to believe, which is simply that I should do everything asked of me at all times. It's not realistic or healthy to have so few boundaries that there is no room left in your life for yourself, your dreams, or your desires.

Let me give you another example of what cycle syncing looks like in my life. In the days before my period, my energy turns inward and I'm less inclined to socialize, start new projects, or power through my to-do list. What do I do? Instead of stressing about how to squeeze it all in, I do something that feels pretty rebellious to me: I glance at my list, pick the two or three things that absolutely *must* get done, and move the rest to another day. That's right. I cross them off the list. Yes, it can feel a little scary to jump off the hamster wheel when we're so conditioned to always do more, but with that one move, I go from super-stressed to relaxed. With less on my list, I'm able to get in the groove on those few very important things. And those tasks I crossed off my list have been shifted to a day when my cycle naturally fills me with more energy and more ability to tackle them.

As a result, I find myself in the flow on a routine basis. It feels like I'm doing less—remember, I crossed things off my to-do list—but I'm achieving more because I'm focusing my efforts and supporting myself physically. I'm more creative and more optimistic, rather than feeling overwhelmed. On days when I do feel like I'm dragging, I know it's because I'm out of sync with my cycle, and it's time for triage. I boost my self-care with strategies you'll discover in upcoming chapters to help me fly through any challenging days. Most important, I look at how choices I made, and boundaries I didn't support, left me feeling burned out.

Tuning in to my cycle opened my eyes to a whole new female-centered way of thinking about time that allows me to achieve more of what I want and enjoy the process along the way by protecting my energy. But if you're like most of the women I've helped over the past seventeen years, your inner dialogue reflects your single-clock lifestyle and its implications for your physical and emotional health. In addition to telling me about their hormonal health issues, women also fill me in on their daily life challenges. You can probably relate to some of the following things I hear on a regular basis.

Check any of the following phrases that sound like you.*

☐ "There aren't enough hours in the day."

☐ "My anxiety is through the roof."

☐ "Sometimes it's hard to stay focused."

☐ "I'm overwhelmed by my schedule."

☐ "I feel like I'm short-changing my kids."

☐ "I feel frazzled."

☐ "I don't have the energy to do it all."

☐ "I don't have enough time for my relationships."

The problem isn't a lack of time. Ignoring your second clock is draining your energy. The secret to achieving more actually lies in *doing less*. It's almost a radical thought in our society, which forces the more-is-better philosophy down our collective throats. The idea of less can seem downright treasonous. But it's backed by science. It's time to let go of these old patterns

---

* Heck, who am I kidding? Just check every box.

and get in tune with a female-centered productivity paradigm that's based on your biology.

Stop Ignoring Your Second Clock

You've been culturally conditioned to unconsciously believe some truly flawed philosophies about time. Let's look at the biggest culprits and cyclical flow blockers and break them down one by one.

FLO Blocker 1:
You're watching only one clock

Time to wake up! Time to go to work! Time for dinner! In our society, we're all chained to the ticking clock. Most of the women who come to me for help with their period problems also suffer from the effects of trying to keep up with the daily grind. Because they aren't living in harmony with their inner cycle, their hormonal systems are crying out for help. When you're dealing with painful periods, headaches, and PMS, it's so much harder to succeed in the male-patterned world where productivity is king. We begin to think we suck at time management.

Our entire concept of time is predicated on the male-patterned 24-hour cycle—a straight shot to an end point. It's time to kick that concept to the curb. Instead of thinking about time in typical chronological fashion, it's time to adopt something I call *right-timing*. The idea is to do things at the right moment, not necessarily sequentially. That daunting to-do list of yours? Instead of adding task after task in no particular order, think about the best time—what the ancient Greeks called *kairos*—for each item, and group your tasks based on the strengths of the phase of your cycle. An upcoming chapter gives specifics on how to do so and provides you with a daily planner geared to help you include both your clocks in your planning.

Ultimately, when you're syncing with your cycle, you can stop trying to master *time* and start thinking about managing your *energy*. This subtle but powerful shift in your thought process will pay off in a big way. The concept is already catching on in the corporate world. In a 2007 *Harvard Business Review* article, some forward-thinking leaders at global consultancy firm The Energy Project explored the effects of managing energy versus time. They wrote, "The core problem with working longer hours is that time is a finite resource. Energy is a different story." They've found that replacing energy-depleting behaviors with self-care practices that recharge and re-energize is the key to sustainable high performance without burnout. I've taken this finding one step further to show that these energy-building strategies are naturally built into your biochemistry and must be managed differently for women in their reproductive years.

Here's what I mean. Think of the male-energy paradigm based on a 24-hour clock as a hockey puck being pushed across the ice. The puck accelerates, decelerates, and eventually comes to a stop. This is the energy paradigm we've been conditioned to adopt: you go as hard as you can, as long as you can, and then crash. The female energy paradigm, based on the 28-day cycle, is cyclical. Which, like a wheel, is arguably more powerful and efficient. When you stabilize it and give it a push, it accelerates and gains speed, gathering momentum naturally as it rolls. In fact, the industrial revolution was powered by cyclical machinery, prized for its ongoing efficiency! This is how your body is intended to work. When you intentionally and strategically support the four phases of your cycle instead of simply pushing through your agenda each day, you'll be gaining energy rather than draining it. Syncing with your cycle keeps you engaged, and you'll arrive at your desired destination faster and might even go farther than you originally intended. Your schedule becomes a reflection of your natural strengths, allowing you to get in the flow and perform at your best.

FLO Blocker 2:
You're living in perpetual productivity

With right-timing, everything has an ideal moment. I learned about that natural rhythm of life in Mr. Bing's biology class when I had to observe a tree from winter to spring bloom. We are meant to live our lives in rhythm with this cycle of creation—from seed to growth to harvest to rest.

Natural Cycle of Creation

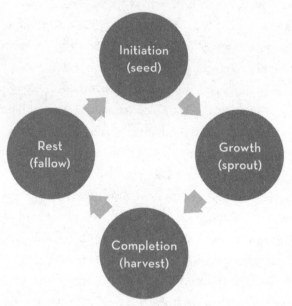

Our culture, however, demands perpetual growth and harvest. Trying to live your life in nonstop growth and harvest mode is taxing for your endocrine system. The message that you need to be in constant production mode puts you in an impossible situation. You are pressured to strive for peak productivity at all times, ignoring your natural rhythm. You feel the need to do more even though your performance falters, your health fails, and your psyche suffers. This relentless pursuit of productivity—at work, at home, and in your relationships—forces you to put yourself last on your to-do list, if you even make it onto your list at all. Self-care goes out the window. You skip lunch, you skimp on sleep, you fuel yourself with double lattes. These make your endocrine system go haywire, and once one of your hormones is disrupted, a cascade of imbalances and a laundry list of symptoms can follow. You can find yourself living with chronic stress, adrenal fatigue, anxiety, insomnia, and more. In a vicious circle, these conditions compound any existing hormonal dysfunction. And somehow, you're supposed to keep producing at top speed anyway. How is anyone supposed to function, let alone thrive, this way?

I'm reminded of something I've heard Oprah say, that life will tap you on the shoulder until it knocks you on your butt. Too many of us have been knocked on our butts. I think Oprah would agree: everything in the right season!

FLO Blocker 3:
You believe being busy is a status symbol or a badge of honor

When I ask women who come to the center, "How are you?," they often answer with something along the lines of "I'm so busy, it's crazy." Think about that answer for a moment. We're so divorced from our feelings that we can't even give an emotional, let alone human, response to a simple question. Instead, we provide a productivity update to connect and commiserate with others. We've been conditioned to believe that the more tasks and activities we have jam-packed into each day, the more valuable we are. That was the conclusion of a 2017 study in the *Journal of Consumer Research*, which found that a busy and overworked lifestyle has become "an aspirational status symbol." We're basing our personal expectations on what our digital tools—computers, cell phones, and other gadgets that can operate 24/7—can do. It's as if we're aspiring to become machines that never power down.

The trend is taking a toll on our health and performance. In her book, *Overwhelmed: Work, Love, and Play When No One Has the Time*, Bridget Schulte dissects how the cult of busyness is leaving us feeling fractured, scattered, and mentally and physically exhausted. We're all jettisoning ourselves from one task to the next, barely taking a moment to breathe. And women may be more susceptible to this, considering our days can be even more jam-packed than men's. Melinda Gates addressed the issue of "time poverty" in the 2016 annual letter from the Gates Foundation. She singled out the gender gap in the number of hours we devote to unpaid work—

think grocery shopping, kitchen duty, and carting the kids around. Statistics show that globally women spend an average of 4.5 hours a day on unpaid work, while men skate by performing much less than half that amount. She wrote, "Unless things change, girls today will spend hundreds of thousands more hours than boys doing unpaid work simply because society assumes it's their responsibility."

Racing through our to-do lists also leaves no time for restorative, relaxing activities. According to the US Department of Labor, men spend thirty-three more minutes per day socializing, engaging in exercise, or watching TV than women do. In a year, this adds up to more than two hundred fewer hours of leisure time for women. No wonder we're exhausted!

A growing number of doctors and scientists are finding that our over-scheduled days are leading to difficulty concentrating, inability to focus, irritability, sleep issues, mental fatigue, physical wear and tear, and more. Suzanne Koven, an internal medicine physician at Massachusetts General Hospital, hit the nail on the head in a 2013 column in the *Boston Globe* when she declared that busy is the new sick. "In the past few years, I've observed an epidemic of sorts: patient after patient suffering from the same condition. The symptoms of this condition include fatigue, irritability, insomnia, anxiety, headaches, heartburn, bowel disturbances, back pain, and weight gain. There are no blood tests or X-rays diagnostic of this condition, and yet it's easy to recognize. The condition is excessive busyness."

This is yet another detrimental effect of living in a society that values relentless productivity more than anything else. Being busy has emerged as the modern-day hero's journey. In mythology, the hero's journey centers on a person heading out on an adventure, facing an obstacle, claiming victory, and returning home a transformed person. Today's hero's journey revolves around endless tasks and efficient production, hour after hour. Sound familiar? It should. Remember that description from my biology textbook:

The testes are powerhouses of efficient production. They produce two to three hundred million spermatozoa daily. . . .

If you're wondering where our society came up with these values, look no further than a man's biology. Seriously! This concept of never-ending production mimics the semen production that takes place in the testicles. It's no surprise that the way we formed our society is based on what we've studied most, which is the male body. We high-five goal achievement and project completion, but we don't reward rest, rejuvenation, or enjoying the ride.

FLO Blocker 4:
You believe success requires suffering

Thanks to trailblazing women, young girls today believe they can be whatever they want to be—president of the United States, an astronaut, a tech CEO, you name it. Anything a man can do, we can do bleeding. We've proven without a doubt that we can do anything. I would just like to see women doing whatever they want without incurring unnecessary health expense. I would like them to have a framework in which they feel supported deeply. Don't get me wrong—working hard for a goal is a very good thing. But what if we could incorporate, from the start, the lessons many learned too late in life, that compromising isn't worth the cost? Women wholeheartedly buy into the belief that we have to suffer in order to succeed—in a way similar to the way we've been conditioned to think we are destined to endure physical pain because of our biochemistry. It's sadistic to think this way. It's time to realize you don't have to suffer from physical ailments, nor do you have to damage your health, relationships, or mental well-being in pursuit of success.

The same way you trim some tasks from your schedule, you may want to readjust your concept of success and productivity. Does productivity equal success? If you have to give up all the things you love in order to rise up the corporate ladder or reach a goal, is it really a win? If your endless pursuit of an objective makes you physically ill—think chronic stress, gut issues, or high blood pressure—is it really an achievement? If you're riddled with anxiety or wracked with worry from constantly pushing, is it really worth it? What are you really trying to accomplish, what void are you trying to fill with this nonstop pursuit?

In Buddhism, there's a concept known as the hungry ghost. I think of the hungry ghost as a sort of black hole within that can never be filled. In our culture, people chase goal after goal or acquire shiny new thing after shiny new thing, but feel increasingly empty inside. In Alain de Botton's seminal book *Status Anxiety*, he describes this constant pursuit of more as a need for love. No matter what people achieve or how much they possess, they still want more. They buy their first condo but still yearn for the big house with the yard. They land a promotion at work but are already plotting their next career move. They lose ten pounds but feel bad that they didn't lose twenty. You probably know plenty of women like this—you could be one of them yourself. Take heart. There's a better way.

FLO Blocker 5:
You expect to feel the same every day

One of the things that blocks your ability to access the gifts of your second clock is the expectation that you should be a static creature. You're not. You're a dynamic being. Like the rest of our body's biochemistry, our emotional energy levels expand outward and then retract inward in a natural rhythm throughout our cycle. Sometimes we're more social and communicative, other times we're more introspective and have a desire to be a homebody. Our society values outward energy more than inward energy, so we tend to think we're being lazy if we putter around the house or that we're self-indulgent if we focus on ourselves. But these ebbs and flows in energy aren't about you being lazy. Feeling withdrawn can be a powerful signal from your cycle to focus inward and take extra care of yourself.

We all have this expectation that we should be able to perform the same way every day so beaten into our heads that when I tell the women who come to me for help that respecting our fluctuations is key to getting in sync, they give me one of those sideways glances. In all my years of health consulting, I've found this to be one of the hardest concepts for women to adopt. I have to reassure them that it's okay—make that *great*—for them to take a break from the grind to check in on personal well-being. In fact, it's mandatory that you rest after a crazy productive period.

FLO Blocker 6:
You have a hormonal imbalance or are taking the pill

I've said it before, but it bears repeating: if you have period problems, PMS, bloating, cramping, or other issues with your menstrual cycle, or if you're taking synthetic birth control, you won't be able to fully access the gifts of your second clock. It's important to address your hormonal health. The Bio-hacking Tool Kit will help you if you need period support.

YES, YOU CAN DO LESS. SERIOUSLY!

If you're thinking the concept of doing less is impossible in your deadline-driven world, think again. I work with a lot of high-powered female executives, business owners, and college students who tend to respond, "Yeah, right," when I tell them about this radical shift in perception. Let me show you more clearly how it can work. When I returned from a recent business trip, I had twenty things on my to-do list. I looked at the arc of my month and thought about what would give me maximum efficiency and creativity while allowing me to maintain a high level of self-care. I also evaluated my task list and carefully curated what was really worth doing based on what would be most enjoyable and rewarding. Most important, I actively ignored the inner voice that said I needed to do everything to get ahead and to do it now. Then I parsed out my task list and mapped it onto my cycle phase by phase. Suddenly, it all seemed infinitely more doable, and I went from feeling overwhelmed to feeling en-ergized.

The Cyclical Secret: Use Your Second Clock

After working for close to two decades with women who are suffering from hormonal breakdown and struggling with their careers, relationships, and motherhood, I've realized their struggles are largely the result of their not factoring in their second clock in a meaningful way. Syncing with your cycle will not only help you overcome your period problems, but also give you the foundation to thrive in every area of your life. When you reframe your understanding of your body's biochemistry and start incorporating your second clock, you can stop pressuring yourself to be in perpetual growth or harvest, stop struggling to manage chronological time, and start pursuing your goals in a sustainable way that makes you feel empowered and confident. And when you approach life from your own inner timing, you will naturally find your way to peak performance that helps you build energy and enhance your health and wellness, not drain them. You'll unlock your creativity, find more pleasure in your relationships, and feel more fulfilled.

Seeing how much of an asset your second clock is, and how ignoring it has cost you so much from a physical, emotional, and even spiritual point of view, can be upsetting. Or this understanding could fill you with excitement and hope, knowing there is a clear answer to your quiet question: "Isn't there a better way?" You may have a visceral reaction—positive or negative—to this information. My advice is to take these feelings and channel them into a new way of living based on the scientific facts surrounding your biology. You don't have to wait for a major societal shift to take advantage of your natural timing, gifts, and talents. You can start today by setting your compass to your true north, and getting in sync with your body's monthly cycle and natural rhythms. I know it can feel overwhelming to make changes on your own, so I've created free resources where you can get in the FLO with all the support you need at www.IntheFLObook.com/bonus.

Remember, finding your way to doing less, achieving more, and being happier isn't just about you. Every time you take up the space you need in your life—for example, allowing yourself to cross something off your to-do list, giving yourself permission to rest and rejuvenate after a busy stretch of time, or planning your day based on your energy rather than your time—it heals your soul and chips away at our cultural conditioning. And it provides an example for other women—our sisters, friends, and daughters. By sharing what we're learning about our bodies, we can start building a global community of women living in tune with our biochemistry. And this female reclamation will continue to grow until the revolution is undeniable.

GETTING IN THE FLO

Want to start practicing the art of doing less, achieving more, and managing your energy so you can get in the FLO? Try these simple cyclical hacks:

1. Take stock at the end of the day: How's your energy? Do you feel exhausted and drained, or invigorated, like you've had a great workout?
2. Keep track of how often you say yes when you really mean no. Boundaries become a problem when you don't fit yourself on your own schedule.
3. Take one thing a day off your to-do list and resist the urge to fill that space with something else to do.
4. Dare to do nothing for half an hour or engage in a small pleasure— take a hike, make a phone call, or catch up with a friend.
5. List three things you can do besides work.
6. When somebody asks you, "How are you?," try answering with an emotional answer—"I'm feeling great today," or even "I'm feeling energized today"—not the default setting, "I'm so busy."

CHAPTER 3

Beyond Your Period—Understanding Your Hormonal Advantages

We must reject not only the stereotypes that others hold
of us but also the stereotypes that we hold of ourselves.
—SHIRLEY CHISHOLM

E ven though I've been helping women heal their hormonal health and unlock the gifts of their cyclical nature for my entire career, I still get excited every time I share the real deal about our female biochemistry with someone new. I was having a session with a college student. As I explained the science of our biology and the concept of the Cycle Syncing Method™, she responded enthusiastically and said, "This makes so much sense. I really want to take care of myself. I want to live this way. And I want my friends at school to live this way too." I am always moved when this concept clicks for a woman, because it is such a reclamation of her personal power. How beautiful that at such a young age, this woman wants to unhook herself from her inherited cultural conditioning, reclaim her body, and encourage her friends to start living a cyclical life. I imagined how much easier life was going to be for her and her friends—enjoying balanced hormones and taking advantage of everything their biochemistry has to offer. As we wrapped up our call, I beamed, thinking about the decades of her life that would not be compromised with the negative effects of imbalanced hormones. If only it had been this way for me and for the countless women who approach me after talks or reach out online and say, "I wish I had known about this sooner"—to which I always respond, "I hope there comes a time when no woman has to say that, when we all know how to thrive in our bodies from the beginning."

If you're like most of the women I meet, "the talk" you received about your monthly cycle probably didn't go beyond the basics. "You're going to have a period once a month, and it's going to be awful. Here are some sanitary products you can use. Whatever you do, don't get pregnant! Here are a few condoms, but it's better if you just abstain from having sex. Do you have any questions? No? Good." It's not much. None of the talk is dedicated to discussing the hormonal fluctuations or the second clock that will impact nearly every aspect of your body, brain, and moods for the next thirty to forty years. Because the talk is so inadequate, we don't have the foundational knowledge to stand on to weather the avalanche of misinformation we're fed about our biochemistry, which leads us to believe our bodies really are a liability. As a result, we don't feel confident discussing our cycles among ourselves, so we tend to avoid the topic throughout our lifetime. The misinformation and avoidance all add up to unnecessary suffering and struggling in silence. Ultimately, this patriarchal wounding forces us to go into survival mode at puberty, disconnecting from our cyclical energy and compartmentalizing our second clock as if it relates only to our period and reproductive heath. Your hormones affect way more than your uterus and ovaries!

It's time to kick those myths to the curb and embrace the beauty and power of our biochemistry. In this chapter, we'll take a deep dive into some legit sex ed that's based on science, not social conditioning. So grab your notebook and get ready for the talk you should have gotten as a young woman and the biology class you should have had in middle school. I am 100 percent convinced our bodies provide us with critical guidance. I realized this long ago when I started listening to my body and formulated the FLO protocol that helped put my hormonal dysfunction into remission and continues to help women struggling with menstrual health issues at www .FLOliving.com. The more research I did, the more I realized science backs up everything I was experiencing in my own body. In this Biology 2.0 lesson, you'll quickly discover these key things:

- **We are not small men!** I'll introduce you to the biological systems—your brain, immune system, metabolism, microbiome, and stress response—that prove our bodies function in vastly different ways from male bodies. You'll discover irrefutable evidence that our biology has given us significant advantages. Although it's true we may not have the same height or muscle strength as the XY chromosome crowd, our bodies function in an exceptional fashion in so many other ways.

- **Our biological systems fluctuate with our monthly cycle.** Not only do all of our biological systems operate differently from male systems, they aren't static. Our systems fluctuate in direct response to the rise and fall of our hormones each month. Balanced hormones can infuse you with energy, spark your creativity, boost your moods, and turn your body into a glorious masterpiece. On an even deeper level, you'll be protecting your biological systems in the long run to preserve fertility and possibly prevent major diseases later in life, such as Alzheimer's, heart disease, and cancer. Yes, your hormones have that much power!

- **Ignoring your female biochemistry and second clock affects far more than just your reproductive health.** As we learned in the previous chapter, ignoring our second clock can lead not only to period problems and infertility, but also to major health issues. Here we'll learn what happens to each biological system when we neglect our second clock and hormonal health.

- **Biohacking the female system requires you to be in sync with your cycle.** Considering our systems fluctuate in response to our hormones, it makes no sense to adopt a self-care routine that is the same day in and day out. Diets, fitness trends, and skin care hacks are guaranteed to fall short if they don't follow your natural cycle. If you want to manipulate your biological systems for optimal performance, you need to biohack like a woman.

Meet Your Hormones

Your endocrine system is a powerful and complex network of glands that work together to secrete hormones that regulate specific body functions. The hypothalamus, the almond-sized brain structure that acts as command central for your endocrine system, receives a steady stream of data about the hormone levels throughout your body. Based on this information, the hypothalamus fires off one of two hormones—releasing hormone or inhibiting hormone—to the garbanzo-sized pituitary gland that is snuggled just below it. The pituitary gland goes into immediate action, sending out chemical messengers—aka hormones—to the other glands and organs in your endocrine system. The pituitary uses a different hormone to communicate with each of them—thyroid-stimulating hormone (TSH) to the thyroid gland, parathyroid hormone (PTH) to the parathyroid, adrenocorticotropic hormone (ACTH) to the adrenals, and follicle-stimulating hormone (FSH) or luteinizing hormone (LH) to the ovaries. The target glands and organs interpret the message from the pituitary and either increase or pump the brakes on hormone production.

Here are the key hormones we'll be learning to balance throughout our cycle.

Estrogen: Produced primarily by the ovaries, but also in small amounts by the adrenal glands and fat cells, estrogen is the superstar of your hormonal cycle. In your reproductive cycle, estrogen participates in ovulation and is responsible for thickening the uterine lining in anticipation of a pregnancy. Estrogen also plays a major role in many other biological systems, and protects you from dementia, bone density loss, heart disease, and high blood pressure.

Progesterone: Production of progesterone kicks in around ovulation, when it gets to work on its main job of controlling and maintaining the buildup of the uterine lining in anticipation of a pregnancy. If an egg isn't fertilized, progesterone levels fall, and the lining is shed through menstruation. Progesterone also counterbalances estrogen and promotes relaxation, improves sleep, and enhances moods.

Testosterone: Produced in the ovaries and adrenal glands, testosterone is present in women in much lower levels than in men. This hormone, which is associated with sex drive, gets a slight surge during and immediately after ovulation—making you feel more sexual at the time you're most likely to get pregnant.

Follicle-stimulating hormone (FSH): Released by the pituitary gland in the brain, FSH stimulates ovarian follicles to mature. FSH imbalances can lead to infertility. As you begin perimenopause, your FSH levels slowly rise to a level that signals the ovary to stop releasing eggs.

Luteinizing hormone (LH): Released by the pituitary gland in the brain at ovulation, LH triggers the release of a mature egg from an ovarian follicle. Abnormal LH levels are associated with fertility issues and PCOS.

Insulin: When you consume carbohydrates, your body breaks them down and converts them into glucose (a type of sugar), which is absorbed into the bloodstream. Your pancreas secretes the hormone insulin in response to the amount of glucose in the bloodstream—more glucose, more insulin. This critical hormone ushers the glucose into your body's cells so it can be used for energy, and it helps keep your blood sugar levels balanced. When insulin levels are off balance, it can lead to blood sugar imbalance, which is associated with menstrual irregularities and reduced fertility.

Cortisol: Cortisol is the body's primary stress hormone. The release of this important hormone is regulated by the body's hypothalamic-pituitary-adrenal (HPA) axis. Small doses of cortisol can be a good thing, but chronically high levels of the hormone can disrupt ovulation, decrease progesterone levels, sap your sex drive, and cause fertility problems.

RESOLVE HORMONAL ISSUES FIRST

When your hormones are working harmoniously, they allow you to unlock all the benefits of your biological systems and feminine energy.

But period problems, such as fibroids, endometriosis, and PCOS, can dampen your experience of your cyclical benefits. So the first thing you need to do as part of the Cycle Syncing Method™ is to resolve any hormonal issues—this is what women do with us at www.FLOliving .com. You'll learn the specific steps to take toward hormonal healing in the Biohacking Tool Kit section at the end of Part II.

Reconnect with Your POWR

Your cycle phases give you tremendous creative force and provide ongoing momentum in your life. In short, they are your power source. To help you connect with your phases and make it easy to remember the special focus in each one, just think of tapping into your POWR—Prepare, Open Up, Work, Rest. In chapter 1, I wrote a brief description of the female hormonal system that I wish I had read in my biology book back in middle school. I used the same positive tone that had been used in my textbook's summary of sperm production. So here, ladies, I offer a breakdown of the four phases of your menstrual cycle using the reverence and awestruck language your cycle deserves. Take note, this will be a radical departure from the description you're used to, which says that your bleed is Day 1 of your cycle. This notion is long overdue for an update. Your bleed as Day 1 is a medical reference that emerged from a time when only men were allowed to practice medicine. It's not the beginning for anyone who bleeds and who lives the experience. Your bleed is the culmination of your hormonal cycle, not the beginning. The only reason the start of the bleed has been referenced as Day 1 of your cycle is that it was assumed that the bleeding phase is the only one you would notice or track and thereby make it easier for doctors to reference. The confusion created by this exogenous labeling diminishes a woman's intuitive wisdom, devalues her physical experience, and robs her of self-authority and self-governance. The imprecise and deficient vocabulary available to describe our physical reality limits our experience of self and breeds doubt. Just as improvements must be made in research to eliminate gender bias, we as women must describe and define this physical experience for ourselves on our own terms as part of healing from patriarchal conditioning, honoring our bodies, and claiming our power.

PHASE 1: PREPARE
Follicular Phase
Duration: 7–10 Days

Phase 1 of your cycle begins directly after your bleed ends. At the outset of the follicular phase, your hormones are in a quiet phase, beginning to increase in concentration in the coming days. The small hypothalamus in your brain has the very big responsibility of kicking off this amazing process, signaling your pituitary gland to shuttle FSH to your ovaries to help some of the eggs inside mature. Your two ovaries, which are each only about the size of a grape, contain your lifetime supply of eggs, each housed in a fluid-filled sac called a follicle. Fueled by the arrival of FSH, the follicles swell in preparation. Estrogen levels begin to rise to initiate the renewal of your uterine lining—the endometrium—so that it can host an egg in an ideal environment later on in the cycle. On a behavioral level, the follicular phase is a time of beginning, a fresh start.

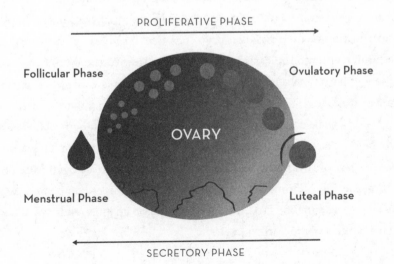

PROLIFERATIVE PHASE

Follicular Phase

Ovulatory Phase

OVARY

Menstrual Phase

Luteal Phase

SECRETORY PHASE

PHASE 2: OPEN UP
Ovulatory Phase
Duration: 3–4 Days

Over just a few days, a dramatic rise in estrogen, followed by a rise in luteinizing hormone (LH), stimulates one lucky follicle to mature fully and
be released into one of the fallopian tubes. The egg diligently makes its
way down the fallopian tube to the uterus where, thanks to rising estrogen
levels, the uterine lining has grown lush and a host of protective immune
system cells have sprouted. In conjunction with the LH that stimulates the
follicle to release an egg, there is also a sharp surge followed by a rapid
decline in testosterone. The ovulatory phase lives up to its popular reputa-
tion—it's a period of feeling social and communicative.

PHASE 3: WORK
Luteal Phase
Duration: 10–14 Days

The corpus luteum (the follicle from which the egg was released) grows
inside the ovary, sparking the production of progesterone. Estrogen levels
continue to rise and promote additional padding of the uterine lining. The
rise in progesterone signals the body to keep the thickened lining in place
in anticipation of a fertilized embryo. The rise in progesterone also signals
the pituitary to stop releasing FSH and LH. Toward the end of the cycle,
if the egg hasn't been fertilized, the corpus luteum is reabsorbed into the
body in utmost efficiency. After estrogen, progesterone, and testosterone
reach their peak concentrations, they begin to fall to their lowest levels
right before your period begins. (PMS is a common—but completely unnecessary—part of this phase and results from too much estrogen in relation
to progesterone.) Think of the luteal phase as a time of completion, when
you're naturally inclined to finish projects and tie up loose ends—you begin
to turn your attention on yourself.

PHASE 4: REST
Menstrual Phase
Duration: 3-7 Days

As the corpus luteum gets reabsorbed, progesterone production drops off in sync. This triggers your uterus to shed the endometrial lining. The consistency, color, and duration of your menstrual period is a powerful sign of your hormonal health. Estrogen peaks and then plummets before the bleed starts as well, signaling your hypothalamus to get prepared for another beautifully rhythmic cycle. This is an ideal time for reflection and looking inward.

28-Day Hormonal Chart—Peaks and Valleys Across 28 Days

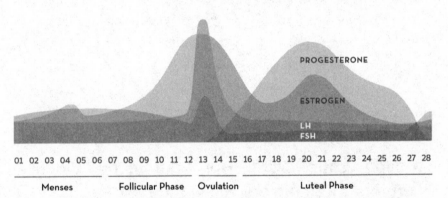

| Menses | Follicular Phase | Ovulation | Luteal Phase |

YOUR MONTHLY HORMONE TEST

Our monthly bleed is a critical biomarker of what is happening in our biochemistry in real time. A few years back, I inadvertently made TV history when I appeared on the Dr. Oz show and used a variety of juices and fruits, including mashed-up blueberries, strawberry jam, cranberry juice, and prune juice, to show the various colors and consistency of menstrual blood and what it means for your hormonal health. Think of it as a monthly at-home hormone test. (You can learn what the color of your menstrual blood means in an upcoming chapter.) In addition, we can thank all of the phases of our cycle for giving us a clear picture at all times of our hormonal health—*remember, it's considered to be your fifth vital sign!* If anything is off-kilter, we know it right away. Cramps, heavy bleeding, missed periods—these are the ways our body tells us our hormones need support. I can't help but think that our hormonal system, so vital to the survival of our species, has been tuned more tightly to give us an immediate heads-up to imbalances and monthly opportunities for improvement in self-care. You can check what the color of your period is telling you about your hormones right now at www.FLOliving.com/what-is-your-v-sign. Unfortunately, as you saw in chapter 1, we turn too often to medications and over-the-counter drugs to mask those symptoms, or we're told that our symptoms are all in our heads and should just be ignored. When we learn to listen to and respect the messages our body is giving us, we can make simple changes that support our beautifully complex system.

Beyond Your Period—How Your Second Clock Affects 5 Key Biological Systems

One reason we don't think we need to seriously consider the care of our second clock is because we've been led to believe that it affects only our reproductive and menstrual experience. Let's end that misconception now—you'll see that the second clock affects every system of your body.

Biological System 1: Brain

If you compared female and male brains in a science lab, you'd probably notice that the female brain is close to 10 percent smaller. Otherwise, you might not detect many surface differences. But when you peer deeper inside with high-tech images of the living brain, things start to get interesting. Thanks to groundbreaking research detailed in neuropsychiatrist Louann Brizendine's seminal bestseller *The Female Brain,* as well as findings in neuroscientist and psychiatrist Daniel Amen's *Unleash the Power of the Female Brain,* we now know the female brain functions very differently, with stronger networks that foster communication, emotional memory, intuition, and anger suppression. Take a look at some of the key ways the research shows our gray matter outperforms the male brain.

Larger prefrontal cortex (PFC): Women have a larger PFC, a region that acts as your brain's CEO and is involved in executive decisions and higher cognitive functions. Located at the front of the brain behind your forehead, the PFC is involved in planning, judgment, and organization. More volume in this area is generally associated with an uptick in empathy, impulse control, controlled risk-taking, and focus. The PFC, which isn't fully developed until our mid-twenties, develops faster in females, which may be the reason young women tend to seem so much more mature than their male counterparts.

Bigger hippocampus: Associated with long-term memory and emotional memory formation, the hippocampus is larger in women, which may explain why we never forget an argument, a wedding anniversary, or a first date.

Smaller amygdala: The brain's fear and anger center is a small almond-shaped group of neurons within the temporal lobes. Smaller in women, this points to a greater ability to defuse tense situations rather than getting into an all-out brawl.

Bigger insula: This area, which houses those gut feelings, is bigger in women and indicates a higher ability to listen to our intuition.

Smaller hypothalamus: Associated with sexual drive, this region is smaller in women, which explains why we aren't as obsessed with thoughts about hooking up at all times.

Bigger anterior cingulate: Greater volume in the female brain's decision-making and anxiety center tends to make us take more time when making big decisions and worry more than men.

Bigger corpus callosum: The human brain is divided into two hemispheres, left and right, with nerve bundles called the corpus callosum bridging the two sides. Women possess more of these nerve bundles, providing greater connectivity between the sides, which allows us to harness the power of more regions of our brain when solving problems.

What's the main takeaway from all this brain science? On a personal level, it means you're brilliant in a uniquely feminine way, and you can thank your female brain that you are wired for leadership, empathy, community building, problem solving, intuition, fairness, and systems thinking.

How Your Cycle Affects Your Brain

Do you ever feel like you aren't the same person day to day—that at certain times during the month you feel energetic and efficient, whereas at other times you feel more inwardly focused? You aren't imagining this. As estrogen and progesterone levels rise and fall throughout your cycle, your brain changes in response. We can thank neuroscientist Catherine Woolley, a professor at Northwestern University who has been studying neuroendocrinology for more than two decades, for some of the most enlightening findings on the effects of estrogen on the brain. Her 1996 study in the *Journal of Comparative Neurology* shows the female brain can change up to 25 percent during the monthly cycle, mainly thanks to fluctuating estrogen levels.

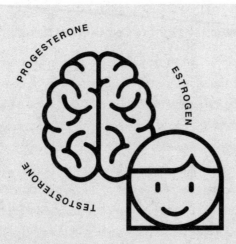

Your hormones affect your brain in brilliant ways each week of your cycle.

Skyrocketing estrogen levels during ovulation lead to a boost in synaptic connections within the hippocampus, which can increase mental sharpness, creativity, and communication skills. According to a 2005 study in *Behavioral and Cognitive Neuroscience Reviews*, an uptick in estrogen enhances the release of serotonin, which is known as the happiness neurotransmitter. This means you're likely to feel more social, verbal, and outgoing in the first half of your cycle as estrogen is increasing. In the second half of your cycle, when estrogen falls, those connections in the hippocampus decrease and serotonin levels fall, causing a shift in your cognitive focus. It would be very easy to interpret these brain changes to mean the first half of the cycle is good and the second half is bad, but that's an old-school interpretation of our cyclical nature. Each half is equally valuable in different ways. Rising estrogen in the first half of the cycle prompts us to be more outwardly focused and to take care of others. Falling hormone levels in the second half of the cycle balance that outward focus by allowing us to turn our attention inward to nurture ourselves. We cannot be in perpetual harvest or constantly in service to others. Nature demands that we take time to rest and attend to our own needs and has built this balance into our hormonal cycle.

What Goes Wrong When We Ignore Our Cyclical Nature

If your hormones are imbalanced or you don't care for yourself in a phase-specific way, the gentle hormonal ups and downs can swing wildly. Out-of-control hormones in the first half of your cycle can cause you to overdo it with all-nighters at work, start too many projects at once, or experience stress and worry. In the second half of your cycle, out-of-whack hormones can lead to brain fog, leave you in a funk, and make you feel like you can barely crawl out of bed in the morning. Because we believe we are destined to suffer from hormonal problems, we accept that we should feel bad and be inefficient during the second half of our cycle, and so we do nothing to reverse this self-perpetuating situation. But life doesn't need to go on this way.

Ignoring period problems—such as cramps, bloating, and missing periods—that signal hormonal imbalance will prevent you from taking advantage of the positive impact your hormones have on your brain. Here's exactly why you need to implement the practices you'll be learning about in the next section of this book, so you can maintain optimal hormone levels to prevent the major negative impact on your creativity. Take severe cramps—one of the most common signs of hormonal imbalance—for example. As if the pain wasn't bad enough in itself, painful periods also lower your ability to perform complex tasks, reduce your attention span, and are associated with abnormal changes in the brain's gray matter, according to multiple studies in the journal *PAIN*. Women with PMS symptoms have hormonal imbalances that primarily impact two areas of the brain: the PFC, and the limbic or emotional center. They may also experience a drop in levels of the feel-good neurochemical serotonin. With these brain changes, you can say good-bye to mental clarity, good judgment, and stable emotions and hello to forgetfulness, trouble concentrating, impulsivity, aggression, moodiness, depression, and irritability. According to the

NIH BioCycle Study, the longer PMS goes untreated, the greater your risk for dementia. This is why it's so important for you to get in sync with your cycle and balance your hormones. It isn't just about getting rid of your cramps and bloating; it's about optimizing your brain function now and safeguarding it for the future.

In the FLO Advantage

When your hormones are balanced, the natural ebb and flow of your monthly cycle has a predictable and positive impact on brain function and allows you to take advantage of your unique gifts and talents throughout the month. Here's what the four phases of your cycle look like when your hormones are balanced.

- **Follicular phase:** The overall hormone effect on the brain is one of openness to new things, creativity, and beginnings. What do you want more of in your life? Where can you set your intentions?

- **Ovulatory phase:** The verbal and social centers of the brain are stimulated by hormones. Talk about what you want with everyone you speak to during this phase. This is a good time for important conversations. Connect with your community and enjoy being magnetic.

- **Luteal phase:** Your brain chemistry is optimized for task and detail orientation and bringing projects to completion. In the first half of this phase, you have some energy to spend with others. In the second half, focus more on taking care of yourself. Speak up for yourself, say no more often, and set your own firm boundaries— otherwise you may become irritated this week.

- **Menstrual phase:** As hormone levels quickly decline to their lowest concentrations, it creates the greatest communication between your two brain hemispheres—the left analytical side and the right feeling side. This means you are best able to synthesize how you feel about situations with the facts and determine the best course of action. Schedule time for analysis and review and think strategically about where you want to go in terms of the big picture of your life. Is what you think you want still feeling good at this point? Do you feel good about what you're doing in the various areas of your life, how you're spending your time, whom you're spending it with? Allow yourself to turn inward to journal or reflect on where you are now. You can get notifications of these phase changes when you download the MyFLO app (www.MyFLOtracker.com).

Biological System 2: Immune System

If something is going around the office, my husband will inevitably get sick, and it will take him some time to recover. I tend to get sick only after a long period of being overstressed. Many of my female friends have noticed the same thing. We seem to do a better job fighting off common ailments, even if the kids bring home nasty viruses from school. A growing body of research is decoding why women have stronger immune systems, and it isn't just when it comes to cold and flu bugs. We're better equipped to fend off shock episodes from infection, sepsis, or trauma. We're less likely to get cancer. In fact, the lifetime probability of developing cancer is 45 percent for the XY-chromosome club and only 38 percent for women, according to 2012 research in *Frontiers in Genetics*. And women ultimately live longer than men.

Our hormones play a role in immune responses. According to 2017 research published in *Hormones and Behavior*, testosterone generally suppresses those responses while estrogen enhances them. Basically, we've been gifted with a genetically and hormonally enhanced immune system that helps us ward off infections and disease—especially during our reproductive years, so we stay healthy for childbearing.

How Your Cycle Affects Your Immune System

Have you ever noticed that you're more likely to come down with a cold right before your period? There's a biological reason. Your immune system responds differently to infections, viruses, and flu bugs throughout your monthly cycle. What you have intuitively noticed about your body's ability to ward off ailments is confirmed by science. An exciting 2018 study published in *Trends in Ecology & Evolution* on the cyclical nature of women's health found that during the first half of your cycle, as estrogen levels rise, your immune system is on high alert and ready to attack, giving you a great ability to fight off infections and fend off illnesses. During the second half of your cycle, when hormone concentrations decrease, your immune system downshifts and is less likely to mount an inflammatory response. I think it's clear these changes in immune response are intended to promote pregnancy. Greater immunity in the follicular phase keeps you in tip-top shape. In the second half of your cycle, your immune system takes a step back so your body won't attack a fertilized egg as a foreign invader. If your hormones are balanced, this shift in immunity should be imperceptible—but if you're imbalanced, you're more likely to feel run down or get that bug that's going around the office during this phase.

What Goes Wrong When We Ignore Our Cyclical Nature

When we're out of sync with our second clock, our supercharged immune system can go into overdrive. With so many women who are suffering from autoimmune diseases, including Hashimoto's thyroiditis, lupus, multiple sclerosis, and rheumatoid arthritis, it's important for us to consider the impact of ignoring this second clock. Scientists have discovered estrogen's role as an immunomodulator affecting some systemic diseases, such as autoimmune and inflammatory conditions. A German researcher writing in *Autoimmunity Reviews* in 2012 found that some women experience more acute symptoms related to chronic conditions in the few days leading up to or during their periods. Let me be clear: your cyclical nature does *not* make you more vulnerable to autoimmune disorders. But if you aren't supporting your reproductive clock by eating, exercising, and living in a cyclical fashion, your hormones may be out of whack, making you more susceptible to immune system stress.

In the FLO Advantage

Understanding the cyclical changes in your immune system gives you the power to biohack your body's virus-fighting ability by fueling up with immune-boosting micronutrients so you won't fall victim to pesky cold and flu bugs in the second half of your cycle. Increasing self-care in the second half of your cycle, when immunity is naturally lower, helps to offset that normal variance. Working with your cycle also prevents estrogen dominance, to protect you from developing autoimmune diseases and to minimize symptoms. I've met with so many women who were suffering from chronic conditions and saw dramatic symptom reduction when they started living in tune with their cyclical nature. The Cycle Syncing Method™ shows you how to feed and care for your body to promote a healthy immune response, ease symptoms, and keep you feeling great all month long.

Biological System 3: Metabolism

For our entire lives, we've been told that having a fast metabolism is the pinnacle of healthy living and the key to weight loss. Decades of research, however, show that women's resting metabolic rate is lower than in men, and the difference isn't attributable to body composition or fitness levels. We've been force-fed the notion that our slower metabolism is a problem we have to overcompensate for with tremendous deprivation and control. It's time for a fresh perspective. Think of it this way: nature encoded women with the ability to create other humans and therefore made our metabolism far more efficient than men's. While men waste nutrients by flushing them out of their systems quickly, women conserve nutrients longer and extract more benefit from the foods we eat to provide a more nutrient-rich environment for the childbearing process.

The evidence is clear. You cannot biohack your nutrition and fitness the same way men do. You need a food and fitness program that caters to your female metabolism. You can access more resources at www.IntheFLObook.com/bonus.

How Your Cycle Affects Your Metabolism

You may think your body should be a consistent calorie-burning machine day in and day out, but your biochemistry doesn't work that way. Your ability to burn calories varies with your hormonal cycle. That's the conclusion a team of British researchers reached when they reviewed existing studies on how the menstrual cycle affects metabolism in a 2007 article published in the *International Journal of Obesity*. In general, rises in estrogen tend to suppress appetite, whereas a dip in the hormone, combined with elevated progesterone, stimulates appetite. As a result, in the first half of your cycle, your metabolism slows down, curbing your appetite and conserving nutrients in anticipation of a possible pregnancy. During the luteal phase of your cycle, energy expenditure jumps anywhere from 8 to 16 percent, according to foundational research from 1986 in the *American Journal of Clinical Nutrition*. That jump corresponds to burning an extra 89 to 279 calories a day. Sounds great—but the British scientists were also quick to point out that this seeming metabolic miracle usually comes with a corresponding increase in appetite, cravings, and intake, amounting to about 90 to 500 calories a day. In the second half of the cycle, our reproductive nature is geared to meet the demands of pregnancy in the event an egg has been fertilized. This is what's behind those food cravings and desire for additional calories.

What Goes Wrong When We Ignore Our Cyclical Nature

If you don't eat in sync with your biochemistry, you may drop pounds in the first half of your cycle and then see the scale tick upward in the second half. Turning to diets based solely on the 24-hour circadian clock to lose weight isn't the solution. They don't take our cyclical nature or second clock into consideration. In fact, as you'll see in the next chapter, many popular diets trends—think intermittent fasting, ketogenic, and paleo—work against our metabolism, and actually prevent us from losing weight.

In the FLO Advantage

You can achieve lasting weight loss by working with your biology through eating and exercising in ways appropriate for each phase of your cycle. This female-centered method teaches you how to compensate for the rise in nutrient conservation in the luteal phase so you can keep extra pounds off all month. All you have to do is focus on eating specific foods that burn fuel more efficiently—you'll learn exactly which foods are ideal for this phase in the next chapter. The British research team mentioned earlier, based on their review of dozens of existing studies, concluded that weight-management programs should be based on tailoring diet consumption, calorie intake, and physical activity level to each phase of the menstrual cycle. Once again, science backs up your body's natural preference to sync with its cycle!

Biological System 4: Microbiome

Your gastrointestinal tract, vagina, and breasts are filled with trillions of beneficial bacteria. When these friendly microbes are balanced, they help keep your body humming in good health and fend off disease. But when they are imbalanced or bad bacteria sneak into the mix, they are associated with conditions such as obesity, rheumatoid arthritis, ADHD, and more. Emerging science is increasingly finding differences between the sexes when it comes to the human microbiome. For example, a 2014 study in *Nature Communications* found that women's and men's gut flora responded differently to the same diet. Other researchers found discrepancies between women and men in the abundance of specific gut bacteria. Researchers also noted differences between the sexes in the proliferation of certain bacteria as weight increased. No wonder your brother can lose weight on diets tailored to his biological rhythms while you don't see the scale budge!

Your gut microbiome also has a unique connection to your female brain. In fact, you have about 100 million neurons in your gut, which is often referred to as the "second brain." Your gut is responsible for pumping out more than 90 percent of the body's supply of serotonin, according to 2015 research in *Cell*. Although the scientists didn't note any differences between the sexes in terms of the gut-serotonin connection, I think it's logical to assume that, with so much of the "happiness neurotransmitter" emanating from your gut, your microbiome health can affect your moods.

Did you know that your breasts also have a microbiome? Or that this bacterial community could modulate your risk for breast cancer? In a 2016 study published in *Applied and Environmental Microbiology*, researchers detected differences in the bacterial makeup between women with breast cancer and those who were cancer free. This finding raises many questions about the breast microbiome's role in the prevention or development of breast cancer, and scientists are in laboratories now trying to determine whether good bacteria could be used as a possible treatment for the disease.

How Your Cycle Affects Your Microbiome

Your microbiome is tightly linked to your hormones and is considered by some to be an additional component of the endocrine system. Science shows that estrogen influences the gut in many ways: promoting the growth and proliferation of good gut bacteria and providing a protective barrier to prevent intestinal permeability, a condition also known as leaky gut that allows contents from the gut to seep out into the body. Leaky gut is associated with bloating, cramps, gas, food sensitivities, and other digestive issues. Estrogen receptors also influence the composition of intestinal bacteria, according to the *Journal of Neuroimmunology*. Considering this research, you might be tempted to think more estrogen is good for your gut and less is bad, but it isn't that simple. As with all your biological systems, balanced hormones are the key to optimal function.

On the other side of the equation, your gut microbiome plays a major role in the breakdown of estrogen and is critical in keeping this key hormone balanced. A certain set of gut bacteria—and more specifically certain bacterial genes, called the estrobolome—produce an essential enzyme that helps metabolize estrogen. Your gut is thus part of the elimination system that is vital to ushering hormones out of the body. This process, when working efficiently, plays an essential role in achieving hormonal harmony.

What Goes Wrong When We Ignore Our Cyclical Nature

Considering the many ways the menstrual cycle impacts the microbiome, it's logical to assume imbalanced hormones can have negative effects on gut, vaginal, and breast health. Likewise, a poorly functioning internal ecosystem can lead to a buildup of excess estrogen. Estrogen dominance is tied to nearly every hormonal imbalance symptom—infertility, PMS, low libido, cramps, heavy bleeding, and PCOS.

In the FLO Advantage

Balancing hormone levels throughout the cycle can promote a more vital microbiome. Better gut health can translate into smoother digestion, easier weight loss, improved neurotransmitter production, and enhanced moods. Balanced vaginal bacteria can reduce the occurrence of yeast infections, improve fertility, increase the chances of a full-term pregnancy, and promote better health for babies. As for the breast microbiome, we still need more research—but I think it's safe to say that hormonal harmony is likely to promote better breast health.

Biological System 5: Stress Response

As you saw in chapter 2, the modern-day quest for perpetual harvest and nonstop production goes against our chronobiology and natural female rhythms and impacts our stress response. It's no surprise that women and men react differently to stress on both a mental and physical level. According to the American Psychological Association's 2010 *Stress in America* report, women are more likely to report having a great deal of stress and are more inclined to say their stress levels are on the rise. We're also more likely to report the following emotional and physical symptoms from stress:

- Headache
- Irritability
- Fatigue
- Lack of energy
- Decreased motivation
- Feeling like we could cry
- Nervousness
- Anxiety
- Sadness or depression
- Upset stomach
- Muscle tension
- Changes in appetite

Emerging research reveals underlying biological and neurological mechanisms that may account for these differences. To understand these mechanisms, let's back up and look at the biochemical underpinnings of the human stress response. Acting as the air traffic controller of this system is the hypothalamic-pituitary-adrenal (HPA) axis. In general, when stressed, your hypothalamus kicks into gear and orders your pituitary gland to start pumping out adrenocorticotropic hormone (ACTH). The flow of ACTH sends a signal to your adrenal glands to open the floodgates on stress hormones, including cortisol and adrenaline. But the HPA axis doesn't always work exactly the same way in women as in men.

The biological responses in men are characterized by a "fight-or-flight" response, in which cortisol channels glucose to the muscles and adrenaline boosts blood pressure and heart rate. Most descriptions of this process involve a look back at our cave-dwelling ancestors, detailing how this response gave them a burst of energy so they could outrun a charging buffalo or fight off encroaching tribes. After they made it safely back to their cave or defeated the other tribe, the danger passed and their internal system returned to normal.

The story about the HPA axis response in women gets a lot less ink (*no surprise here!*). Prior to 1995, most research on the stress response had been done almost exclusively on males, which is part of the reason why the fight-or-flight response earned a place in our cultural conditioning. Newer research, including a 2000 study in *Psychological Review*, suggests that our biology doesn't always follow this same male pattern. Instead, women are more inclined to have a "tend-and-befriend" response to stress. During these times, we are more likely to tend to young ones and befriend others for support as a way to enhance the odds of survival—not only our own survival but also that of our offspring. Just look at how women rush to social media to support crowdfunding for disaster relief—organizing donations to victims of hurricanes, earthquakes, and even terror attacks. On a biological level, our female sex hormones may dampen the adrenaline rush that men typically feel when faced with an outside threat or a stressful situation. In times of stress, the female brain may also release the feel-good neurochemical oxytocin, which is known as the bonding hormone. Estrogen promotes the release of oxytocin, while testosterone blocks it. Women and men don't secrete the same levels of these hormones, which activate different areas of the brain.

How Your Cycle Affects Your Stress Response

During the week before your period, do you feel more stressed? Is it harder for you to deal with that extra work assignment? Do you wake up in the middle of the night worrying about that fight you had with your sister? You're not alone, and no, it's not all in your head. Science backs up what you've known all along. Your biology is programmed to heighten your stress response in the second half of your cycle compared with the first half, according to a 2017 study in the journal *Physiology & Behavior.* Earlier research from a 2013 issue of *Psychoneuroendocrinology* found that females release a greater amount of the stress hormone cortisol during the second half of the cycle compared with the first half. It's likely this heightened response is nature's way of helping you protect a fertilized egg in the event you're pregnant.

What Goes Wrong When We Ignore Our Cyclical Nature

Stress can do a real number on your brain. According to a 2015 paper in the *Journal of Endocrinology*, stress hits the neural circuitry responsible for cognitive function, decision-making, and moods, which in turn can alter other biological systems, including the nervous system, immune system, and metabolism. A 2011 review in *Industrial*

Psychiatry Journal found that the stress response sparks activity in different regions in women (the limbic system) and in men (a region of the prefrontal cortex). A receptor in the brain's hypothalamus, which is involved in appetite and satiety, also reacts differently in women and men when stress hits. Appetite drops in women but not men, which could be a reason women tend to be more prone to eating disorders, according to 2016 research in *Cell Metabolism*.

Too much stress can also disrupt your sex life and fertility. The chemicals released during times of stress interfere with your body's production of estrogen, progesterone, luteinizing hormone, FSH, and prolactin. Too much stress can really throw off your hormone levels, leading to irregular periods, fertility problems, and a lukewarm libido. A 2013 study in the *Journal of Sexual Medicine* revealed that the impact of chronic stress goes deeper than decreasing the desire to get frisky in the bedroom. Chronic stress hits us on a physiological level too. In fact, women with high levels of chronic stress have lower levels of genital sexual arousal.

Exposure to chronic stress can deplete your body's resources, make you feel tired all the time, and lead to burnout. You might think chronic stress will eventually cause adrenal fatigue, but traditional physicians don't recognize this as a legitimate ailment. Make no mistake, though— the symptoms are very real. If you ask your doctor to check you for adrenal fatigue, you might get the "You're fine—it's all in your head" speech. Some standouts in the health field, such as Dr. Aviva Romm, however, suggest adrenal fatigue could actually be something called allostatic load. Researchers say allostatic load is a biomarker measure of the "wear and tear" on the body and brain that affects overall health. In 2017, a paper in *PLOS ONE* concluded that the higher your allostatic load, the poorer your health.

The stress response–hormonal cycle is a two-way street. Just as your hormonal cycle influences your stress response, your period can be disrupted when your stress response gets out of control. Here are five ways a rise in cortisol can affect your monthly cycle.

- **It interferes with insulin:** Increases in cortisol levels disrupt insulin's ability to control blood sugar levels. In turn, this disruption messes with ovulation and menstruation.

- **It decreases progesterone:** Cortisol gets in the way of progesterone production, which can disrupt your cycle. When your body is stressed, it uses progesterone to crank out more cortisol rather than what it is intended to do. If you're trying to conceive, be aware that insufficient progesterone levels can decrease your chances of getting pregnant and make it more difficult to sustain a pregnancy full-term.

- **It delays ovulation:** If stress hits when you're nearing the ovulatory phase, increased levels of cortisol can delay or even prevent an egg from being released into the uterus. From a biological standpoint, you can understand why your body wouldn't want to promote pregnancy during a period of heavy stress. This is your body's way of conserving your energy to handle the stress, which it sees as an immediate threat. Once that threat is gone, your body can set the stage for conception to take place.

- **It changes the length and timing of your period:** Stress that occurs after the ovulatory phase can cause a hormonal imbalance that may lead to a number of changes in your period. These may include spotting, an early arrival for your next period, a bleed that's thicker or more watery than usual, or a change in color or duration. This imbalance can also set you up for symptoms like cramps, even if you don't usually experience painful periods. A 2004 study in *Women's Health Issues* determined that women with high stress levels have a shorter cycle interval and shorter duration of bleeding compared with women who don't have increased stress levels.

Other studies show that common stressors like going to college can trigger longer cycles, according to research in the *American Journal of Epidemiology*.

- **Your period can go MIA:** After a particularly stressful time, you may start bleeding later than usual. But did you know that a late period might not be a real period? If you skipped ovulation, your hormones didn't go through the usual dance to cause menstruation. In this case, it's more like a breakthrough bleed to shed any endometrial lining that built up in the uterus. If you didn't ovulate, it's not a physiological period. However, your uterus will still shed any lining that had been built up. Your late period isn't just a nuisance you can ignore; it's your body's way of telling you it's under constant or chronic levels of stress and unable to operate optimally. In order to perform all the countless functions necessary to keep you alive, your body shuts down ovulation in an effort to conserve resources and energy. If you're not trying to conceive, maybe you think this lack of ovulation is no big deal. But think again: when your body doesn't ovulate, the stage is set for more hormonal symptoms and period problems—everything from PMS, to acne, to cramps. A late period due to excess stress is more than just an inconvenience—it's a precursor to a long list of other serious health issues.

In the FLO Advantage

You don't have to let stress dominate the second half of your cycle or develop into a chronic condition. You can take control of stress instead of letting it control you. In the following section of this book, you'll see how the Cycle Syncing Method™ helps you tame stress in the luteal phase, how honoring your second clock puts the brakes on chronic stress, and how biohacking like a woman keeps cortisol from getting out of control.

The Feminist Take: Different and Equal

When you're struck with the scientific evidence of all these fundamental biological differences between women and men and how they affect you in so many ways, it can feel very validating. You may feel a little tinge of concern, however, because we certainly have been fighting for decades to prove we're all equal as human beings. Of course, we're equal, and deserve to be treated equally at the workplace, in the political realm, and in society at large. Nothing about our distinctive female biology prevents us from standing on an equal footing with men or having access to the same opportunities. But from a health standpoint, now we deserve even more. Medicine is already moving toward a bio-individual treatment approach. The concept of one-size-fits-all treatments is becoming a thing of the past. For example, cancer treatments are increasingly targeted to a person's genetic expression and individual form of the disease. What needs to happen next is the health care arena finally adding our female biology and fluctuating hormonal cycle into the equation when it comes to our health care and wellness.

It also might seem that men and women have less free will than thought if our hormones govern so much of our experience. The reality is that you enhance your ability to express yourself by working with these biological rhythms, and the inverse is also true: your experience can become increasingly negatively limited by not supporting your biological rhythms. This is the reality for both men and women. When I first experienced this powerful shift in understanding, I found it to be incredibly liberating. Finally, I could let go of this notion that I needed to somehow force myself to be the same every day, which got twisted into an idea that I needed to be perfect. In working with many women over the years, I know that this feeling of relief is a common reaction. Learning about my female biochemistry gave me more compassion for myself, and I developed a greater understanding and love for the way my female body, brain, and biological systems operate. And one thing became absolutely clear: once you accept your biochemical nature and how much it influences your life, you're left with a simple choice—are you going to fight your nature, or are you going to work with it? Your day-to-day lifestyle and self-care choices either work against your cyclical nature and lead to symptoms, or they support it and enhance cognitive skills, rev up your energy, and boost your moods. It's a no-brainer.

IN THE FLO MANIFESTO

I acknowledge my cycle has four distinct hormonal patterns.

Each of these phases requires different nourishment and self-care.

Supporting each phase is the key to optimizing my health.

Syncing with each phase allows me to tap into creativity to optimize work, motherhood, and relationships on my own terms.

Living according to my biological rhythmic timing restores my sovereignty and makes me more free.

Now that you understand your beautiful biological reality, it's time to discover the phase-specific foods, fitness routines, and energy-management strategies that will help you biohack your nutrition, workouts, and calendar. The next section of this book will unveil the simple steps to begin syncing with your cycle, so you can start optimizing your health and life now!

PART 2

GETTING YOUR BODY IN THE FLO

And I said to my body, softly, "I want to be your friend." It took a long breath and replied, "I have been waiting my whole life for this!"

—Nayyirah Waheed

CHAPTER 4

Never Diet Again

When we give up dieting, we take back something we were often
too young to know we had given away: our own voice. Our
ability to make decisions about what to eat and when. Our belief
in ourselves. Our right to decide what goes into our mouths. . . .
Your body is reliable. . . . If you listen, it will speak.

—GENEEN ROTH

A re you ready to become a cyclical biohacker? Think of biohacking as
an ongoing experiment in which you track biomarkers so you can
modify your diet, fitness routines, and lifestyle habits to find the best
ways to optimize your hormonal health, biological systems, and creativity.
Long before this trendy term became part of the everyday lexicon, I was
desperately trying to biohack my way to better health by trying to balance
my hormones and heal my PCOS symptoms. I spent thousands of dollars on
products that promised to clear up acne, and I went on every diet under the
sun. A practitioner I worked with had me follow a morning regimen that involved drinking carrot juice with powdered greens added—the juice looked
like pond scum—and after a few months it turned my skin orange! The juice
didn't help my acne, and I didn't lose weight on any of those diets. It was so
frustrating, and I felt like a failure. I couldn't understand why nothing was
working for me. I wish I had known then what I know now. All those remedies I was trying were not factoring in my monthly hormonal patterns. As

you saw in the previous section, women have long been viewed as diminutive versions of our male counterparts. Aside from our anatomical parts and sex hormones, it's been largely assumed that our bodies operate and respond similarly. This has led to the prevailing belief that what's good for the gander is good for the goose. *Wrong!* As my early biohacking experiments showed, many "surefire solutions" simply didn't work for me because they were designed with men and their 24-hour clock in mind. Those solutions are especially unhelpful for any woman trying to lose weight.

Nothing clicked until I realized that even though we have proved we are capable of doing anything men can do and more, we are not the same biochemical creatures as men. And in addition, because of our hormonal fluctuations, we are not even same creatures from day to day ourselves. It was crazy to think I should be doing the same self-care routine every day or following biohacking strategies created with men in mind. The answer lay in finding tools that worked with my female biochemistry, my body's cyclical rhythm, my feminine biological systems, and the hormonal changes taking place over my 28-day clock. But what are these tools?

Many things in the current biohacking sphere—think intermittent fasting and ketogenic diets, to name just a couple—fall short for women. Why? These biohacks are all geared to the 24-hour clock and helping men enhance their energy, concentration, and stamina day in and day out. Women, with our second 28-day clock, need something different and less extreme. The key for us to optimize our system and access its gifts is to simply support and nurture our natural cyclical rhythms. With some simple tweaks, you can biohack your way to a symptom-free period, enhanced productivity, better overall health, happier moods, more creativity, and more loving relationships—and you can achieve these results in a very short amount of time. In this part of the book, rather than thinking about biohacking the way men do—using outside sources to boost energy within a 24-hour period—we're going to adopt a female-centered concept of biohacking, in which you're supporting your natural inner energy and unlocking your biological gifts by replenishing your micronutrient levels and syncing your diet, exercise, and lifestyle with your cyclical nature.

This part of the book will show you step by step how to use the Cycle Syncing Method™. This chapter shows you how to use food to support your hormones and biological systems during each phase of your menstrual cycle. Chapter 5 reveals the secrets to exercising in rhythm with your body so you can get better results with less sweat. Chapter 6 introduces you to the right-timing planning tools that will help you achieve more with less effort. These are the foundations of the Cycle Syncing Membership. And I'll also help you find simple ways to get started syncing with your cycle, even if your hormones are unbalanced or you have irregular or missing periods. Adopting a cyclical way of living is the most revolutionary and empowering shift you can make to overcome the miseducation and cultural conditioning you have faced throughout your life. It is the most effective way to nourish your two biological clocks and is the gateway to living in tune with your body's inner rhythm so you can unleash your creativity, reclaim your power, and build momentum in your life.

Think of the Cycle Syncing Method™ as the "undiet" that puts you in touch with the natural biofeedback system your brain and body are inherently equipped to provide. At the center of the Cycle Syncing Method™ is something no other wellness, diet, or exercise program you've tried has: *you*! This is a whole new mindset, in which you take the driver's seat. Getting healthy and feeling good by partnering with your body goes against what you've been taught—to control your body because it's unpredictable and unreliable. The cyclical self-care practice outlined in this part of the book heals your relationship with your body. You have to live inside your female body—to care for, feed, rest, move, and love it.

The only way to get the results you want is to get in tune with your biology. Any time you don't feel good, you need to stop, examine what's going on, and start troubleshooting. This is the guiding principle behind female biohacking—to be in a deep and continuous observation-and-response mode about your own body, or what I like to call active listening and compassionate response. Remember, your body is the container for the experiment; you are the citizen scientist interpreting the results of those experiments. Your energy levels, performance at work, moods, and hormonal symptoms are the experiment's results that will guide you through the process. In a short amount of time, it will become second nature for you to understand what's happening in your body and how to support it in the best possible way. After all, no one can know your body as well as you do.

Special note: *If you've been diagnosed with a hormonal condition, such as PCOS, endometriosis, amenorrhea, or fibroids, be aware that you need to do some foundational work before you start syncing with your cycle. See the Biohacking Tool Kit section for a step-by-step process to help you take the path from problem periods to syncing with your cycle.*

The Food-Hormone Connection

In this chapter, I'll map out the first part of the Cycle Syncing Method™ by exploring food—the ultimate medicine for your body, brain, and hormones. Most of my clients begin their cyclical lifestyle journey with food. And even if you change only one food per phase or focus only on adopting the foods recommended for a single phase, you can start to see some big payoffs. For example, look at Allie. At twenty-six, she quit the pill and her periods went MIA. As an organic chef, she was drawn to the idea of a food-focused approach to balancing her hormones. In general, she was already eating many of the healthful foods I recommend, but she used caffeine, chocolate, and sweets whenever she needed an energy boost, even though she hated the crash that usually followed. When she decided to give cycle-based eating a try, she swapped out those three foods for more nutrient-dense options that provide lasting energy rather than a quick fix, and started tailoring her meals to the phases of her cycle. With these minor changes, it took only about two months for her period to return to a regular 28-day cycle, and she noticed less bloating and less breast tenderness during her luteal phase. And the discomfort she used to feel in her lower abdomen? She says it now feels more like "a buzzing, singing sensation rather than cramps"—all from changing a few things in her diet. These are the kind of results you can see when you eat for your cycle. It's possible because what you eat provides the foundation your body needs to keep your hormones balanced. Eating the wrong foods or eliminating entire categories of macronutrients from your diet can rob your system of the raw materials it needs to produce healthy hormones, which play a critical role in our physical health, cognitive function, moods, and longevity.

Food has profound effects on your menstrual cycle and fertility, but when we have issues with our hormones, we're often told there's nothing we can do about it other than take synthetic birth control, have surgery, or invest in expensive fertility treatments. Nobody tells us the foods we're consuming could be contributing to the problem or that we can fix our symptoms simply by changing our eating habits. But science proves it's possible. Want proof? Here are just a few examples of the way food influences our hormonal health.

Menarche: Several studies have clearly linked consumption of certain dietary items—including meat, caffeinated drinks, sugar-sweetened sodas, and beverages—with artificial sweeteners to an earlier age of menarche, the onset of your first period. In one study in a 2015 issue of *Human Reproduction*, researchers followed 5,583 girls for five years to determine the effects on age of menarche of drinking sugar-sweetened beverages—uncarbonated fruit juice, sodas, and iced tea—and guess what? Girls who gulped more than 1.5 servings of sugary drinks per day started their periods an average of 2.7 months earlier than those who drank less.

The age when you get your first period is important: it is one of the first signs of your hormonal well-being, and early menarche has been associated with an increased risk of cardiovascular disease, diabetes, obesity, and breast cancer.

PMS: The foods you eat have also been linked to premenstrual symptoms. In the late luteal phase just before your period arrives, falling estrogen levels can cause a drop in serotonin levels, which can ratchet up your cravings for simple carbs. But science shows us these foods are likely to exacerbate your PMS symptoms. For example, gobbling a bag of salty pretzels to satisfy your PMS cravings makes your body retain water to counteract all the additional sodium swimming in your bloodstream and ends up bumping up the bloat factor. Giving in to your cravings for cookies, pastries, or candy can feel like a quick fix for a mood boost because the body uses carbs to produce serotonin, but the quick fix is followed by a sharp decline in blood sugar levels and energy. This puts you on a veritable blood sugar roller-coaster ride that can increase PMS symptoms of moodiness, irritability, and nervousness, and crank up those cravings. On the flip side, certain foods can help calm your PMS symptoms. For example, a 2005 study in the *Archives of Internal Medicine* found that women whose diets included foods with higher amounts of calcium and vitamin D had less of a risk for PMS than women who got less of these micronutrients from their foods.

Fertility: If you're one of the more than six million women ages fifteen to forty-four who have difficulty getting or staying pregnant, it's important to look at your diet along with other potential causes. Researchers at the Harvard School of Public Health followed 17,544 married women for eight years as they attempted to become or succeeded in becoming pregnant. In their 2007 study published in *Obstetrics & Gynecology*, these researchers found that women who adhered to a "fertility diet," along with engaging in physical activity and keeping their weight under control, experienced 69 percent less of a risk of infertility due to ovulatory problems. According to the study, ovulatory problems make up 18 to 30 percent of infertility cases. The fertility diet included the following eating habits:

- Higher consumption of monounsaturated fats (**olive oil, avocados, pumpkin seeds**) rather than trans fats (**margarine, crackers, doughnuts**)
- Higher consumption of low-glycemic carbohydrates (**beans, lentils, broccoli, spinach**)
- Consuming more protein from plants than from animal sources
- Eating more iron (**spinach, shellfish, legumes**)
- Eating more fiber (**chickpeas, artichokes, Brussels sprouts**)
- Consuming more high-fat dairy products compared with low-fat dairy—*this one surprised the researchers* (if you're going to consume

dairy, make sure it is sheep, goat, buffalo, or camel dairy, which contains A2 proteins, as opposed to A1 proteins that have been associated with leaky gut)

- Taking more multivitamins
- Having a lower body mass index (BMI)
- Engaging in longer periods of physical activity each day

Perimenopause and menopause: Food impacts your hormonal cycle on the other end of the menstrual spectrum as well. The number one complaint I hear from most of the women I see who are entering the perimenopause zone is hot flashes. Most women associate hot flashes with postmenopause, but they can start years or even a decade or more before your periods stop. In fact, I've heard from several younger women that they get hot flashes right before their monthly bleed begins. This timing makes sense because your body experiences its biggest dip in estrogen right before the lining sheds, which means you can have a temperature change that bumps up the heat factor. Food can come to your rescue! A 2015 review of existing research in *Climacteric* found that phytoestrogens—plant-derived compounds that mimic natural estrogen—significantly reduce the frequency of hot flashes. Adding phytoestrogens—found in tempeh, miso, and flaxseeds—to your meals during the right phase of your cycle is the key to keeping hot flashes in check. We'll learn more about this topic soon.

All of this research validates what I have been witnessing firsthand throughout my career—your diet can have a real impact on your hormonal function. As more research continues to support the real-life results I've already seen in my clients, the concept of using food rather than synthetic hormones to balance your hormones will become more commonplace. It's exciting to envision a day when nutrition therapy, like the kind we offer at FLO Living and that you're learning about in this chapter, will be a routine complement to your annual gynecology appointment. Most important, this research unravels the toxic period mythology that we are victims to our hormones. You do not have to suffer from hormonal imbalance. You can eat your way to a better period for longer in your life. Syncing with your cycle is the way to do it.

Eating for Each Phase of Your Cycle

Your body isn't the same every day, and your diet shouldn't be either! Yes, eating at regular intervals to honor your 24-hour clock is important, but as your ovaries and uterus engage in distinct functions each week of your cycle, your micronutrient needs vary. You need to eat foods that support each phase of your cycle. These phases aren't separate siloes; your cycle flows from one phase to the next, and each one influences the others. Eating the right foods in one phase offers immediate rewards, but that's not all. Think of it as the gift that keeps on giving. Eating the right foods in that phase also helps lay the foundation to optimize your biology for the next phase and even to provide benefits in the other phases that follow. Consuming phase-specific foods not only eliminates period problems, but also gives your biology the boost it needs to support your cyclical hormones and become the best version of yourself by maintaining and increasing the energy you have available to do what you want. This information is the opposite of what we've been taught, that these hormones hinder us and we need to shut them down—*not true!*

The concept of eating in sync with your cycle is simple. Each phase of your menstrual cycle correlates to a different set of proteins, grains, vegetables, fruits, and other foods that support the hormonal changes your body is experiencing. Certain foods are included in specific phases based on their ability to metabolize estrogen, support progesterone production, or stabilize blood sugar levels. Throughout the month, you'll be eating a wide variety of nutritious foods, and you'll have a lot of flexibility when it comes to meal planning. The Cycle Syncing Method™ is intended to be convenient, and it helps you save money, too. Forget about diet plans that suggest you eat half a grapefruit for just one meal, on one day of the week. I always wondered, what the heck am I supposed to do with the other half of that grapefruit? Perhaps best of all, this way of eating is radically freeing. You won't be counting calories, because this method is not about how much you eat but about eating the right foods at the right times. Once you get the hang of it, this way of eating becomes intuitive. You'll be able to listen to your body to know what it needs, and you'll naturally crave healthy foods instead of foods that sabotage your systems. Let's look at how to eat your way to hormonal health in each phase of your cycle.

Origins of the Food Chart

Based on my research into Chinese medicine and functional nutrition, which uses micronutrients, foods, and herbs to support and nourish the body, and its organs—including the endocrine glands and hormones—I was able to create this cyclical eating program. In this ancient system, organ systems have a dominant season during which they are more active and most receptive to support. As I was doing a deep dive into the four phases of the hormonal cycle, I saw the parallels between these seasonal foods and the four "seasons" in our monthly cycle. The foods recommended on this program represent the intersection of the Chinese medicine theory of using foods to support bodily organs and the seasonality of the cycle to support your hormone levels throughout the entire month.

For example, the foods in the follicular phase are reflective of our inner spring. These foods tend to be lighter, which fits with this phase when metabolism is naturally a bit slower. Follicular foods also have a bit of astringency, making them particularly good for liver function and detoxification. In the ovulatory phase, which is our inner summer, the foods help our bodies balance out the spike in estrogen and support the heart. In the luteal phase, which corresponds to our inner fall, the fiber-rich foods support the large intestine to increase transit time, which is critical during the luteal phase, when progesterone levels increase and slow digestion. The nutrient-dense foods here also correspond to the fact that your body's metabolism naturally speeds up in this phase. During menstruation, which reflects our inner winter, it's important to stock up on micronutrients that build up the blood, because you are losing blood as you shed the lining of your uterus. These foods also support the kidneys and help balance hormones as their levels drop during your monthly bleed.

Rotating foods based on the inner seasons of the body, or the hormonal phases, makes a lot of sense. The biochemistry of how our hormones actually work requires certain foods on many different levels—from eating foods that help support the production of our hormones, eating foods that help support their elimination, eating foods that help us navigate the changes in our metabolism, eating foods that help us stabilize our blood sugar, and eating foods that replenish our micronutrients. It just makes so much sense that you would not want to eat the same way, day in and day out.

Follicular

Fresh, vibrant, light foods make you feel more energized during this phase, when all hormone levels are beginning to rise. This week you'll want to focus on those phytoestrogens that I mentioned earlier—plant-based compounds that mimic the body's natural estrogen. You wouldn't want to eat them when you already have high levels, but during this period of lower estrogen, they can be balancing and beneficial. Think pressed salads (**kimchi** and **sauerkraut**): plenty of veggies (**string beans, zucchini, carrots**); lean proteins (**chicken, trout**); sprouted beans and seeds; and nutrient-dense, energy-sustaining grains like **oats**. Emerging research suggests that probiotic supplementation—and, I would argue, probiotic-rich foods like those you're eating during this phase—help balance the estrobolome. In addition, the foods you consume in the follicular phase set the stage for ovulation. By eating fermented foods packed with beneficial bacteria, you're priming the microbiome and estrobolome to be ready when ovulation occurs.

Ovulatory

Thanks to surging estrogen, your energy levels should be high, and your moods should be stable during the ovulatory phase of your cycle. However, without the right dietary support, that surge may go too far and make you vulnerable to experiencing the symptoms of excess levels of estrogen, such as acne. According to traditional Chinese medicine, this is a hot phase of the cycle because of the temperature change from ovulation, so you can sustain the most raw foods during this phase. Fill up on veggies (**red bell pepper, spinach, tomato, leafy greens**) and fruit (**raspberries, strawberries**) for their cooling effect and fiber. These foods also provide high levels of glutathione, a powerful antioxidant that will help your liver metabolize excess estrogen from your body more efficiently. Remember, your metabolism is slower in the first half of your cycle, so you don't need as many calories and will feel good with lighter meals. You don't need as many carbohydrates, so you can feel satisfied with lighter grains, such as **quinoa** and **corn**. Ovulatory foods promote antioxidative well-being and provide vascular support for your ovaries so your body can create the healthiest egg possible. These foods will also ward off estrogen-driven symptoms, such as acne and bloating. By eating a lot of fiber-rich foods in this phase, you're also supporting your large intestine to increase transit time and help flush the estrogen that the liver is working hard to metabolize.

Luteal

In the luteal phase, your body needs more calories—remember, as you saw in the previous chapter, the *American Journal of Clinical Nutrition* found that your metabolism naturally speeds up during this phase—along with B vitamins to pump up the production of progesterone and to stabilize blood sugar levels. Not following these guidelines can trigger sugar cravings. To curb cravings, you need to proactively eat slow-burning carbohydrates (like **brown rice** or **sweet potato**) throughout the day, and shift your diet to emphasize foods rich in B vitamins, calcium, magnesium, and fiber. Eat cooked leafy greens such as **collards, mustard greens,** and **watercress,** which are high in calcium and magnesium to reduce fluid retention, something that affects many women in this phase. Consuming high-fiber foods like **chickpeas, pears, apples,** and **walnuts** will help your liver and large intestine flush out estrogen more effectively, reducing the effects of estrogen dominance. In the second half of the luteal phase, when estrogen levels dip, boost your intake of healthy, natural sugars, such as roasted or baked root veggies. Be sure to keep filling up on complex carbohydrates, such as **millet,** to stabilize serotonin and dopamine levels and help prevent mood swings. Eating more nutrient-dense foods that provide more calories in the luteal phase will help prevent any energy dips during your period. The foods recommended for this phase offer another unexpected bonus—better bowel movements! The rise in progesterone during the second half of the cycle slows transit time and can lead to constipation.

Menstrual

Your hormone levels are at their lowest levels during menstruation, but you can compensate by increasing your intake of protein and healthy fats. Doing so will keep your energy and moods stable while your brain adjusts to the downshift in hormones. Protein is rich in amino acids, which are involved in hormone synthesis. In addition, eating these foods now can help set you up for a healthier ovulatory phase during your next cycle. The reason is that dietary fat intake has been linked to increases in progesterone and testosterone, and a reduced risk for ovulatory problems, according to 2016 research in the *American Journal of Clinical Nutrition*. And a 2013 trial on animals in the *European Journal of Experimental Biology* found that dietary fats and fatty acids increased the release of estrogen and progesterone and improved egg and embryo quality. When your body is involved in the intense process of menstruation—shedding the built-up lining of the uterus—it's especially important to turn your focus to nutrient-dense foods, such as **red meat, kidney beans,** and **buckwheat**. According to traditional Chinese medicine, this is the coldest part of the cycle, so warming foods are ideal during this phase. Protein, fats, veggies, and fruits with a low-glycemic index—think **blueberries** and **blackberries**—keep your blood sugar steady while adding fiber and antioxidants. **Seafood, kelp,** and **nori** can help re-mineralize your body with iron and zinc, which you lose during menstruation. These foods are deeply restorative to the blood and kidneys and are ideal while you're bleeding. If you find that you have looser bowel movements when your period begins, it's due to the absence of progesterone to slow down transit time in the bowel and the introduction of prostaglandins to stimulate the uterus. Modulating your food cyclically will also help alleviate the weird period poop experience.

The Cycle Syncing Method™: Food FLO

	Follicular Phase	Ovulatory Phase	Luteal Phase	Menstrual Phase
Grains	Barley Oat Rye Wheat	Amaranth Corn Quinoa	Brown rice Millet	Buckwheat (kasha) Wild rice
Vegetables	Artichoke Broccoli Carrot Lettuce: Bibb, Boston, romaine Parsley Pea: green Rhubarb String bean Zucchini	Asparagus Bell pepper, red Brussels sprouts Chard Chicory Chive Dandelion Eggplant Endive Escarole Okra Scallion Spinach Tomato	Cabbage Cauliflower Celery Collard Cucumber Daikon Garlic Ginger Leek Mustard greens Onion Parsnip Pumpkin Radish Squash Sweet potato Watercress	Beets Burdock Dulse Hijiki Kale Kelp Kombu Mushrooms: button, Shiitake Wakame Water chestnut
Fruit	Avocado Grapefruit Lemon Lime Orange Plum Pomegranate Sour cherry	Apricot Cantaloupe Coconut Fig Guava Persimmon Raspberry Strawberry	Apple Date Peach Pear Raisin	Blackberry Blueberry Concord grape Watermelon
Legumes	Black-eyed pea Green lentil Lima bean Mung bean Split pea	Red lentil	Chickpea Great northern bean Navy bean	Adzuki bean Black soybean Black turtle bean Kidney bean
Nuts & Seeds	Brazil Cashew Flaxseeds Lychee Pumpkin seeds	Almond Flaxseeds Pecan Pistachio Pumpkin seeds	Hickory Pine nut Sesame seeds Sunflower seeds Walnut	Chestnut Sesame seeds Sunflower seeds

	Follicular Phase	Ovulatory Phase	Luteal Phase	Menstrual Phase
Meat	Chicken Eggs	Lamb	Beef Turkey	Duck Pork
Seafood	Fresh-water clam Soft-shell crab Trout	Salmon Shrimp Tuna	Cod Flounder Halibut	Catfish Clam Crab Lobster Mussel Octopus Oyster Sardine Scallop Squid
Other	Nut butter Olives Pickles Sauerkraut Vinegar	Alcohol, moderate Chocolate Coffee Ketchup Turmeric	Mint Peppermint Spirulina	Bancha tea Decaf coffee Miso Salt Tamari

Note: You can dive deeper on the MyFLO app (www.MyFLOtracker.com)
and at www.cyclesyncingmembership.com/bonus.

How Cyclical Eating Supports Your Five Biological Systems

The beauty of a cyclical "diet" is that eating phase-specific foods that support your hormones also helps you eliminate PMS, protect fertility, achieve and maintain a healthy weight, have clearer skin, experience easier periods, improve moods, and boost energy. Think of cyclical eating as priming your physical body, brain, and mental fortitude so you can be your most productive, creative, and happy self. Here's the science behind what food does for each of your biological systems:

Biological System 1: Brain

Estrogen in the brain has profound effects on memory, learning, and moods. As you've seen, during the ovulatory phase, high estrogen levels enhance your verbal and social skills. You may wonder, if higher levels of estrogen boost these beneficial traits, why would you ever want to reduce estrogen levels? Well, with hormones, it is possible to have too much of a good thing. It's a Goldilocks situation: Too much estrogen can make you anxious and foggy. Too little can leave you feeling irritable. You need just the right amount to keep you in the sweet spot. What you eat can impact where you fall on the hormonal spectrum—too much, too little, or just right. For example, that kale smoothie you drink because you think it's good for you? It is *great* for you during the ovulatory phase, when your estrogen levels are high, but it works against you during the menstrual phase, when estrogen levels dip. Your diet also affects the production of those mood-inducing neurotransmitters, such as serotonin. When serotonin levels naturally dip during the luteal phase, you may be tempted to go for a quick fix like chocolate chip cookies, a handful of caramel popcorn, or a red velvet cupcake. But research in the *Indian Journal of Psychiatry* and *Public Health Nutrition* found that poor food choices are linked to mood disorders, such as depression, and may be due in part to lower levels of serotonin. If you don't eat in a cyclical fashion, your food choices could mess with your neurotransmitter levels, affecting your thinking, impulsiveness, and moods, especially during the second half of your cycle. This effect helps explain why so many of us believe the myth that we're destined to feel good in the first half of our cycle and lousy in the second half. As you saw in chapter 3, this myth just isn't true. Excess estrogen makes you feel anxious when it surges in the ovulatory phase; you then can feel depressed when estrogen dips in the luteal phase. You can balance these highs and lows just by being smart about your food choices.

The cyclical advantage: Syncing your food with your cycle helps optimize your brain chemistry. In the follicular phase, you'll be eating foods that promote estrogen metabolism to prevent a buildup of the hormone in the gut, which plays such an important role in serotonin production. When estrogen peaks in the ovulatory phase, you'll be focusing on consuming raw vegetables to flush the hormone from your body and calm anxiety. During the luteal phase, you'll be eating slow-burning, complex carbohydrates (aka "mood foods") that stabilize blood sugar levels and help boost the feel-good neurotransmitter serotonin, which acts as a natural appetite suppressant and mood stabilizer. One of the main priorities of the endocrine system is to safeguard the transport of glucose to the brain, so if you want to have a fighting chance at having healthy moods, you've got to make sure your brain is getting an adequate supply of glucose from complex carbohydrates.

Biological System 2: Immune System

Food plays a vital role in your immune system's ability to keep you healthy. Research shows that your immune system operates at full throttle during the first half of your cycle, helping you ward off viruses, then downshifts during the second half of your cycle. If you aren't compensating for these shifts by eating in sync with your cycle, you could be more susceptible to the cold that's going around the office. According to a 2002 study in the *European Journal of Clinical Nutrition*, deficiencies in micronutrients—especially zinc; selenium; iron; copper; and vitamins A, C, E, B_6, and folic acid—can reduce immunity.

The cyclical advantage: The nutrient-dense foods you'll be eating with this cyclical program provide the micronutrients you need to boost your immune system. These are especially critical during the late luteal phase, when your immune system needs the most support.

During this time, you'll be bypassing raw foods—goodbye, salads—in favor of more cooked fare like **soups** and **steamed broccoli,** because the cooking process makes micronutrients more bioavailable and easier to absorb. Bonus: If you suffer from an autoimmune disorder, eating in tune with your cycle balances estrogen, which may help ease symptoms.

Biological System 3: Metabolism

As you saw in chapter 3, your ability to burn calories depends on the phase of your cycle. In the first half of your cycle, when estrogen levels are increasing, your appetite decreases and your metabolism slows. During the second half of your cycle, when estrogen drops and progesterone rises, your body naturally burns 8 to 16 percent more calories, but this change comes with an increase in appetite. Restriction diets, crash diets, and diets that force you to eliminate major food groups—especially carbohydrates and fats—prevent your body from producing the hormones it needs to keep your metabolism humming along and burning effectively. Those restrictive diets actually work against your fat-burning system.

   The cyclical advantage: To fire up your body's fat-burning ability, you need to feed it the right kinds of foods and the optimal amounts of food during the right phases. During the first half of your cycle, rising estrogen curbs your appetite and stabilizes your blood sugar levels, so you can eat lighter—think salads and smoothies—and focus on slow-carb meals like chicken with spinach and lentils. In the second half of your cycle, however, you have to eat enough to meet your additional caloric needs. Trying to starve yourself during this phase will backfire; your body will rev up its fat-storing mechanisms. This is the time you want to reach for richer proteins and lots of slow-burning carbohydrates like beans, grains, and root vegetables.

Biological System 4: Microbiome

When you don't eat in sync with your cycle, you may alter the balance of your microbiome, which can lead to a host of issues, including estrogen dominance, period problems, digestive issues, increased susceptibility to illnesses, fuzzy thinking, anxiety and depression, and more.

The cyclical advantage: The fermented foods recommended for the follicular phase help seed your microbiome with good-for-you bacteria. Balancing your blood sugar by shifting away from refined sugars and simple carbohydrates, and by opting for complex carbohydrates (oats, barley) and low-glycemic index fruits (grapefruit and plums) and veggies (carrots and green peas), protects you from developing harmful gut bacteria and keeps your microbiome working for you rather than against you. Keeping your microbiome balanced leads to better hormonal health and a reduced risk of estrogen dominance, helping you eliminate PMS problems and enjoy clearer thinking, better moods, and sustained energy. And because you're cycling foods in and out of your meals from week to week and transitioning from raw foods during the ovulatory phase to cooked foods during menstruation, your gut is never overexposed to any particular food that may be causing an inflammatory response. It's as if you're rotating crops—and it is one of the keys to better gut health.

Biological System 5: Stress Response

Scientific studies have concluded that certain foods and nutrients are key to stress management. In particular, complex carbohydrates, proteins, vitamin C, vitamin B, magnesium, and selenium—all plentiful in this cyclical eating plan—play an important role in reducing stress by lowering cortisol and adrenaline levels, according to research in a 2016 issue of the *Journal of Nutrition & Food Sciences*. When you ignore your body's cyclical needs, you might not be getting the proper amounts of these micronutrients at the right times, which could ramp up your stress levels, especially in the second half of the cycle when women naturally release more cortisol. When you aren't eating in a cyclical way, your body will create cortisol spikes to compensate for fluctuating blood sugar levels when insulin can't keep up. Some women who don't metabolize estrogen efficiently may feel anxious during ovulation, when hormone levels are at their highest. And as estrogen recedes dramatically leading up to your period, you can feel depressed. Eliminating certain food groups, as is common in many popular diets, limits your exposure to key micronutrients, also creating stress in the body.

The cyclical advantage: When you tap into your cyclical nature by eating the right foods for the right phases, you ensure that you're giving your body the micronutrients it needs to keep stress at bay—even during those premenstrual days. When you're feeling frazzled, seafood, avocado, and dark chocolate will soothe your stressed-out system.

YOUR GENETIC BLUEPRINT

Your individual genetic makeup can tell you so much about your health. These days, thanks to companies that offer genetic testing, it's easy to discover predispositions for diseases, such as breast and ovarian cancer, Alzheimer's disease, and celiac disease. What you may not realize is that these tests can also reveal clues to your hormonal health. For example, researchers in a 2016 edition of the journal *PAIN* pinpointed a genetic variant associated with severe menstrual cramps. Genetic scientists writing in a 2009 issue of *Nature Genetics* have identified ten gene variants that determine when you'll get your first period, and thirteen other gene variants tied to the age you'll shift into menopause. Certain gene mutations may point to a predisposition for hormonal sensitivity. The consumer DNA company 23 and Me tests for a genetic risk for blood clots, which may indicate you aren't a good candidate for synthetic birth control. In her book *Sweetening the Pill,* Holly Grigg-Spall detailed how health care professionals dole out prescriptions for hormonal birth control without much of a warning that it might not be safe for you based on your genetics. With genetic testing these days, you can even discover if you'd be better off avoiding caffeine. (I'll explore the caffeine-gene connection in greater detail below.)

Imagine having this knowledge *before* your hormones get totally out of whack, *before* the pill has wreaked havoc with your system, and *before* you've become a caffeine junkie. The earlier you have this knowledge, the sooner you can start taking steps to support your system to avoid hormonal symptoms from developing. Research also shows that you can positively impact gene expression with diet and lifestyle. And if you're already suffering from period problems, exhaustion, or any number of physical or mental health issues, genetic testing can give you the hard evidence you might need to inspire you to start getting in sync with your cycle.

Caffeine: Biohacking Wonder or FLO Blocker?

Coffee, especially the kind made with a dollop of butter or ghee, has recently emerged as a high-performance, fat-burning, energy-boosting, cravings-busting tool for biohackers, and if you're going to have it, that way is helpful. But much of the research in this arena, once again, has been done on men and doesn't factor in our cyclical hormonal reality. So, what's the real deal on caffeine and women? Let me share a story that forever changed my relationship with caffeine. I was twenty-something and went to my gynecologist for my annual checkup. During my breast exam, my doctor found a lump and asked a couple other doctors to come in to examine it. If you've ever had your doctor tell you there's a lump in your breast, you know how terrifying it can be. After what seemed like an eternity, they informed me it was just a cyst. A cyst is a benign fluid-filled sac that can be found in women of any age. I was so relieved it wasn't serious, but I wanted to know what might have caused it. "Do you consume a lot of caffeine?" she asked me. I was a college student studying for my finals. Of course I was drinking a lot of caffeine! When she informed me caffeine increases the tendency of breast tissue to produce cysts, I cut out all forms of caffeine cold turkey and have been caffeine-free ever since. And based on the research that continues to emerge, I'm so glad I listened to that early warning signal from my body.

We all know not to consume caffeine when we're pregnant or breast-feeding, but science shows coffee and other caffeinated beverages, such as energy drinks and sodas, are terrible for the female ecosystem at any stage. Here are five reasons women should avoid coffee and caffeine in general, especially if you have PMS, are trying to conceive, or have a diagnosed menstrual issue.

1. *Caffeine may lead to the development of breast and ovarian cysts.* For women with PCOS, fibroids, endometriosis, ovarian cysts, or fibrocystic breasts, consuming caffeine is a sure-fire way to fuel the development of benign cysts. For women who haven't been diagnosed with a hormonal condition but who have hormonal sensitivity, drinking beverages that give you a buzz may not produce cysts, but it can disrupt your monthly cycle.

2. *Your genes impact your ability to metabolize caffeine safely.* Are you one of those people who can have a double espresso after dinner and sleep like a baby, or does a single latte keep you up all night? It depends on your genetics. Emerging research on genetics has zeroed in on a gene called CYP1A2, which controls an enzyme of the same name that breaks down caffeine in the liver. Variants of this gene dictate how well your liver is able to break down and eliminate caffeine from your system. Based on your gene variation, your body will either produce a lot of this enzyme, making you a "fast metabolizer" (and a successful caffeine imbiber), or only a little, putting you in the "slow metabolizer" category. Less than

half the population produces an abundance of this enzyme, according to genetic testing company 23 and Me. What does this information have to do with your cycle? The CYP1A2 gene is also involved in metabolizing estrogen. If you're a slow caffeine metabolizer, you're probably a slow estrogen metabolizer, too. When you drink coffee or energy drinks, your liver has to work overtime to eliminate the caffeine and may not have the micronutrient reserves available to flush excess estrogen out of your system. If you're a slow metabolizer, take note. A 2006 study in *JAMA* showed slow metabolizers who drink two or more cups of coffee a day have a higher risk of a nonfatal heart attack. With an increased risk for excess estrogen and a heart attack, it's a good idea to find out whether you're a slow metabolizer before you get hooked on caffeine.

3. *Caffeine decreases fertility rates.* The negative impact caffeine has on fertility—in both women and men—is alarming. If you're trying to conceive, you need to kick the habit now! Here is some of the latest research linking caffeine intake to infertility and miscarriage:
   - Caffeine increases cortisol levels and stresses the adrenals, interfering with ovulation.
   - Caffeine depletes vital vitamins and minerals—including B vitamins and folate—needed for ovulation and healthy fertility.
   - Drinking three or more caffeinated beverages a day prior to conception increases the risk of miscarriage by 74 percent, according to 2016 research in *Fertility and Sterility.*

4. *Caffeine depletes micronutrients essential for hormone balance.* Caffeine may reduce the absorption of key nutrients and minerals—such as magnesium and B vitamins—that are critical for hormonal balance.

5. *The acidity in coffee can alter the microbiome.* Coffee's high acid content can cause an imbalance in your gut flora, reducing your body's ability to absorb micronutrients. So even if you're eating healthful foods, your body may not be benefiting from all the vitamins and minerals they contain. Without adequate micronutrients, it's harder for your endocrine system to balance your hormones.

Now that you know the science behind that cup of coffee, are you still hesitant to give it up? Rest assured: getting off the caffeine-energy roller coaster is much easier when you're syncing with your cycle, because you're stabilizing your blood sugar and energy levels. For my clients who are hooked on caffeine, I generally recommend a gradual step-down approach to quitting, downshifting to half-caf, replacing with decaf, then switching to rooibos. This approach works even if you're drinking eight cups of coffee a day, as my client Lucinda was. She was experiencing a whole host of hormonal symptoms, and when she learned that caffeine could be contributing to those issues, she wanted to kick the habit. She started syncing with her cycle and at the same time began tapering down her intake; within a few months she was caffeine-free. She was so happy to find that as her caffeine intake decreased, so did her hormonal symptoms.

Getting in tune with your cyclical biochemistry naturally boosts your energy reserves, so you don't need to look to outside sources like coffee or energy drinks for a quick buzz. And when you do feel your energy waning, you'll realize it's just your body's way of telling you that it's time to rest and recharge. If you ignore that signal and slurp up a caffeinated drink to stay in productivity mode, the caffeine can have short- and long-term hormonal and inflammatory impacts on your overall health, moods, and fertility.

Let's Cook!

It's not just about what and when: *how* you prepare your food matters, too. According to traditional Chinese medicine, foods are believed to have warming or cooling effects on the body. These effects play into your hormonal cycle. When estrogen levels rise during follicular and ovulatory phases, the body becomes warmer. When you're following this cyclical program, it's best to counteract this tendency by consuming cooling foods, such as raw vegetables. On the flip side, when estrogen levels decline during the late luteal and menstrual phases, you can support your system by focusing on warming foods and cooking methods.

- **Follicular:** As estrogen levels begin to rise during the follicular phase, opt for light cooking methods, such as steaming or sautéing.
- **Ovulatory:** As estrogen surges, your body is at its warmest during ovulation. This is the ideal time to enjoy fresh, raw foods, such as veggies, fruit, and salads. Juices and smoothies are also great cooling options. When cooking, stick to lighter preparations, such as steaming or poaching.
- **Luteal:** When estrogen levels dip during the luteal phase, opt for warming cooking methods, such as roasting or baking.
- **Menstrual:** Your body is at its coolest level during menstruation, so prepare warm, hearty foods such as soups and stews.

Weight Loss and Why Diet Trends Leave You Feeling like You've Failed

Are you one of those women who has tried every diet, without success? Or maybe you managed to lose some weight, but you felt miserable in the process, started having period problems, and ended up gaining back all the weight you lost? I hear stories like these on a regular basis from the women who seek me out for help. Weight loss can be tricky for women for a number of reasons—*which have nothing to do with willpower!* Here's the truth:

- **Popular diets don't take hormonal fluctuations into consideration.** They expect you to eat the same way every day. As you've seen in this chapter, it makes no sense to consume the same foods day in and day out. Many trendy diets—think low-carb, intermittent fasting, and keto—were not created with women's biochemistry and hormonal cycles in mind. Just look up studies on intermittent fasting, and you'll discover that most of them have been done on males or postmenopausal women. And you'll see later that the few studies that do include women—or female rats—clearly show we do not get the same results as our male counterparts. In fact, some of these diets can disrupt your cycle, interfere with your biological systems, and set you up for failure.

- **Your caloric needs shift throughout your cycle.** In the second half of your cycle you naturally burn 89–279 more calories per day and have an increased appetite, but diets don't account for this difference.
- **You have a greater opportunity to burn fat in the first half of your cycle.** Leveraging this advantage is key to lasting weight loss.
- **You have to heal your hormones first.** If you're struggling with any menstrual conditions, you need to focus on balancing your hormonal levels *before* you think about cutting calories, eliminating carbohydrates, or any other method of dieting. Otherwise, you won't get rid of that stubborn fat and are likely to make your period symptoms worse. As a former PCOS sufferer, I know firsthand how important it is to balance hormones before trying to lose weight. At one point I weighed more than 200 pounds, and I tried every diet I could find. I followed them to the letter, whether the diet involved counting calories, weighing my food, or eliminating entire food groups from my meals. But nothing worked. I couldn't drop the weight, and my hormonal symptoms got worse. It was so frustrating, and for a long time I thought *I* was the problem. What I learned is that the whole premise of separating out weight, skin issues, period issues, mood issues—or any other health issues, for that matter—just does not reflect how the body works. All aspects of our health are interconnected with our hormonal cycle and our natural biological rhythms. Trying to solve one issue without addressing the underlying hormonal issues is a recipe for failure. When you give your biochemistry the support it needs, your systems start to hum—it might even feel like magic—and your weight, energy, and skin issues will no longer be such a struggle.

Don't get me wrong: many popular diets have benefits for women—*if* you take your biology into account. If you're still interested in trying one of the current diet trends (keto, intermittent fasting, grain-free, raw vegan, macrobiotic, or calorie restriction), let's first look at how they impact your hormones and how you can use these diets to your advantage.

The Ketogenic Diet

The ketogenic diet is a low-carb, high-fat plan. Its primary goal is to trigger ketosis, a natural metabolic state that occurs when you don't take in enough carbohydrates, which are your body's number one source of energy. When your body doesn't have carbs to burn for energy, it switches to burning fat as a fuel source. The concept is simple: burn fat, get leaner, lose weight. There are several variations of the keto diet, but the most common one— the Standard Ketogenic Diet—recommends eating 75 percent fat, 20 percent protein, and no more than—*gulp!*—5 percent carbohydrates. That ratio typically means consuming less than 50 grams of carbs (or even as little as 20 grams in some cases) a day. To put those numbers into perspective, consider that one cup of cooked oatmeal provides about 30 grams of carbs. The keto diet is like an extreme version of the paleo diet or the Atkins diet, both of which emphasize protein and fat over carbs.

- **Advantage:** Filling up on protein and fat helps keep you feeling full, and focusing on fresh, whole foods reduces the amount of processed junk you'll be eating.
- **Hormonal disadvantage:** Burning fat sounds like a good thing, but the keto diet may not be so good for women. Animal protein–heavy diets can also lead to liver congestion and estrogen dominance, which is the biggest culprit in hormonal dysfunction. Mark Sisson, author of *The Keto Reset Diet*, says, "Women need to take special precautions when implementing a ketogenic diet." He understands that women's biology is more sensitive to calorie restriction, because our bodies are finely tuned to conserve nutrients for fertility. To adapt a keto diet for your feminine biochemistry, he says to avoid intentionally restricting calories, combining keto and intermittent fasting, or being too strict. Another reason to think twice before going keto is the potential impact of the diet on thyroid health. Research is mixed, but much of it suggests that the diet affects T3 production. It's important to take this issue into consideration because thyroid problems are five to eight times more

common in women than in men, and many women struggle with hypothyroidism, making weight loss even more challenging.

Intermittent Fasting

Intermittent fasting (IF) is a popular diet that involves cycling between periods when you consume food and others when you skip eating. The concept draws on the notion that our cave-dwelling ancestors went through periods of feasting—after a successful hunt—and fasting. Advocates claim this is the way our bodies were naturally intended to operate and say it can help regulate blood sugar and burn fat. IF can take many forms. A few of the more common strategies involve fasting two days a week and eating normally the other five days, or eating during an eight-hour window during the day and fasting the other sixteen hours.

- **Advantage:** Some studies have linked IF with increased weight loss, reduced body fat, enhanced insulin sensitivity, improved cognitive function, a lower risk for various diseases, and improved new cell growth.
- **Hormonal disadvantage:** IF takes a toll on your hormonal and biological systems in a number of ways. For example, Sara Gottfried, a physician and author of several books, including *The Hormone Reset Diet*, explains that IF may cause adverse effects in people with blood sugar issues. Fasting causes blood sugar to plummet, and feasting causes it to spike. Anything that causes blood sugar imbalances is harmful for hormonal health.

But what about those studies that show all those benefits of IF? As you might suspect, most of the studies on intermittent fasting have been done on males, and the few that include females tell a very different story. A 2005 study in *Obesity Research* concluded that IF enhanced insulin sensitivity in men but worsened it in women. A 2013 study on intermittent fasting in rats in *PLOS ONE* found that females experienced a reduction in the size of their ovaries, stopped ovulating, and had sleep problems. The bad news keeps coming. In 2018, researchers found that fasting for two days caused moderate stress in overweight women. *The Keto Reset Diet* author Mark Sisson concluded that compared with men, "As it stands right now, I'd be inclined to agree that pre-menopausal (and perhaps peri-menopausal) women are more likely to have poor—or at least different—experiences with intermittent fasting (at least as a weight loss tool)." In my opinion, the only fasting schedule that is safe and effective for women is to avoid food for a 12-hour period daily, from 7 p.m. to 7 a.m.

Gluten-Free/Grain-Free

These days, it's common to find restaurants that offer gluten-free menu items, and grocery store shelves are stocked with gluten-free products. Gluten—the protein found in wheat, barley, and rye—has been villainized in recent years for its potentially detrimental health effects. Although its connection to celiac disease is well known, and an increasing number of people are becoming aware of gluten sensitivity, what isn't common knowledge is gluten's negative impact on hormonal health, which is why I recommend eliminating it from your diet when you're syncing with your cycle. Many popular diets, such as paleo, advocate excluding all grains to promote weight loss. Of course, you should stick to grains you can tolerate.

- **Advantage:** Some people find that removing gluten or all grains provides relief from stomach pain, bloating, and even brain fog, while others go gluten-free or grain-free for fast weight loss. If you have leaky gut or other allergies, limiting these gluten or all grains can be beneficial.
- **Hormonal disadvantage:** I meet with many women who think going grain-free will put an end to their cravings and binge eating, only to discover that being grain-free actually increased cravings and made the women even more vulnerable to binge moments. This pattern results in irregular insulin levels, which can interfere with ovulation, disrupt metabolism, and put the brakes on fat loss. A grain-free diet can also be

problematic in the second half of your cycle, when women's blood sugar levels are lower. During the luteal phase, we need to consume more complex carbs to help stabilize glucose, insulin, and estrogen levels. If you've been following a grain-free diet and the notion of adding grains during your luteal phase concerns you, experiment with root vegetables and try a grain like buckwheat that is very easy to tolerate to see how you feel.

Raw Vegan

A vegan diet is based on vegetables, fruits, nuts, seeds, and other plant-based foods. It excludes all animal products—no meat, no fish, no eggs, no dairy. A *raw* vegan diet dictates that you can't heat any of the plant-based foods you eat over 104 to 118 degrees. You also need to avoid any foods that are pasteurized, refined, treated with pesticides, or processed. Advocates of raw veganism believe cooking destroys important enzymes and reduces the nutritional content of foods.

- **Advantage:** It's always beneficial to consume lots of organic, fiber-rich fruits and veggies. Plant-based foods provide many health benefits, including better digestion, improved heart health, lower cholesterol, and reduced inflammation. Rich in antioxidants, they can clear up acne, reduce signs of aging, and according to some research, contribute to cancer prevention.
- **Hormonal disadvantage:** A raw vegan diet can disrupt your cycle. In a trial published in *Annals of Nutrition & Metabolism*, about 30 percent of women on a raw food diet experienced missing periods. If your gut microbiome is out of whack, it's harder for your body to absorb the healthy nutrients found in raw foods. Over time, this difficulty can lead to a micronutrient deficiency. A lack of the essential nutrients for hormonal balance can wreak havoc with your cycle, cause your period to go MIA, and increase PMS symptoms. A lack of those nutrients can also lead to weight gain, which is the exact opposite of what you're

trying to achieve on a diet. Sticking solely to raw foods throughout your entire cycle is too cooling, according to Chinese medicine, and can cause your reproductive system to get sluggish—think late periods and delayed ovulation. You can even experience lighter periods as a result. Veggie-heavy raw vegan diets also typically lack the adequate amino acids necessary to produce sufficient hormone levels.

Macrobiotic Diet

Steeped in ancient Eastern tradition and rooted in yin-yang theory, macrobiotic diets were popularized in Western society in the 1960s and focus on whole grains, vegetables, beans, and bean products, such as soy and tempeh. Things that don't get the green light on a macrobiotic menu include meat, processed foods, refined sugar, sodas, and coffee.

- **Advantage:** Plant-based, high-fiber, low-fat diets have been found to lower inflammation and reduce the risk of heart disease and cancer. These diets are also high in micronutrients.
- **Hormonal disadvantage:** Processed soy is one of the worst foods for women. Soy products contain high levels of phytoestrogens that mimic the body's natural estrogens. Women with estrogen-dominance hormonal imbalance conditions—including endometriosis, PCOS, fibroids, and ovarian cysts—are particularly sensitive to the phytoestrogens in processed soy. Processed soy is found in substitute products, such as soy milk, soy meat, soy cheese, and soy yogurt. Fermented, organic, unprocessed soy—known as tempeh, miso, and natto—can be very helpful when consumed *in small amounts.*

Calorie Restriction

Extreme calorie restriction (CR), which typically involves reducing your caloric intake by 25 to 50 percent, encourages people to simply eat less for the rest of their lives.

- **Advantage:** Restricting calories has been associated with lower risks of major diseases and increased longevity.
- **Hormonal disadvantage:** You might lose weight during the first half of your cycle, but you may gain it back during the second half, putting you right back at square one. Also, when your BMI drops below a certain number because of calorie restriction, your cycle may be completely disrupted—preventing ovulation and eliminating your period altogether. Female rats experienced a drop in fertility, ovary shrinkage, increased menstrual cycle irregularity, and enlarged adrenal glands related to calorie restriction in a 2006 study in the *American Journal of Physiology*. CR has also been linked to bone density loss in women.

Cycling Through Popular Diets

Do the potential disadvantages mean you need to steer clear of all of these diets? Not necessarily. But as you've seen throughout this book, you need to make sure you're getting the whole story as it relates to your female biochemistry. All of these diets completely ignore our cyclical, fluctuating hormones and are geared solely to the 24-hour biological clock. Diets that advocate eating the same foods day in and day out don't sync with our cyclical nature. And diets that restrict or eliminate essential macro- and micronutrients prevent you from getting the adequate nourishment your body needs for hormonal balance. Restricting any food group can set you up for micronutrient deficiency, which can be exacerbated if your microbiome is already compromised, you've been on the birth control pill, or you have any kind of hormonal imbalance. And restricting in one area generally means overdoing it in another, which can throw your body off balance as well. It is possible to benefit from these trendy diets without the hormonal downside—if you vary the diets based on the phases of your menstrual cycle. Here's a look at how you could include popular diets in a cyclical way to maximize their effectiveness and support your hormones.

A Cyclical Diet Plan

Phase	Diet	Why It Works
Follicular	Calorie restriction/ IF	During the follicular phase, appetite is suppressed, so it's easier for your body to handle a reduction in calories, which can help with weight loss in the first half of your cycle.
Ovulatory	Raw vegan	As estrogen peaks, vegetables aid in metabolizing the hormone to prevent an excessive buildup and to avoid estrogen dominance. As your body temperature rises during this phase, it is an ideal time to consider a raw vegan diet.
Luteal	Macrobiotic, complex carbs	Your body needs more calories during this phase, and slow-burning complex carbs and beans provide calories while stabilizing blood sugar.
Menstrual	Keto, paleo, or grain-free	As hormone levels and your body temperature drop during this phase, skip the foods that promote estrogen metabolism and stick to warming foods. A keto, paleo, or grain-free diet can give your body what it needs during your monthly bleed.

Syncing with Your Cycle in the Kitchen

Cooking: Keep It Simple, Smarty!

You don't have to be a master chef to make the Cycle Syncing Method™ work for you. I don't really like to spend a lot of time in the kitchen, and I wouldn't call myself a gourmet chef. For me, cooking is more about focusing on phase-specific nutritional value, not culinary skills or pretty plating. In general, I like to keep things as simple as possible. The concept of syncing with your cycle is based on this philosophy—simplifying your life while amplifying your health. Here are some things I do to make meal prep a breeze and what we suggest to our members in the Cycle Syncing Membership:

- **Sync your shopping:** Before I go grocery shopping, I check the Foods for Your Cycle chart included earlier in this chapter and make a short list of phase-appropriate ingredients for the week.

- **More prep, less cooking:** I've devised a strategy so I only have to "cook" twice a week in big batches. On Sunday I focus on prepping and assembling the main ingredients for meals for the next few days; then, if necessary, I'll repeat this process on Thursday. Then it's so much easier to quickly put things together for lunches and work-night dinners. I'll always make a grain, a bean dish, a protein, and two veggies—and from there, the potential leftover combinations are varied and easy.

- **Cook in big batches:** I like to find ways to stretch my cooking so it lasts for several days. For example, if I roast a whole chicken on Sunday, I will use it in soup, sandwiches, and salads throughout the week. I will also use it to make a healthy, nutrient-dense bone broth.

- **Simplify your pairings:** I like to keep our meals to no more than two or three main elements. For example, in my luteal phase, I might prepare turkey, sweet potatoes, and mustard greens. To make cooking even quicker, I prepare the elements all the same way, whether I'm baking, boiling, roasting, or sautéing. See—I told you it was simple!

Sample Daily Meal Plans for the Four Phases of Your Cycle

Check the end of this book for daily meal plans for each phase of the cycle and for sample recipes from the Cycle Syncing Membership.

Stop Stressing! Syncing with Your Cycle Is Easier Than You Think

"Do I have to be totally precise?"

"Do I have to do everything to get results?"

"If I eat a food that's off-phase, will it mess everything up?"

"I have a full-time job and kids. Is this going to require a lot of time-consuming effort?"

I often hear these questions from women who are new to a cyclical approach to life. The answer to all these questions is *no!* You can stop stressing about trying to be perfect at syncing your cycle, and stop worrying that it won't fit into your schedule. In fact, adopting just a few of the suggested tweaks is enough to start seeing and feeling the benefits. And because the nature of your cycle is fluid, with one phase flowing gradually into the next, you can give yourself some wiggle room. For example, even though you're only in the ovulatory phase for three to four days, your body is still in transition for a few days before and after, so it's okay to dedicate a full week to the foods that support ovulation. Even if you're transitioning from the follicular or into the luteal phase, you can still benefit from the ovulatory-phase foods for their various liver-supportive and estrogen-metabolizing benefits. There's no need to berate yourself with thoughts like, "Oh no! Did I eat an extra day of follicular food when I'm actually ovulating?" It's okay to be experimental and see what works for you. The goal of the Cycle Syncing Method™ isn't to try to be perfect or to be worried that you'll screw it up. The whole point is for you to learn about your body and what it needs, so you can do better with your next cycle. If you want more recipes, shopping lists, and support as you adapt to syncing with your cycle, you can dive deeper with a community of women who are using this revolutionary "un-diet" approach at www.cyclesyncingmembership .com/bonus. You'll also find a number of helpful tools and additional information, including phase-specific meals, workout videos, planners, live coaching, and support.

Of course, if you have any food intolerances or struggle with autoimmune disease, you can omit any foods that are on your personal no-go list. This cyclical program is very different from traditional diets that dictate what you can and cannot eat. This method—*remember, it's a method, not a diet!*—is intended to increase your intake of foods that support your hormonal fluctuations. At its core, this program is *additive*, not *reductive*. This approach is reflective of your feminine energy—abundant, generous, and nurturing. Syncing with your cycle should never make you feel deprived; it should make you feel good.

A NOTE ON EATING DISORDERS

Many women with anorexia, orthorexia, or binge-eating disorders have told me that cycling their foods helped them finally unhook from disordered eating. Some women develop eating disorders following puberty, which could be in response to society's overarching message that we should feel the same and act the same every day. When menarche unlocks our cyclical nature, we feel the need to find ways to deny our biological reality, and some of us begin controlling our food intake. Syncing your food with your cycle gives you permission to unravel the thinking that pushes you toward unhealthy eating patterns.

Five Quick-Start Strategies to Ease into the Cycle Syncing Method™

When you're just beginning to sync your food with your cycle, you don't have to change everything at once. It's okay to take baby steps. In fact, I've found that many women are more successful when they make just a few small changes at the outset and gradually fine-tune things while growing more accustomed to the program. Give yourself time to get used to this new way of thinking, cooking, and eating. It will take some thought at first, but before long it will be second nature. If you want to dip your toe into a cyclical way of eating before diving in head first, try one of the following strategies. I created these quick-start plans for women like me who are busy building a business or a career, tending to their families, and struggling to find "me" time.

Quick Start 1: Rotate your veggies only. Veggies are such an important way to help your body get the micronutrients it needs, which is critical for optimal hormone production for your biological systems. Just choose a few of the options from the list below based on the phase you're in. What could be simpler than that?

- *Follicular:* Artichoke, broccoli, carrot, green peas, parsley, string beans, zucchini
- *Ovulatory:* Asparagus, Brussels sprouts, chard, escarole, scallion, spinach
- *Luteal:* Cauliflower, collard greens, daikon, onion, parsnip, radish, squash, sweet potato
- *Menstrual:* Beet, kale, kelp, mushrooms

Quick Start 2: Sync when PMS strikes. Many women begin syncing their cycle by focusing on the most troublesome part of their cycle—the late luteal phase, when PMS symptoms tend to kick in. Add more complex carbs—think sweet potatoes, brown rice, chickpeas, and apples—to your diet on the days when PMS usually hits, and see how you feel. Do you feel happier? Do your headaches disappear? Are you sleeping better?

Quick Start 3: Sync to curb cramps. If cramps are your main period problem, focus on changing the fats you eat during the menstrual phase. For example, foods that are high in omega-3 fatty acids, such as wild salmon, are beneficial for combating period cramps.

Quick Start 4: Sync your cooking methods. I've worked with many women who begin syncing their cycle by focusing solely on the way they prepare their foods to balance the body's natural cooling and warming rhythms. Here's a cheat sheet for you:
- *Follicular:* steaming, sautéing
- *Ovulatory:* raw foods, salads, juices, smoothies, steaming, poaching
- *Luteal:* roasting, baking
- *Menstrual:* soups and stews

Quick Start 5: Try seed cycling. Some women have experienced a reduction in hormonal symptoms by consuming certain seeds as part of their cyclical routine. Here's how to do it:
- *First half of your cycle:* When estrogen levels are rising, consume one tablespoon each per day of flaxseeds and pumpkin seeds. Flaxseeds are high in lignans, which act as estrogen blockers to reduce excess

estrogen. Pumpkin seeds are high in zinc, which sets the stage for progesterone production in the luteal phase.

- *Second half of your cycle:* When progesterone levels rise, switch to one tablespoon each per day of sesame and sunflower seeds. The lignans in sesame seeds—not as abundant as in flaxseeds—help prevent the buildup of excess estrogen while their high zinc content promotes progesterone production. The high concentration of selenium in sunflower seeds supports liver detoxification, while an abundance of vitamin E contributes to healthy progesterone levels.

Keep Yourself in the FLO

The Cycle Syncing Method™ isn't a quick fix that you adopt temporarily, then quit. It is a long-term solution and a proactive way to live in harmony with your hormones. I created this program because after I resolved my own issues with PCOS, I wanted to make sure I didn't have any relapsing symptoms. I never wanted to have cystic acne, extra weight, or irregular periods again. If I reverted to my former diet and lifestyle—dairy, gluten, sugar, caffeine, disconnection from my body and stress—my symptoms would absolutely come back. I wanted to make sure that didn't happen because it was such a hard-earned victory, and syncing with my cycle gave me that protection.

For you, syncing with your cycle is a way to heal hormonal issues and so much more. When you adopt this way of living, you'll feel the positive effects in so many areas of your life. You'll be reaching a healthy weight, improving overall well-being, building energy, achieving more, getting in the flow, and feeling happier. The Cycle Syncing Method™ is the ultimate insurance policy for living your best life.

CHAPTER 5

Work Out Less, Get More Fit

It's time to acknowledge, treat, train, and fuel women
as the different physiological beings we are.
—STACY T. SIMS, PHD

S everal years ago, a woman named Alicia arrived at the center. Frustrated, she told me she had been training for a triathlon as a way to lose weight, but it was having the opposite effect. "I don't get it," she said. "I'm working out more than ever, but I've gained twenty pounds! What's happening?" Alicia wasn't the only woman with this problem. I started seeing client after client complaining of packing on pounds despite logging hours and hours exercising. These women wanted to know why they were gaining weight when the prevailing wisdom seemed so simple: if you work out harder and more often, you'll lose weight. Their experiences didn't add up, and my curiosity was fired to figure out why this was happening. As I delved into science for the answer, what I discovered revolutionized my thinking about women and exercise.

If you're like most of the women I meet, you try to exercise regularly, and you may have tried several of the trendy, intense exercise classes that are available right now. You probably feel that if you could just make it to one more boot camp class a week, or if you just sweated it out at cycling class more, you'd finally reach your fitness goals. But often, even if you can find the time, money, and motivation to get to those classes, you still don't see the results you're hoping for. If you've been busting your butt at the gym only to find yourself feeling exhausted, not losing weight, or worse, somehow *up* a pants size, it's time to learn why the no-pain-no-gain strategy is holding you back. This should come as no surprise now, but the predominant "go hard or go home" mindset is geared to the 24-hour biological clock and maximizing the male physique. It's part of the perpetual harvest concept you read about in chapter 2. But just as our bodies aren't intended to be in endless go, go, go mode, neither are they supposed to be engaged in intense workouts every day. Doing the same routines week in and week out doesn't work with our 28-day clock. As you now understand, your body isn't the same every day, so it makes no sense to stick to the same sweat-inducing workout routine day in and day out. It's time to learn how to exercise in rhythm *with* your cyclical nature, not against it, so you can hit peak physical performance, feel more energized after your workouts, and get off the weight loss–weight gain roller coaster.

The Truth About Female Hormones, Metabolism, and Exercise

As you might suspect, when I was digging into the research for answers to why my clients were gaining weight when they increased their workouts, I found that most exercise studies were performed on men or postmenopausal women. Consequently, most of the expert advice we get on exercise—how often to do it, how much to push yourself, which types are best—is geared toward optimizing male fitness. This advice is just not applicable to female biochemistry, which is why you don't get the results you expect. Fitness trends and training regimens simply don't take the female hormonal cycle into consideration. In part, we can blame the shortage of research on the relationship between the metabolic and physiological effects of exercise and the menstrual cycle. A 2017 *British Journal of Sports Medicine* review of 1,382 sports and exercise–related studies from 2011 to 2013 confirmed that women are underrepresented in the research. This review revealed that only 39 percent of the more than six million participants involved in those studies were women. And among the studies that did include the double-X chromosome crowd, participation was often limited to women who were in the early follicular phase of their cycle, when hormone levels favor fat loss. This underrepresentation of women results in a skewed view of the effects of exercise and contributes to the collective belief that women should push harder and do intensive workouts every day.

In the first half of your cycle, you burn fat more easily and gain lean muscle. With normal blood sugar levels, your body more easily accesses carbohydrates for fuel. This all adds up to greater energy and stamina, so you can crush it in spin class, boot camp, or high-intensity interval training (HIIT) and feel great afterward. A 2017 study in *PLOS ONE* on female soccer players concluded they had better endurance during the first half of the cycle than in the luteal phase. Another bonus during the follicular phase is that higher testosterone levels help your body build muscle more efficiently. In fact, some studies, including a 2014 trial in *Springerplus*, have found that when you strength train during the follicular phase, you get stronger and gain more lean muscle than when you train during the luteal phase. The follicular phase is when you can crank up the intensity, hit it hard at the gym, and see the weight melt off.

But you can't do high-intensity training throughout your entire cycle. A study published in a 2008 issue of *Biological Rhythm Research* concluded that too much intense exercise may lead to irregular or missed periods, which are a clear sign of hormonal imbalance. On the flip side, hormonal imbalances were found to have a negative impact on exercise endurance, muscular strength, and metabolism. This vicious circle can leave you feeling exhausted and prevent you from getting the results you want.

In the second half of your cycle, your metabolism speeds up and you naturally burn more calories, but intense exercise works against this effect by pumping out the stress hormone cortisol, which leads to fat storage and muscle wasting. Estrogen, testosterone, and your blood sugar levels dip. This saps your energy, causes you to sweat more, and makes that spin class or boot camp feel a lot more challenging than it did just a few weeks earlier. I'm here to tell you: it's not you—it's the workout! Research in a 2003 study in *Sports Medicine* shows that women reach exhaustion faster during the midluteal phase than in the first half of the cycle. Endurance activities aren't the only area that suffers during the second half of your cycle. You don't make the same gains from strength training, and you're actually more likely to experience an athletic injury during the luteal phase and first few days of menstruation than during the first half of your cycle. If you suffer from PMS, you may be at even greater risk for injury during the premenstrual days, according to a 2003 study in *Gynecological Endocrinology*. Trying to "just do it" during the second half of your cycle, even though your body is telling you to take it down a notch, can sabotage your exercise efforts. All that hard work you put in during the follicular phase just goes to waste, and you end up right back where you started.

Nutrition scientist, exercise physiologist, and triathlete Stacy T. Sims discovered the luteal slump when she was competing in the grueling Ironman Kona race. In her book *Roar: How to Match Your Food and Fitness to Your Female Physiology for Optimum Performance, Great Health, and a Strong, Lean Body for Life*, Sims recounts how she developed a headache and swelling during the second half of the race, clear signs of hyponatremia, a condition in which the sodium concentration in the blood falls below normal. She managed to complete the race but wasn't happy with her finish time. What went wrong, she wondered? She had trained to acclimate to the heat and followed the same gender-neutral nutrition regimen as most racers. When she polled her fellow female participants, she made a surprising discovery. The ones who were in the late luteal phase of their cycle, as Sims was, also experienced issues that cramped their performance. The women who were in the follicular phase of their cycle had no problems and finished with great times. Sims realized she needed to start tweaking her training regimen to work with her cyclical biochemistry, not against it. "I went to work researching how hormones impact thermoregulation, macronutrient usage, hydration, performance, and recovery," she says. "Right out of the gate, it was apparent that sex differences extend far beyond ponytails and sports bras." How right she is!

You don't have to be a triathlete to benefit from some exercise optimization. But if you want to get the most out of your workout, it is essential to plan your exercise with each phase of your cycle in mind. And just as you saw in chapter 2 how our body's biochemistry naturally drives us to alternate between periods of productivity and rest, your workouts also need to honor this rhythm. Going hard all the time is what our culture admires, and many women interpret that to mean doing intense cardio on a daily basis. But cardio is only one aspect of the fitness equation. Gaining lean muscle, improving flexibility, and recovery are equally important. Adopting a well-rounded routine requires shedding the cultural conditioning we have around what "fitness" looks like—starting with the idea that the path to a healthy body lies in sweat and suffering.

When Less Is More—Seriously!

Like me, you've probably been indoctrinated into the exercise cult of "more is good, harder is better." We all look at professional female athletes with their lean physiques and think they are the picture of health. But even though they may look great on the outside, they aren't necessarily hormonally balanced on the inside. Ironman champion and professional triathlete Meredith Kessler, who was already running long distances as a teenager, admitted she hadn't gotten her first period by the time she was nineteen, and she had developed borderline osteoporosis due to lack of estrogen. There's nothing healthy about that! Thankfully, she says she has since fixed those issues. Extreme exercise and dieting can lead to serious consequences and something health care experts call the female athlete triad: inadequate nutrition for the amount of training, irregular or missing periods, and prematurely low bone density. It's clear that more and harder exercise isn't the answer for women.

In fact, doing *less* can be the key to getting the results you want. When I finally realized that in addition to adapting my eating patterns to my cycle, I needed to sync my exercise, I easily dropped 60 pounds without having to work out aggressively. I started working out less—*seriously!*—and the extra pounds melted away. Even better, I felt energized, alert, and motivated. The same thing happened after I gained 40 pounds while pregnant with my daughter. After giving birth, I stopped doing all high-intensity training and switched to short walks—no more than half an hour—and gentle Pilates. The extra pounds melted away, and I'm back down to my feel-good weight. I was finally able to end the war with my body. I was thrilled, and a little bit shocked, because it went against everything I had ever learned about fitness and weight loss.

Our female biology shines a light on why the less-is-more approach works for us. When you get your heart pumping, your body burns the glucose in your bloodstream for energy. This supply lasts only about thirty minutes; after that, your body needs to find a replacement to keep your energy up. Where does your body turn? It calls on your adrenal glands, and they jump into action by pumping out the stress hormone cortisol, which converts stored fat into usable glucose so you have the energy to continue working out. Although the fat-burning part of this process may sound like a win-win for you, it comes with some serious side effects. If you have unresolved hormonal issues, such as excess estrogen—the most common hormonal imbalance I see among my clients—the cortisol spike and fat burning lead to something counterproductive. The estrogen overload programs your body to convert any circulating glucose back into fat. And estrogen tends to cause your body to hold on to the fat cells in your midsection and hips. Your body doubles down on the action when those fat cells, which are hormonally active tissue, pump out even more estrogen into your body. The more fat cells you have, the higher your estrogen levels. And the more estrogen, the more your body hangs on to those fat cells. So instead of becoming a fat-burning machine, you become stuck in an ugly cycle of burning stored fat with cortisol, only to have your high estrogen levels send the fat right back to all the wrong places. This is especially likely to happen in the luteal phase of your cycle, when your body naturally pumps out more cortisol.

Even worse, if you're suffering from adrenal fatigue, exercising too hard or too long will cause your adrenal glands to become overstimulated. Going all out at the gym when you're already dealing with the effects of chronic stress will leave you feeling even more depleted and further strains your adrenals. Eventually, adrenal fatigue can spiral to a point where you can barely crawl out of bed each morning, you struggle to get through your workouts, and you feel more exhausted than ever. It's a no-win situation. You force yourself to work out because you think you're doing something healthy for your body—but really, you're just compounding your hormonal issues.

Don't worry. There is a solution.

Work Out Smarter, Not Harder

Your rhythmic biochemistry provides a clear road map to plan your best workouts. During each phase of the menstrual cycle, the female body is primed and prepped to respond to different kinds of exercise. The first half of your cycle is the ideal time to focus on cardio and building lean muscle. In the second half of your cycle, you'll benefit more from skipping intense cardio and shifting to resistance training, flexibility, and recovery. You may even want to skip the gym altogether on some days—and that is not only okay, it's recommended! Finally, you can stop beating yourself up for not doing enough. You can stop feeling guilty if you walked out of your dance class after half an hour. You can do less, get better results, and feel better, too.

Letting go of the "more is good, harder is better" mentality can be hard. In fact, you may be asking yourself, "Won't I gain weight if I don't exercise with the same intensity every day?" Women ask me this all the time. I promise you, the answer is a resounding no! In fact, when you begin syncing with your cycle and give yourself permission to scale back your workouts during the second half of your cycle, you'll start to see results within a month or two. For example, instead of trying to make PMS bloat go away by sweating it out on the treadmill, you'll find that you no longer feel bloated in the first place. So there's no need for that high-intensity workout. Why keep swimming upstream?

That's the lesson Emily, a twenty-eight-year-old fitness and yoga instructor, finally learned after a lifetime of giving in to the more, more, more mentality. She taught about twenty classes a week and would push through her period pains out of fear she might gain weight if she took time off. Eventually, her stressed-out body began screaming for a break, and she realized she needed to make a change. After learning about this cyclical program, she made a commitment to start honoring her body in a way that would support her cycle. She started by taking off the first day of her period from teaching and simply doing a few restorative poses on her own. Then she began to notice that her body craved different types of movement and intensity depending on the phase of her cycle. By listening to that inner wisdom, she developed routines that fueled her cycle and left her feeling energized rather than deflated. "I've come to a place where I feel balanced," she says, adding that she doesn't even bother weighing herself anymore.

(DON'T) JUST DO IT

You might be saying, wait a minute, weren't we raised to think that we should absolutely never let our periods get in the way or hold us back from going to gym class in high school, from playing sports, or from training for a marathon? Let's unpack two problematic aspects of this thinking:

1. The assertion that your period is a liability you must overcome with willpower is toxic.
2. Enforcing a cultural norm—the belief that you should work out no matter how you feel—further forces a woman to practice actively ignoring her inner wisdom and feel more disconnected from her body.

Why is the standard that we should go to gym class when we're not biorhythmically primed for it? It's because male biology responds well to daily exercise, and we feel compelled to model our behavior after theirs so we can be taken seriously, respected, and valued. Why would any woman who has learned the truth about her biological rhythms do high-intensity training during a hormonal phase that would turn on muscle wasting and fat storage?

Biological common sense requires women's different needs to be acknowledged and respected. Can't we reimagine our cultural narrative so our differences are celebrated and we are equally respected and valued regardless of our differences? We should be free to pursue whatever activity we feel like doing in any phase of our cycle. We should *not* be making choices as a reaction to the cultural conditioning that dictates we must never acknowledge our hormonal fluctuations for fear of being considered weak. There's a big difference between forcing yourself to work out—pushing yourself to ignore your biological rhythms—and gaining strength from your workouts by syncing with your biological rhythms. When you take a cyclical approach to exercise, you can "just do it" when it works best for you.

When you sync your activities with the fluctuations of your hormonal cycle, you support your biological systems, energize your body, fire up healthy metabolism, boost your moods, shore up overall health, and prevent injury and boredom. Want more details? No sweat—check out the handy guide of phase-specific exercises below. And if you want your fitness routine to honor your 24-hour clock, too, try exercising in the morning during the first half of your cycle and in the afternoon during the second half of your cycle—*if that routine would fit your schedule and feel right for you.*

Getting in the FLO with Your Workouts

Follicular phase: In the first few days after your bleed has finished, your energy begins to rise again, so this is the time to wake up your body with some fun cardio. And because you are more open to new experiences during this phase, mix up your old routine with a new class. As your follicular phase continues, your body will react more efficiently to hardcore workouts to boost metabolism, help you shed weight, and build lean muscle. However, if your hormones are imbalanced or you're trying to lose weight or struggling with anxiety, fatigue, or depression, you must keep your workouts to no more than thirty minutes. Going beyond half an hour will overstress your body and push it into fat storage mode.

Workout suggestions: running, biking, dance, hiking, jumping rope

Ovulatory phase: In this phase, estrogen and testosterone are at peak levels, giving you energy to burn. This is the time for you to crush an intense workout and to choose group workouts that feed your desire to be more social.

Workout suggestions: interval sprints, HIIT, indoor cycling, boot camp, kickboxing

Luteal phase: During the first five days of the luteal phase, you still have elevated estrogen and testosterone levels, and progesterone enters the picture. You'll still have a good dose of energy, but not as much for high-impact activities. Use this energy to maximize lean muscle gains by focusing on any kind of strength training. Once you hit the second half of the luteal phase, all three of your reproductive hormones begin to diminish in concentration, shifting you out of muscle-building mode. To align with this phase, switch to workouts that focus on flexibility.

Workout suggestions: first half of the luteal phase: strength training, intense yoga; second half of the luteal phase: Pilates, barre, gentle yoga

Menstrual phase: While you're bleeding, your hormone levels are at their lowest, and so are your energy levels. Any form of high-intensity exercise during this phase will backfire by turning on fat storage, causing muscle wasting and putting stress on your cardiovascular system. Engage in activities that feel restorative to you. Don't forget that deep, restful, uninterrupted sleep helps with weight loss, so focus on getting some good shut-eye. It's completely okay to consider napping a workout on these days!

Workout suggestions: walking, foam rolling, yin yoga, mat Pilates, breath work, napping (really!). Quick tip for cramps: yoga can help. *The Woman's Yoga Book: Asana and Pranayama for All Phases of the Menstrual Cycle*, a beautiful book by Bobby Clennell, suggests triangle pose, standing forward bend, downward dog, and fish pose (sitting cross legged and leaning back on a block so your back is arched) to calm cramps.

The Cycle Syncing Method™: Fitness FLO*

This chart offers suggestions for weekly workouts, but it can be tailored to your individual fitness level, phase timing, and hormonal reality. If you're fit and hormonally healthy, you may want to work out every day, but if you're in the process of rebalancing your hormones, it's better to start with just three days a week. And remember, the phases flow gradually from one to the next, so there may be some overlap. For example, the ovulatory phase typically lasts three to four days, but you may still have an abundance of energy in the few days immediately following, so go ahead and enjoy a few more intense workouts. And each phase isn't exactly one week long, but this plan can help you move through your cycle smoothly. The best advice is to listen to your body and go with what makes you feel good.

	Follicular	Ovulatory	Luteal	Menstrual
Monday	Cardio dance	Kettlebells	HIIT	Rest
Tuesday	Rebounding class	HIIT	Pilates	Rest
Wednesday	Dance class	Indoor cycling	Weight lifting	Yin yoga
Thursday	Jumping rope	Boot camp class	Pilates	Walking
Friday	Indoor cycling	Kickboxing	Barre class	Mat Pilates
Saturday	Hiking	Power yoga	Yoga	Walking
Sunday	Rest	Rest	Rest	Rest

* If you're in the early stages of syncing your cycle and trying to heal hormonal imbalances, it is critical to keep your workouts to no more than thirty minutes. This time limitation will prevent excess cortisol production and adrenal fatigue, and will gradually lead you to an energizing cycle. And always check with your physician before starting any exercise program.

To help you keep track of which phase you're in and which workouts are best for your current phase, try the MyFLO app (www.MyFLOtracker .com). The app makes it super simple to sync your fitness activities with your cycle, so you're always getting the most out of your workouts—and you can learn more about workout videos tailored to each phase of your cycle at www.cyclesyncingmembership.com/bonus.

GO FOR THE GOLD

The US women's soccer team players follow the unique timing of their individual cycles to map out the most effective training and resting schedule, as well as a dietary approach to maximize their energy and recovery.

Four Steps to Get in Sync with Your Workouts

Making the shift from feeling you need to "go hard or go home" every day, to accepting that you can do less and allow your body to guide your workout intensity levels, can be deeply triggering to our fears about our bodies being out of our control. To help transition to a more cyclical mindset and to keep from reverting back to your old conditioning, try this four-step approach.

1. **Note where you are in your cycle.** Understanding how your hormonal fluctuations impact your performance will allow you to make smarter decisions about your fitness routines. If you've tried to power through a boot camp class during your monthly bleed, and it left you feeling fatigued, you'll know for yourself that you need to switch to a more restorative activity during that phase. I have found noticing where you are in your cycle to be one of the most empowering and liberating pieces of syncing with your second clock. You'll understand why you can zoom through dance class one week but feel like you're dragging another week. And you'll stop beating yourself up when you're dragging. You're

not a slacker; you're just doing the wrong workout for your biochemistry at the wrong time! By educating yourself about your body's unique cyclical nature and how it affects your performance, you can avoid the frustration and hurtful inner dialog that can be so misery-making. You can track your progress with the MyFLO app so you feel good about yourself every day and achieve lasting results—*no pain required!*

2. **Have an exit plan.** If you're healing your hormones and need to limit your workouts to thirty minutes, but you're taking a class that's an hour long or you're meeting up with friends for a hike, craft an exit plan before you start. Many of us are so conditioned to follow along, be polite, and avoid rocking the boat that we'll risk injuring ourselves or harming our hormonal health by overdoing it rather than leaving halfway through a class. Use this strategy: Tell the instructor beforehand that you need to bow out early, so she is prepared to see you leave before the class is over. And find a spot at the back of the room where you can make a quick exit without disrupting the class. If you're going out with your workout buddies, give them a heads-up that you'll have to peel away after thirty minutes. Let them know you're in the process of healing your hormones. You'll be delightfully surprised at what opens up in the conversation among your friends when you talk about your hormones. This should be a matter-of-fact conversation women can easily have together. Just as we'd mention needing to make choices based on the weather, we should mention needing to make choices based on our biological rhythms without feeling any shame.

3. **Be flexible.** Are you in the first half of your cycle but feel like taking it easy with a gentle stretching class? That's 100 percent okay! You can always take it down a notch if you feel like it. Your hormonal cycle is fluid, which allows you to take some flexibility with your fitness routines. But what if you're in the second half of your cycle and have a burning desire to lace up your running shoes and hit the road for some hardcore sprints? You may want to give it a try to see how your body reacts. I've been following this cyclical program for close to two decades now, and I still like to experiment to see how my body responds. Recently, while I was in the early stage of the luteal phase, I got a strong urge to do some interval jogging. Keep in mind, I don't run often as it's not an ideal workout for me, but this

desire was so intense I decided to give it a go. I cruised around the loop in the park, alternating between walking for a few minutes and ratcheting up the speed to a full jog for a minute. The first two times I did this workout right after my ovulatory phase, I felt fantastic. But when I did it a third time on the fifth day of my luteal phase, I felt drained. When I got home, I hit the couch, and it took me until the next day to recover my energy. It was a powerful reminder that even though an activity made me feel energized a few days earlier, I needed to honor my cycle and skip the high-intensity interval training that late in the second half of my cycle. The science is the science: I can't get away with going against my biochemistry.

4. **After your workout, ask yourself how you feel.** Do you feel energized and awesome? Do you feel drained and depleted? Examining your body's response to exercise will give you invaluable insight into what your biochemistry needs to thrive. For example, if you feel exhausted, and it takes you hours to recover your mood and energy, it's a clear sign you may be overexercising. You may have used up your adrenal and glucose reserves, pushing your body into survival and fat storage mode. Without judgment, make a mental note of this outcome, and don't go quite so hard next time. Remember, the goal is to *feel good* after you exercise.

THIS ALL SOUNDS GREAT, BUT . . .

"I don't want to get bulky." Why should you care about strength training? Lean muscle—the kind that makes you look toned and defined, not big and bulky—is a key element in your body's metabolism. The more lean muscle on your bones, the faster your body burns calories and fat. Research shows that starting at about age thirty, you begin to lose muscle mass each year. And unless you actively engage in strength training to counteract this, that lean muscle is often replaced by fat, which kicks out estrogen, increasing your risk for estrogen dominance. More lean muscle and less fat can put the brakes on excess estrogen production.

"Stretching is a waste of time." Taking the time to stretch can be very beneficial in helping you reach your fitness—and weight— goals. Stretching primes your muscles for your workouts so you can perform better, prevents injury, soothes stress to reduce cortisol levels, and even helps you sleep better (and sleep is critical for balancing your body's hunger and satiety hormones!).

"Taking a day off is lazy or throws me off." After intense workouts and during certain times of your cycle, your body needs rest so it can recover. If you're caught up in perpetual productivity mode and continually work out without a break, you could stall or completely derail your progress. You need to listen to your body when it tells you to push harder and also respect it when it asks for some rest and recovery.

Let's Talk Our Way into a New Normal

Earlier in this chapter, I told you about triathlete Meredith Kessler, who had the courage to share her story about her missing periods. I applaud her for going public with her experiences and am thrilled with the growing number of professional athletes who are talking about their periods on Twitter and in the media. British pro tennis player Heather Watson attributed a loss at the Australian Open to low energy levels during her period and told the press, "I have nightmares about getting my period at Wimbledon." Olympic gymnast Aly Raisman has spoken openly about her struggles with her cycle and told *Allure*, "You can't tell the judges you want to compete tomorrow or wait a few days." The gymnast, who bravely spoke up about being sexually abused by former USA Gymnastics physician Larry Nassar, is encouraging women to stop feeling uncomfortable or ashamed of our periods and to start talking about them. I couldn't agree more. I think everybody involved in the fitness industry and in high school, college, and professional sports should be talking about periods. Professional coaches, personal trainers, and fitness instructors should make allowances for women's cycles. How great would it be if your personal trainer knew you were on Day 1 of your bleed and scaled back your workout to focus more on stretching and flexibility rather than pushing you to run sprints in between heavy lifting when you're already feeling blah? Imagine the day when group exercise instructors make an announcement at the beginning of an hour-long class that any women in the second half of their cycle should feel comfortable staying at the back of the class and leaving early after thirty minutes. Wouldn't you love to go to a yoga studio that offers classes based on the phases of the cycle? And please, can coaches finally stop overtraining women to the point that their periods go MIA? This practice is harming our biochemistry as a direct consequence of ignoring our second clock.

I understand that at the professional level, athletes may not be able to reschedule their tournaments to sync with their cycle, but you can do so in your everyday life. That said, syncing with your cycle doesn't mean that being on your period should be an excuse to avoid engaging in physical activity. Instead, syncing with your cycle will make your period easier—you'll have fewer cramps, less fatigue, and more energy—so you'll have more "get up and go" to enjoy your favorite activities.

Losing the Postpartum Baby Weight and Breastfeeding

After we give birth, we feel intense pressure to get our bodies back into sexy pre-pregnancy shape and to bounce back to our former selves without a hitch. But as Kimberly Ann Johnson wrote in her book, *The Fourth Trimester*, it takes time to recover from the life-altering physical changes while also adjusting to the significant emotional, neurological, and relational upheaval that birth brings. This is an extremely important time to recover from pregnancy and birth by nourishing and resting the body. We need to treat the twelve weeks after birth like an extended menstrual phase and support it with nutrient-dense foods, such as bone broth, homemade chicken liver paté, and bison burgers. You can find some amazing postpartum recipes in Heng Ou's book, *The First Forty Days*. This phase also requires lots of rest with some gentle movement sprinkled in—think easy walking, soothing yoga, and Pilates geared to helping realign your bones and muscles.

In the first year after I gave birth to my daughter I basically took a break from exercise. I went for a walk—more of a stroll, actually, *not* a power walk!—three or four times a week in the park pushing my baby in her thirty-pound stroller. And I worked with a postpartum physical therapist at home. And I didn't do anything for more than thirty minutes. And guess what? I lost forty pounds in six months without feeling deprived and without wearing myself out with intense exercise. I was able to lose the weight because I was tuned in to my second clock and honored my hormonal reality during this postpartum stage of my life. Our cultural conditioning tells us that after giving birth we ought to diet and work out to drop the baby weight. But that's bad advice. We need to respect our body's biochemical needs. I needed to make sure I was consuming enough calories to handle the energy- and nutrient-heavy process of producing breast milk for my baby. My body was healing from the massive nutrient requirements that accompany pregnancy and the delivery of a tiny human. Like all new moms, I was sleep-deprived and needed to get rest whenever I could. I listened to my inner guidance system and understood that if I wanted to provide for my child and keep myself healthy and happy, I needed to support and nourish my body.

Many women think the calorie-burning magic of breastfeeding is the key to getting your prebaby body back. While women who breastfeed exclusively for three months lose over three pounds more than women who use alternative feeding methods, according to a 2014 study in *Preventive Medicine*, I've had many clients tell me they have actually gained weight while breastfeeding. I usually ask them what they're eating and how much they're exercising. In most cases, they're not eating enough and they're exercising too much, a combination that stalls metabolism. The American College of Obstetricians and Gynecologists recommends consuming 450 to 500 extra calories a day to make up for energy expended on milk production.

If you don't listen to your body and try to lose the baby weight by going on some low-calorie diet and heading straight to boot camp, your body will fight back by going into fat storage mode. Pushing yourself too hard also depletes your stores of nutrients, energy, and hormones and can lead to adrenal fatigue or thyroid issues that can linger for years. This is one of the most critical times in your life, when you absolutely must work with your body to give it the rest and nourishment it needs.

Your Body Is the Boss

This chapter has given you a framework to help you choose workouts that sync with your cycle, but the framework isn't intended to be restrictive or prevent you from doing what you love. Ultimately, syncing your exercise with your cycle is about experimenting to find what feels good for you. You're the one who's living inside your body; only you know what feels right and what doesn't. Work on fine-tuning your sense of self-awareness, so you can hear your body's inner voice communicating with you through sensations and feelings, and make adjustments accordingly. There is no right or wrong—simply what your body needs in the moment. Listening to your body, you regain the power nature instilled in you.

CHAPTER 6

Your Blueprint to Do More with Less Stress

For most people, creativity is a serious business. They forget the telling phrase "the play of ideas" and think that they need to knuckle down and work more. Often, the reverse is true. They need to play.
—Julia Cameron

As a young girl, I naturally gravitated to all things creative—I loved to dance, sang in choir, played piano, sewed some of my own clothes, and even made jewelry. But around age fifteen, right about the time when puberty should have been kicking in, I abandoned my artistic side and disconnected from the feminine energy it nurtured. I thought if I was going to be successful in this world, I needed to leave my creative hobbies behind and get serious. Nobody had ever directly told me that dancing or making jewelry was frivolous, but those ideas had somehow seeped into my unconscious mind and reflected my interpretation of our cultural values: I believed that I had to finish all of my work before I could play, and that the path for success in life seemed to require continuous pushing; I grew up in a home that valued productivity. So all of my creative pursuits and the desire to explore my interests didn't seem to fit into the things I was observing about how to be an adult. I began to work more, play less, and rest less. I abandoned the rest, play, grow, learn/work pattern of childhood (which, interestingly, is a nice balance of feminine and masculine energies). We all go through this shift in our own way: we begin to over-rely on our masculine energy of constant doing, we develop anxiety around fallow time, and we become experts in ignoring the body's cries for rest, nourishment, and pleasure. I shifted my focus to the things I thought would put me on the fast track to the traditional concept of success—a big job, a big salary, a big house. In high school, I loaded up my schedule with AP classes and clubs. I started working in the summers for different businesses, small at first, then larger and more corporate as I went from high school to college. I thought this approach would help me get a head start in my career. I didn't realize that all the pressure I was putting on myself to constantly push as hard as I could was exacerbating my hormonal issues, long before I eventually got diagnosed with PCOS. Not only did I not have time for my creative pursuits, but I also found myself increasingly anxious and overwhelmed, and I developed a habit of procrastinating to unofficially give myself a break and then rushing at all hours of the night to meet deadlines. This was exhausting, and I was miserable. Things on my to-do list were falling through the cracks, and I felt like I was floundering. I hadn't been diagnosed with PCOS yet, so I didn't know why I felt so bad all the time. This feeling that I needed to continually push myself carried over into my career, until I finally began actively searching for ways to gain control of my life, feel better, reclaim that creativity I had abandoned, and have more energy for the things I wanted to do.

Jocelyn, 29, knows what it's like to feel drained. She was experiencing bad PMS—cramps, breast tenderness, full-body bloating, feelings of despair, and fatigue to the point that she couldn't work. She felt that her body was failing her. She had energy for only seven days out of the month and didn't feel like she could accomplish anything. Syncing with her cycle turned that situation around and helped her regain her energy. She began to re-identify what gave her pleasure, and instead of listening to other people's plans and feelings, she started tuning in to her own. "It totally turned my life around," she says. "The cramps are gone, the clots are gone, and I have energy all through the month. Even when I'm bleeding, I have energy. I don't have to stop and check out."

The Time Management Myth

I thought learning time management would be the key to making every-thing better. I convinced the people at one of my summer jobs to send me to a conference on time management. It turned out this wildly popular pro-gram involved using an elaborate time management planner that was very repetitive—the same habits every day that ensure you can meet your daily appointments by the hour, lists of tasks, and so on. I was so excited about it, and started filling in my to-do list, but as much as I tried, I just couldn't stick with it. There was also no real structure or guidance around self-care—just that one should do it daily. Each day, I would start with the best of intentions, attempting to accomplish all I had planned out the night or week before, but instead of feeling like I was breezing through my to-do list, and feeling less stress and more satisfaction and confidence, I felt worse about myself than before! And when I planned activities a couple weeks in advance, by the time I got to that day in my schedule, my to-dos were absolutely not what I felt like doing. What I thought I wanted to focus on two weeks earlier now felt stifling and wrong for my frame of mind. For example, I would plan to finish a project, to do a group fitness class, or to go out with friends on a certain day, but when that day arrived my head was in a completely different space, so I didn't follow through. I began to feel I couldn't stick to my plans and commitments. Within a few months, I tossed the planner aside, telling my-self, "I can't do this. I'm a huge failure. I'll just never be able to manage my time." I even stopped wearing a watch. I literally broke up with time.

Finding My Feminine Energy

By my midtwenties, when I was finalizing my research on what would be-come the FLO protocol, I was still struggling with trying to manage ev-erything I wanted to do in life and preserving the hormonal health I had recently fought hard to recover. Something key was missing. I had an unex-pected source of inspiration to guide me to ask the right question that eventually led me to create the Cycle Syncing Method™. A group of girlfriends and I had decided to travel to India to visit a female zen master, because she was the only one we could find who was a woman. We stayed nearby at an ashram and got to participate in various meditation classes that were so different from all the meditation I had experienced before. These classes were all movement-based. This practice of reaching higher states of conscious awareness through engaging the body, not ignoring it, countered every bit of conditioning I had ever received. I became aware of a whole new perspective on feminine and masculine energy, and that's when I realized the key that was missing. Instead of trying to fit my body and its biological rhythms into a paradigm clearly suited to male physiology, I needed to create a paradigm that included my physiology at the center. I realized there must have been a connection between that decision I made to abandon my creative expression at puberty and my body's blocked ability to perform its own version of creative expression—having a functioning cycle. By buying into our cultural conditioning, which says that relying on our masculine energy is the path to success, I had unconsciously disconnected from my feminine energy. Dr. Christiane Northrup writes in her book *Women's Bodies, Women's Wisdom* about the many ways women divorce themselves from their feminine energy, whether it's as a result of cultural conditioning or an abusive relationship that makes you turn it off, and how this manifests in our bodies in conditions like PCOS and fibroids (more on this in the Biohacking Tool Kit). Many of us have some version of my story of shutting down our feminine energy to try to survive in a culture that devalues such energy.

When I returned from India, I felt like I had awakened to a larger truth about life, and I realized I wanted to create a practice that would do more than just keep my hormones balanced. I asked myself a new question. My old question was always something like, "How can I do more to achieve happiness and success?" The new question was radically different: "What does it look like to live as an embodied woman, connected to my inner wisdom and creativity?" I wanted to heal from the wounds of our patriarchal conditioning in every way—physically, emotionally, and spiritually—so I could live with a better balance between my feminine and masculine energy. And then something clicked: I had only to look to my menstrual cycle for the perfect road map for my new vision for success. My biological rhythmic pattern laid out the ideal way to support my whole life—not only by taking care of my physical body with nutrition and exercise that supported the phases of my cycle, but also by adopting a phase-specific approach to my everyday activities that fueled my feminine energy and creativity. My goal wasn't to be able to get more stuff done so I could chase the masculine ideal of success. My goal went much deeper. I wanted to feel satisfied each day and not have to wait until I did or achieved something to feel successful. I wanted to be in a more consistent state of flow.

So when I began my own cyclical journey, I started tracking how I was feeling each day—how the foods I ate, the exercises I did, and the way I scheduled my days affected my moods, energy levels, and sense of satisfaction. And more important, how this new approach to my life strengthened my connection to my feminine energy. I experimented until I created the Cycle Syncing Method™, the principles of which are detailed in this book. At first, I noticed the weight loss and regulated periods—encouraging milestones that let me know the first three steps of the FLO protocol, outlined in *WomanCode*, were working. Then I began tuning in to more subtle things— feeling more energized throughout the day, getting into a state of flow on a more regular basis, hearing my inner guidance system and heeding its intuitive messages. The more I honored my feminine energy, the more enthused I was to take on the projects I was interested in and the more fulfilled I felt. I also regained confidence in stopping, resting, and making space as a safe and necessary part of the creative process. After syncing with my cycle for a few months, my health, my body, my moods, and my energy levels had all transformed. I used to feel like I was grinding away, just trying to check things off my to-do list to feel a little relief. Now, I woke up feeling excited about what the day would bring, and I found myself more often in the right place at the right time, ready to receive opportunity and abundance. I also noticed that instead of continuously draining my energy "bank account" and feeling exhausted in the second half of my cycle, I was adding to the account daily to offset any natural dips in energy that are a healthy part of the cycle.

With this feminine-based energy practice, you're always connecting to your body and inner wisdom rather than obsessing on what you think you should be doing. It's a big shift in your mindset, but you'll know you're doing it right when you get off the hamster wheel of doing and start feeling connected to your body and desires.

FEMININE AND MASCULINE ENERGY

Both men and women have both feminine and masculine energy. Both forms of energy are good, and you have to find your own balance. However, engaging one exclusively can lead to burnout.

Masculine Energy	Feminine Energy
linear	cyclical
goal-oriented	process-oriented
competitive	collaborative
static	flexible

The Value of Rest

In the beginning, I was more comfortable doing all the active parts of syncing with my cycle because I have more of that dominant masculine energy, as many of us do: navigating within a patriarchal environment causes many of us to rely more on our linear masculine energy of continuous doing and pushing. So when I first came to the Cycle Syncing Method™ as a way to heal this imbalance in my energies (among other things), I noticed that what felt easier to do first was the *doing* part, and what was more challenging was the *not doing*. When I'm in my menstrual phase, I'm not doing a lot of things that my outward self of the first half of the cycle (the follicular and the ovulatory) would love to be doing. I was, of course, under the impression that I should be *doing* every day. It's the gift of the luteal and menstrual phases, when you align with and let yourself be guided by the energies of those phases, to heal you from this toxic concept that you must have the same "doing," masculine energy every day. It lets you have some healing for your feminine aspect of the give-and-take, the resting and the receiving. The dynamic in the masculine is binary (on or off), and in the feminine it's additive (cyclical).

There is tremendous value in committing to the practice of going inward, of connecting to your feminine energy, of doing less, of observing that you're okay and that things are not going to fall apart—and doing this over and over again, every month. For me, it has provided tremendous rebalancing. I am a first-generation citizen, and anyone who shares this experience knows that immigrant families share a culture of constant work. In addition, like most of us, I had no perspective on feminine energy. I was, as the only female child, surrounded by brothers and male cousins, and the women in my family, like women everywhere, were all very wounded by the patriarchy, too.

There was no modeling for me of what it looked like to be an embodied woman or integrated with my feminine energy. I used the Cycle Syncing Method™ as a healing practice for this psychospiritual wound that we all receive as women in this unbalanced environment, and to unhook from the conditioning that our value is based on what we do. I've been able to prove that resting and taking care of myself, slowing down, being authentic with my emotions, and including my needs is the key. It's cleansing and it's healing, and I look forward to it now—but it took me many, many repetitions of working with the ritual of my cycle to really integrate these energies.

Managing Your Life

In this chapter, we're going to look at your relationship to time, energy, creativity, and productivity. If you're like most women, you probably assume this will be directed specifically at your work life (chapter 7 is devoted to work); but because syncing with your cycle is about managing your energy versus managing your time, it extends into your relationships, parenting, home life, social life, and more. When you're managing your schedule effectively, you stop feeling drained by all that you do, freeing up space that allows you to flourish creatively in a natural, organic way in every area of your life.

First, we'll explore the negative effects of our culture's frantically flawed pace and master a more intuitive way of planning and scheduling. Then, we will focus on how you can take advantage of your cyclical strengths to create a more sustainable, fulfilling life. My hope is that by the end of the chapter, you'll see that the secret to success is not figuring out how to do it all—rather, it's about defining your own success and focusing your energy on the things that matter most to you at the right time, feeling good throughout the day, and continuously building energy rather than draining it.

The Cost of an Energy Leak

We live in a culture that encourages us to push continuously. To keep up with the demands, we try to extend our energy and increase our focus by exogenous means—think double espressos and energy drinks. But the fact is, creating more energy is an inside game, won by supporting our biological rhythms. It's similar to saving money—you'll have more money if you spend less of it. Likewise, you'll have more energy if you're thoughtful about where you're letting it go. Where is your energy leaking? Is it due to the foods you eat? A lack of movement? Not getting enough rest? Not setting up healthy boundaries at work and in relationships?

It's a fact that you can't create more time, but you can create more energy by plugging the leaks.

Because we've been so conditioned, however, it can be hard to let go of the feeling that we should be in perpetual go-mode. I say, listen to the science. A wealth of research has proven pretty definitively that pushing too hard for long periods of time actually diminishes your productivity and creativity and sets you up for burnout. The grind is real. In May 2019 the World Health Organization (WHO) officially recognized burnout as a legitimate health diagnosis.

So, let's go back to the big energy leaks in your life. You can see now that these energy leaks can impact your productivity and creativity, but did you know that they can also take a toll on your body's biological systems, creating a negative biofeedback loop and more deeply draining your energy? Take a look at how trying to operate as if you only have the one 24-hour clock ravages your biological systems and disrupts your 28-day clock.

IDENTIFY YOUR ENERGY LEAKS

Where is your energy leaking? Our energy gets drained when we are unconscious about all the little ways we compromise what we need in order to be in our peak flow state. Over time, this accumulates not only into mental overwhelm, but also into measurable stress and inflammation in the body. Check off all that apply to you on a regular basis:

☐ not getting enough rest

☐ skipping exercise

☐ skipping meals or not eating nutrient-dense foods

☐ not maintaining boundaries, or saying yes when you mean no

☐ not asking for help, and doing too much

☐ not managing your money and feeling stressed about it

Evaluate where your energy and time are going, and plug those holes!

The Productivity Toll on Your Biological Systems

Biological System 1: Brain. Chronic stress can lead to long-term changes in the brain that affect cognitive function, including changes in memory, learning, and mental health. For example, did you know that stress shrinks the brain? Researchers at Yale University found that stress reduces gray matter volume in key areas of the prefrontal cortex and limbic regions, areas involved in emotional stability, impulse control, and reward regulation. In a 2012 study in *Biological Psychiatry*, these researchers suggested that brain shrinkage in these areas may increase the risk of depression and addiction, among other mental health issues. How are you supposed to perform your best when your brain isn't operating at optimal levels? Chronic stress also alters the way neural stem cells develop in the hippocampus, a region associated with memory and learning, according to a 2014 study in *Molecular Psychiatry*. These cells typically develop into neurons, but under chronic stress these cells instead transform into a protective coating called myelin. The excess myelin growth disrupts the timing and communication of neural networks and could increase the risk for depression, anxiety, and other mental disorders. When you're feeling anxious or depressed, it's hard to feel focused or enthusiastic about your to-do list. With unrelenting stress, you may also have trouble concentrating, making a decision, or keeping things organized. And since your brain is critically involved in supervising your body's hormone production, too much stress can increase production of the stress hormone cortisol, which has the effect of suppressing progesterone production, which can lead to more severe PMS symptoms and other period problems (more on this in chapter 7).

Biological System 2: Immune system. Stress can take a toll on your immune system, leaving you more vulnerable to routine colds and flu bugs, as well as flare-ups like itchy skin, rashes, hives, acne, or cold sores that can distract you and get in the way of your creative flow. When you're regularly fighting a cold or flu or dealing with symptoms, you can't possibly feel up to the task of running errands, attending meetings, or working on your side hustle. When your immune system is constantly under attack, it can also lead to systemic inflammation, which has been linked to painful cramps and PMS. In 2016, researchers reported in the *Journal of Women's Health* that women with elevated levels of the inflammation bio-marker CRP had up to a 41 percent increased risk for PMS symptoms, such as cramps, bloating, and breast tenderness.

Biological System 3: Metabolism. When you get stuck in perpetual work mode, your metabolism goes haywire and you're more likely to gain weight. We all know that when we're feeling stressed, we're more likely to reach for some chocolate, cookies, or ice cream. The biological mechanism behind this tendency is the rise in cortisol, which ramps up insulin levels and can cause blood sugar levels to drop. When blood sugar levels drop, cravings for sugary, fat-laden fare increase. A 2017 study in the journal *Obesity* involving 2,527 women and men showed that having chronically elevated cortisol levels was associated with higher weight, larger waist circumference, and a great risk for obesity. As you've seen, fat cells also secrete estrogen, so being obese can contribute to estrogen dominance, which can then increase PMS symptoms and lead to heavier bleeding. Every woman who's had to deal with heavy periods knows that this doesn't leave you in the most energized creative space. Low blood sugar can also make you feel nervous, anxious, irritable, impatient, or confused, among other things. These feelings can also sabotage your interactions with friends and family, colleagues, and the innocent person in front of you in the checkout line.

Biological System 4: Microbiome. Feeling stressed from nonstop productivity? The stress might make you queasy, give you heartburn, cause ulcers, or give you an embarrassing bout of diarrhea. The consequences of chronic stress go even deeper. A 2010 study showed that after subjecting mice to ten days of stress, their gut microbiome became significantly less diverse when compared with whiskered critters that didn't undergo stress. When you're under stress, hormonal changes disrupt your gut microbiome and cause it to become unstable and behave erratically, according to 2017 research in *Nature Microbiology*. This instability may increase your vulnerability to mood disorders, irritable bowel disease, obesity, and type 2 diabetes. Other researchers suggest that a healthy microbiome is associated with mental toughness; compromised gut health could add to difficulties coping with everyday challenges at the office or in your personal life. A stressed-out and compromised microbiome can also disrupt your 28-day clock by causing excess estrogen, which can leave you foggy-headed, tired, bloated, and depressed, and completely derail your creative process.

Biological System 5: Stress response. When a crazy schedule, big demands at work, and self-induced pressure to perform don't subside, your stress response works overtime just as you do. Eventually your stress response gets stuck in high alert mode, and you feel as if you're under threat at all times. As a result, your adrenal glands can become overtaxed, leading to adrenal fatigue, which makes it harder to function at your best and can stop ovulation, decrease fertility, and lower libido.

There's got to be a better way—right?

Stop Managing Your Time and Start Managing Your Energy

Are you struggling to stay on top of everything—multitasking to the max, juggling multiple schedules, finding time for family, squeezing in a social life—and feeling stretched to the limit? If so, you're probably (and rightfully) frustrated. And being the proactive woman that you are, you've probably set out to try and solve the situation. Maybe you've downloaded a few different to-do list apps. Maybe you bought a planner that promised to keep you organized and focused. Maybe you turned to an inspiring daily journal. Or maybe you went to a time management seminar as I did. Like me, you were probably hoping your efforts would help you gain control of your life. But none of those apps or planners did the trick—and I have to tell you, they never will. Why? Because traditional time management tools don't work for women who have the 28-day hormonal clock running. With most time management systems, we're expected to make to-do lists, check things off as the day goes by, and then wake up the next day and do it all over again. Every day, every 24 hours, the same thing. Rinse. Repeat.

When I finally got in sync with my own biochemistry, I realized I never actually had a problem with time or time management. I understood that those linear planning tools correspond with the 24-hour clock. And they didn't work with my cyclical nature. Don't get me wrong— they're magnificent tools for anyone who's operating solely on a daily circadian clock. But they aren't suited to the pattern changes of the female hormonal cycle or the concept of right-timing. When we schedule our lives without taking our natural 28-day hormone clock into account, we don't get to access the gifts provided by our cyclical nature, and we experience constant energy drains. I needed to stop managing my time and start managing my energy in a way that aligned with *both* my 24-hour and my 28-day clock. As you saw in chapter 2, this subtle but powerful shift in your mindset gets you off that endless treadmill of tasks and onto a path to achieving more of the things that are important to you while seemingly doing less.

The Cycle Syncing Method™ is working for Larissa. When this graphic designer started managing her energy according to the phases of her cycle rather than simply scheduling her time, she said, "It felt like the fog lifted." Even though she has been syncing with her cycle for some time, she occasionally finds herself getting sucked back into thinking, "I wasn't productive enough this week." When she flips the script and honors her cycle by saying no to certain things or taking a step back during her menstrual phase, for example, she experiences a real payoff. "I find that the next week, I'm just unstoppable and it's effortless," she says. "The things on my to-do list are just bam, bam, bam, done, versus forcing and trying to push and trying to make it happen all the time."

Self-help guru Tony Robbins has helped millions of people, including me, learn how to trigger a flow state that puts you in peak performance mode. He points out that a major stumbling block to achieving a flow state is the disconnect that occurs when your core beliefs and expectations for your life don't match with your reality. If you believe what our culture has told you, that you should be able to perform nonstop and ignore your biology, you're going to suffer. Robbins explains you need to change your inner blueprint to match your reality so you can enjoy your life and optimize your performance. Among his many teachings, he wants you to identify what motivates you, establish daily physical habits that prime you for achievement, let go of your fears, and take massive daily action in the direction of your dreams. I believe that for women a critical key to unleashing our inner power comes from patterning our creativity and productivity according to our hormonal biological rhythms—a practice that leads to a fulfilling and sustainable life.

When you stop thinking about time management and start managing your energy according to your cycle phases, you're going to reduce stress, support your biological systems, optimize communication, build energy reserves, and enjoy sustainable productivity. Everything in your life will start to feel easier, and you'll accomplish more of what you want to do with less effort and stress. Letting science and the principles of this cyclical program be your guide, you will decrease multitasking, increase your focus on the projects you care most about, and take more restorative breaks, and the payoff will be keeping end-of-day exhaustion at bay, a more positive mood, and fired-up creativity. And what about that natural pattern of creation—initiation, growth, completion, and rest—detailed in chapter 2? You will realize you have this same pattern reflected in your hormonal cycle. By nurturing each of these phases, you will unlock the creative matrix within. I'm not necessarily referring to the traditional sense of creativity—dancing, playing piano, or jewelry making—but rather the sense that you can bring to life the big ideas, projects, and plans you dream about. You'll be able to optimize your creative output according to the predictable nature of your cyclical patterns (when your hormones are balanced). Following this rhythm will be so deeply nourishing, you will never fall into an energy hole and will no longer feel disconnected from your creative force. For me, a woman who had made a conscious decision to disconnect from my inner creativity at a young age, cycle syncing opened the door to tap into that creative matrix to bring more of what I wanted into my life. Valuing my creative process over mere productivity ended up making me more productive and less stressed!

Choosing to Feel Good

I used to be someone who struggled with decision-making. I would be stuck in my head, arguing back and forth, generating pros and cons lists, and never getting anywhere. I would drive myself and my friends crazy asking for their thoughts. I'm sure you've had conversations like this where you don't get anywhere, instead agonizing over any decision—whether it's staying in a relationship or buying a new pair of shoes. I really struggled with knowing *how* to know what felt right for me, and it wasn't until I really committed to the Cycle Syncing Method™ that I was able to engage a different process to make decisions.

I now had the opportunity, for example, to reconsider attending an event. Every time I thought about going to this event, I had opposing thoughts about what I might miss out on by not going, and what I might not be able to get done on my own agenda if I went. So I checked in with my body and how it felt while envisioning the activity. The whole process of traveling to and attending this event felt tight and stressful in my body. Then when I leaned in to feeling my body doing the things on my project list for that same time period, I felt centered and grounded. When I do this process of asking my body, I'm always reminded that my thoughts and emotions will always be multifold, but my body holds a clarity and certainty that allows me to make a decision with confidence.

Adding in the practice of syncing with my cycle, I see that I'm given opportunities to build confidence in putting my preferences first. When I allow myself to do less each month in my menstrual phase, for example, I'm experiencing more moments of feeling grounded and good in my body. Then I can reference this feeling when I'm making decisions in general. I know what being aligned feels like, versus the sensations of confusion, stress, and anxiety that are my body's ways of letting me know when I'm out of alignment with my optimal flow. This practice keeps me coming back into my body and feeling safe about being my own reference point for decisions. It's hugely freeing.

I'm only now appreciating how much being disconnected from my cycle and my body has created so much anxiety throughout my life. I remember feeling a low level of anxiousness as a teen about homework, deadlines, and social situations. My hormonal imbalances during that time added to it as well. Now, almost two decades into cycle syncing, I find that I'm more at ease with things and I am able to navigate occasional anxiety better. For example, if I wake and feel a flood of stress, I'll check in about why—asking myself about whether I'm getting enough sleep, where I am in my cycle, and what's happening in my life in general. I'll shift my self-care to prioritize helping myself address the anxious energy with food and exercise that are phase-specific.

I am committed to being at ease and choosing to feel good. And it is, for me, a personal revolution. I can only imagine that if we all as women committed to choosing to feel good what kind of cultural shifts could be created. We can do more of creating ease and balance in the world the more we practice it internally for ourselves. Even though it is a small thing to choose feeling good, to take a walk, to do what's aligned for us in our cycles, the ripple effect from this on our families and communities would be powerful.

Managing Your Creative Process According to Your Cycle

Women can—and do—create differently depending on which gifts are brought forward by each phase of our cycle. As those strengths fluctuate from week to week, you don't have to feel like a hormonal victim, as if you're being hit unexpectedly by waves that toss you around and threaten to pull you under. By tapping into your hormonal shifts, you can become a steady, predictable powerhouse, and surf those waves for greater performance with less effort and more satisfaction. Once you understand how your hormones influence your strengths throughout the month, it becomes very simple to leverage that knowledge for more successful project planning and performance.

Research from 2017 dispels the myth that our cycle has a negative effect on our cognitive function at certain times of the month. You can do anything at any time during your cycle, but just because you *can* do it doesn't mean you *ought* to do it. Going with your own FLO is where you start to experience your peak state more often.

When we match our activities with our unique skill sets during each of the four phases of our cycle—instead of expending all our energy trying to force ourselves to focus on similar tasks day in and day out—we can accomplish more of what we truly want to be doing and prioritize what's right for our bodies with less effort. All of a sudden we shift from feeling like we don't ever have enough time, to feeling like we have plenty of time to do all that we want and need to do. We have more space to get things done. We can perform at our highest levels and feel more energized at the end of the day.

This same four-step creative matrix plays out in all the projects we undertake and in our business cycles. Let's say you need to update your website. You'll start with a brainstorming session (initiation), then produce all the copy and images you'll need (growth), then input all the new material and changes (completion), then sit back and evaluate any final tweaks that could be made (rest). Whichever phase of the project you're in, you can bring forth the best of your cyclical phase at the moment. The same goes for business cycles. For example, in my own business, sometimes we are in what I would call an ovulatory phase. Our main objective would be spreading the word about what we do through marketing. At other times, we're in more of a luteal phase, tackling behind-the-scenes tasks such as updating our systems. Although these tasks are more luteal in nature, I can bring the strengths of my follicular, ovulatory, luteal, and menstrual phases to the projects at different times.

The Cycle Syncing Method™: Creative FLO

Phase	Duration	What's Happening Hormonally	Strengths	Activities to Schedule
Follicular PREPARE	7–10 days	Estrogen is on the rise.	Creativity	Dream big, brainstorm, initiate, prepare, and plan. Research, be curious, explore, interview people, take courses, gather resources, and chart your strategy. Set your intentions for the week, month, or year ahead. Clarify your vision and get new projects off the ground. Fill in your planner with what you want to accomplish in the coming weeks.
Ovulatory OPEN UP	3–4 days	Estrogen is at its highest point.	Communication and collaboration	Socialize, pitch ideas, and be seen. Talk about your plans, collaborate with others on projects, schedule dates and meetings, go to lunch with girlfriends, host a party, and connect with others. Have important conversations.

Phase	Duration	What's Happening Hormonally	Strengths	Activities to Schedule
Luteal WORK	10–14 days	Progesterone is at its highest point.	Completion, nurturing, tending	This is your get-it-done phase! Don't procrastinate. Get organized. Accomplish the projects and goals you planned during your follicular phase. Feel good about wrapping things up. Attend to your home, finances, and administrative tasks. Do your deep work. Celebrate how powerful you are.
Menstrual REST	3–7 days	All of your hormones are at a low point.	Evaluation and intuition	Relax and reflect on the past month. Be kind with yourself as you review all the good things you've accomplished, and note any areas of your life that feel less than optimal or that need attention. It's especially important to trust your instincts during this phase. Is your gut telling you something? Spend time journaling, reviewing, and noting what you might need to let go of and what you might need to shift in the coming month. Use this as a starting point for setting intentions during your next follicular phase.

Plan-Her: A Cyclical Approach to Managing Your Energy

After I latched on to the concept of scheduling in accordance with the natural rhythm of my hormones, I began teaching a right-timing / energy management program to women in corporations. I present them with a female-centered planning tool (see page 172) to help them get in the FLO on a personal level and on a team basis in the workplace. As someone who has tried almost every time management system possible, I created one that adopts the best practices from each of them and aligns with your female biology so you can be productive in a healthy, balanced, and sustainable way. This planner is special because it's not just a place to write your to-do list, but a tool to help you incorporate your body, mind, energy, and mood into the projects of your day, week, and month. The planner not only ensures that you prevent burnout and energy leaks but also ensures that you have more time to focus on the things that really matter to you, so you can feel more fulfilled and centered each day regardless of what life throws at you. Of course, I think the planner I've created is ideal for scheduling in a way that maximizes our cyclical nature, but you can always create your own planner using these same principles. The Daily FLO Planner I created is organized into the following sections:

Current phase: Keep track of the phase of the cycle you're in so you ensure you curate the right projects each phase and stay connected to your body.

Monthly theme: Make note of which monthly theme you're focusing on. Choose monthly themes based on the natural seasonal cycles of the year. I use these themes as a way to ensure I'm touching all the most important aspects of my life throughout the year. For example, March is a cleansing and detoxing month for me. This theme might translate into a weekend of cleaning out my closets or switching out my winter wardrobe for my spring and summer clothes. This way, I don't get to May 1 and think, "Oh, no! It's already spring, and I still haven't put my winter coats away." You can experiment with your own monthly themes and you can follow along with our monthly themes in the Cycle Syncing Membership.

Tasks or work focus: In this section, you can plan out what you're doing and when. Be sure to note the focus of the phase as a whole, whether it's creativity, communication, completion, or evaluation. Outline your top three points of focus for the day. What is really essential for you to accomplish today? How does it all fit into the routine of your day? Use morning, afternoon, and evening sections to write out a plan for the day in as much detail as possible.

Food plan: This section helps you organize your meal plan throughout the day with phase-specific recipes.

Self-care focus: In this section, you can keep track of specific ways to nurture yourself, based on your current cycle phase combined with what want or need to accomplish on this day.

Energy check-in: Here you'll assess how you're feeling with your energy, mood, sleep, and any symptoms. Do you feel energized, or do you feel drained by the end of the day? This is such an important question to ask yourself each and every day. If you consistently feel zonked, it's a big red flag that you're probably overstressing your adrenals and taxing your system.

End-of-day reflections: Jot down anything that helps you check in with yourself. Ask yourself how you feel about how your day went. How did you do with your cyclical planning? What worked for you? Many of the women I see really love this part of the planner because it lets them dedicate some space and time to their emotional self. Here you can pump yourself up with some positive reinforcement. These are some examples of what women jot down in this section:

- *"It feels so good to give myself permission to do the things that are right for me when I need to do them."*
- *"I took some 'me' time today, and the world didn't fall apart like I thought it would."*
- *"I'm not gaining weight even though I didn't do a hardcore workout."*
- *"Wow! I haven't had PMS all week. This is really making me feel better!"*
- *"I'm feeling so energized!"*

These statements are in stark contrast to the way we typically talk to ourselves. Think about it. Prior to understanding your body's need for a cyclical lifestyle, you had to motivate yourself through fear, guilt, and anxiety. I remember reading words of singer and poet Vanessa Daou that stopped me in my tracks: "There's no greater beating than that of the fine lashing of woman's tongue upon her own mind." When I read this, it hit me right between the ovaries. It called out my own masochistic behavior in response to trying to be the same day in and day out. We tend to berate ourselves at the end of every day with negative thoughts like these:

- *"I didn't push myself hard enough at the gym today. I suck."*
- *"I didn't get enough done today. I'm such a slacker."*
- *"I ate super unhealthy foods today. I have no willpower."*

As a recovering perfectionist, I used to be a big offender in this category. To this day, there are still times when I have to remind myself to shift my mindset from this negative space to one of compassion and gratitude. One of the most beautiful things I notice when women begin syncing with their cycle is their ability to stop this emotional self-abuse and start opening their hearts to self-love.

Here are some additional tips to make your planner work best for you.

Red-flag demands on your time and energy: Each day, ask yourself, "Are there demands on my time that are out of sync with my cycle?" For example, if you're on a tight deadline at work and have so much to do, but your body is in the menstrual phase and needs more down time, make a note of this misalignment, because these work demands are not ideal for this phase of your cycle. In this case, add in an extra piece of self-care to ensure you're balancing out your body's needs and giving it the nourishment it requires so that you don't burn out. I realize we don't live in a perfect world where everybody and everything around us can sync to our personal hormonal cycle. (Wouldn't that be nice, though?) But we still don't have to abandon ourselves. When this happens to me—and as a busy entrepreneur, wife, and mother, you can bet it happens more frequently than I would like—I immediately get strategic. If possible, I move work demands to a different phase. But if something can't be shifted or delayed due to a deadline or other obligation, I come up with a plan to upgrade my self-care on that day or in the days leading up to that date to offset or compensate for the extra energy requirement.

Schedule downtime: Remember, right-timing relies on the natural ebb and flow of your hormones and energy levels. Time for rest and relaxation is required to balance the periods of activity. Block out R&R time in your planner just as if you were scheduling an appointment with a client. When that time is blocked out in your schedule, you're more likely to follow through, and you've given it equal importance with the other items on the day's to-do list.

Give yourself some wiggle room: Remember that your cycle phases are not distinct. They transition gradually from one to the next, so it will never work out perfectly that each week of the month starts and ends exactly with your cycle phase. This is a good thing! It means you don't have to be "perfect" or "precise" throughout this process. Instead, you can feel your way into your schedule and flow with your own energy and phase awareness. You know your body best. The idea is that the more you practice living cyclically, the more in tune you'll get, the more you'll learn to trust your body, and the more your life will flow.

Less Doing, More Being

When I returned from my trip to India, my entire perception of success and happiness had changed. I no longer felt tethered to the notion that doing more is better, or the belief that if I had a particular thing, then I'd be happy. And it became painfully obvious that the idea of trying to make it to the top by doing *more! more! more!* even if it was hurting my health no longer made any sense at all. For example, while I was working on this book, I was invited to speak at several local events by some friends and colleagues. Our cultural conditioning tells us we should just say yes—women are taught

The Cycle Syncing Method™: Daily FLO

Date: _____   Phase of Cycle: _____

Main Tasks to Focus On:

1 _____   2 _____   3 _____

Plan for the Day:

Morning _____
_____
_____
_____
_____

Afternoon _____
_____
_____
_____
_____

Evening _____
_____
_____
_____

**Are there demands on your time
that are out of sync with your cycle?***   YES | NO

*If you mark yes, pay attention to starred notes
in the next section.

End of Day . . . Energy Check-In:

Energy?   ●————●————●   Mood & Symptoms? _____
           0   5   10   _____

Sleep?   < 8 hrs | 8 hrs | > 8 hrs   _____

○ Reminder to set up tomorrow's plan   _____

POWR Phase: Prepare / Open Up / Work / Rest

Current Creation Cycle: Initiating / Collaborating / Producing / Evaluating

Theme of the Month: _____

Food Plan:

*If you marked yes, remember to take your supplements!

Breakfast

_____
_____
_____

Snacks

_____
_____
_____

Lunch

_____
_____
_____

Beverages

_____
_____
_____

Dinner

_____
_____
_____

Supplements

_____
_____
_____

Self-Care Focus of the Day (Pick at least one!):

*If you marked yes, please add one extra piece of self-care today!

◯ Movement

◯ Self Pleasure

◯ Social Time

◯ Home Spa (Facial, Manicure, etc.)

◯ Sleep

◯ Other: _____

Reflections:

_____
_____
_____
_____
_____

to be people pleasers—but I knew that I needed to conserve my energy so I could be optimally creative and focused on writing. So I said no and explained why. And you know what? No one was upset. But I was proud of myself. This represented success to me—advocating on my own behalf and looking out for myself. I relish these little wins just as much as the big projects at work.

When you say goodbye to the productivity treadmill patterned after the 24-hour clock and hello to a paradigm based on the dual clock that includes your female biological rhythms, you open the doors to happy hormones, healthier biological systems, and the path to more sustainable success and creativity in your personal life and at work. What is work anyway? Essentially, it's creating something from nothing. Work starts with an idea of how to fill that void. Think of work—whether it's in your personal or professional life—as the process of bringing those ideas to life. We create projects. We develop presentations. We launch new products. Women are ideally wired to create out of a blank space. A fertile void exists within the womb, and from this empty space springs new life. In nature, all living things adhere to that seed-growth-bloom-rest cycle that fascinated me so much in my first biology class. Your body is attuned to create in this same pattern. You have brainstorming sessions to plant the seeds of a new idea. You nurture that concept as it sprouts. You launch it and make it grow. You wrap it up and evaluate its performance before moving on to the next cycle of creation.

Similarly, all living things go through periods of activity and rest, expansion and retraction. Think of the growth pattern of a field. Farmers understand that they need to rotate their crops, allowing the harvested soil to rest and replenish itself, or it will not produce. We need to follow these same patterns to optimize our hormones and biological systems so we can reach our greatest potential. I love the way Julia Cameron, the bestselling author of *The Artist's Way*, writes about the importance of "fallow" time being nonnegotiable for the creative process. Our current perpetual productivity model, when applied to farming—demanding continuous harvest and maximum output—relies on toxic biohacking, with harmful fertilizers, pesticides, and GMO seeds. Perpetual productivity isn't sustainable, and it's damaging our environment and making us sick.

These same patterns hold true for our bodies. If you're constantly "doing," you aren't giving your brain and body the rest they need to restore your creative juices. We need to have fallow days to reenergize our minds, bodies, and creativity. Instead of expecting to add ever more on to your overwhelming to-do list every day, and relying on artificial energy boosters, take time to connect to your body and get grounded. Look for inspiration. Take a walk in nature. Watch your dog or cat playing. Dance to your favorite song. Stretch your body. Give your brain and body time to explore possibilities you never imagined. In this way, you refresh your hormones and biological systems rather than draining them so you can feel more energetic and be on top of your game.

TAKE THE EGG APPROACH

Once a month, when a mature egg is released by your ovaries, it waits calmly in the fallopian tube for fertilization. The egg doesn't chase the sperm; it doesn't need to. The chemicals it radiates make it so irresistibly attractive, the sperm go into a wild frenzy trying to reach it. Millions of sperm swim upstream on their quest to find the alluring egg. Most will get lost along the way, but a few hundred of them will make it to the gorgeous orb, with only one lucky swimmer being selected by the egg and earning the honor of fertilizing her. It's a great analogy for us to learn from. We don't always have to chase. If we position ourselves properly like the egg, more things can flow to us. This applies to the creative process. Both pushing and receiving are essential to the success of the creative process. And if conditions are not optimal for fertilization, the egg passes via the period, and another cycle and opportunity can be expected. You don't have to compensate for your cyclical way of being: focus on showing up fully energized, trust the timing of your body, and choose to feel good.

WHAT ABOUT SYNCING WITH THE LUNAR CYCLE?

My social media feeds are filled with women sharing their new moon rituals and asking if they should be bleeding during the new moon or the full moon. So many women feel a pull to tap into the goddess culture by syncing their cycle with the lunar phases. This is a completely natural desire considering that the light our eyes were designed to take in—moonlight and sunlight—affects our pineal and pituitary glands, which stimulates our circadian rhythms and hormone production. It's reasonable to imagine that in the past, many women who lived in communities might all bleed at the same time during the new moon and follow the rhythm of the lunar cycle because they were all exposed to the same light—waking with the sun in the morning, sleeping when the sun went down, and being exposed to powerful and changing moonlight at night. This is the reason fertility festivals were held on the full moon; that's when a woman was most likely ovulating. People observed the connection between the cycles of the earth, the moon, and women's bodies, and created rituals that worked in harmony with them. In our modern world, however, we live in a light-polluted environment with perpetual brightness. Many of us can't even see the moon at night. And we have all this blue light from our tech devices further disrupting our circadian rhythms. We're so detached from the lunar-based cycles of our female ancestors, we have to gradually work our way back to the way nature intended our bodies to work. The first step is to restore your own menstrual rhythm by syncing with your cycle. Then start reducing your exposure to blue light and make it a practice to go out and see the moon and stars at night.

This can work even if you live in a big city. I live in a city and can manage to do it if I'm diligent. At first my cycle would rarely sync with the lunar phases, but then I moved to a different apartment where I can see the moon transiting every night. And it has deeply affected my cycle. More often, I'll ovulate on the full moon and bleed on the new moon. But you don't have to move to get in tune with the moon.

I also keep a lunar calendar where I can see it, and I do my best to use blue-light blockers to minimize circadian disruption. I think of syncing with the lunar phases as a bonus that I enjoy, but it definitely isn't a requirement for optimal biological functioning. If your phases aren't following the lunar cycle, don't let this stress you out. Take advantage of all the benefits of syncing to your own cycle and then explore syncing with the lunar cycles if that's something you would like to experience. And take note that if you are not cycling for any reason—if you're postmenopausal, if cancer treatment has eliminated your period, or if you're transgender, for example—you can use the lunar patterns to remain connected to a cyclical energy.

After reading this chapter, you now know that you're uniquely wired to create in a way that reflects your inner hormonal patterns and that following a rhythm will heighten your efficiency and productivity, and give you greater access to your creativity. You may even have intuitively felt this way at times without having anyone define it or put a frame around it. And you may have recognized yourself within the pages of this chapter and thought, "Yes! This is my reality." Even so, you may still be hesitant to dive in to this new way of scheduling your energy and your life. It might seem risky, as if you'll be swimming against the tide. Can you really succeed in today's perpetual productivity culture if you're operating on a cyclical pattern? The answer is yes! You simply need to be willing to experiment with this female-centered way of living, so you can see for yourself how good it feels. When you give it a chance, it will allow your body to sustainably accompany your imagination on the ride toward creating a life you love.

In the FLO Four-Week Quick-Start Plan

- Determine which phase you're in.
- Decide if you'll start with food or workouts.

- Week 1: For the phase you're in, sync either just your food or just your workouts.
- Week 2: For your next phase, sync both your food and your workouts.
- Week 3: For the third phase, while maintaining the food and workout elements, look at your schedule and task list and see what activities are in sync with that phase, note how many are out of sync, and make some decisions about what can stay and what should get moved to another phase.
- Week 4: Take out your daily planner, look at the next four phases, and plan your ideal schedule for the next whole cycle.

How to Get in the FLO When Your Hormones Are Out of Balance

When women take care of their health,
they become their own best friend.
—MAYA ANGELOU

When you understand the science behind it, syncing with your cycle makes so much sense. Of course you want to balance your hormones so you can get rid of cramps, bloating, and heavy periods, or more serious conditions like endometriosis or PCOS. But that's just the starting point. When your hormones function optimally, they become a force that enhances every biological system in your body—boosting your moods, creativity, energy, and so much more. When you feel great, your productivity, relationships, and ability to be a great mom all improve. Feeling good helps you achieve your life goals without all the suffering. Learning about all these advantages may make you want to jump right in to syncing with your cycle. But what if your period doesn't arrive like clockwork every month? What if it's irregular, or even MIA, some months? What if you're suffering from hormone hell? How do you start syncing with your cycle when you don't even know what phase you're in? I've got you. This section is dedicated to all you women who are dealing with hormonal issues, the same way I was when I was diagnosed with PCOS. And it shows you that when you have symptoms, doing nothing is *not* an option. You can and must hack your symptoms to promote healing. This Biohacking Tool Kit will show you how to do it. It will help you understand why you're having the symptoms you're experiencing, what the research shows about what works to alleviate them naturally, and how to biohack your way back into balance quickly now or whenever you might find yourself out of optimal hormonal flow. If you need to dive deeper for your specific condition, I've added individual biohacking guides that you can download whenever you need.

WHAT IF I DON'T HAVE HORMONAL ISSUES?

If you don't have any serious hormonal issues, feel free to skim this chapter or go straight to the sections that interest you. For example, if you're on the pill or you're a mom with a preteen or teenage daughter and are considering putting her on oral contraceptives for period problems, I highly encourage you to check out the section on hormonal birth control. If you have PCOS, fibroids, endometriosis, heavy painful periods, missing periods, or severe PMS, then read on.

I first want to say that I truly understand your frustration! When I was dealing with my PCOS issues, I was always looking for spot treatments for my acne, diets to try to lose the weight I'd gained, and some medication that would regulate my period. I went to one doctor for my skin, another to help me with my weight, and yet another to deal with my missing period. You've probably done the same thing in trying to eliminate your cramps, mood swings, or acne. The medical industry generally takes the same symptom-focused approach to our period problems, offering over-the-counter pain relievers, hormonal contraceptives, antidepressants, or surgical interventions to treat individual symptoms. But this way of thinking about how to treat our hormones needs updating with a more functional medicine–based approach.

Many treatments for individual symptoms have significant side effects. Several over-the-counter pain relievers contain caffeine, which isn't ideal for women for all the reasons you read about in chapter 4, or affect the liver, further compromising estrogen metabolism. Other medications impact your hormonal system in negative ways. And when these medications fail to do the job, what comes next may be prolonged suffering or surgery. Historically, we have been given two options: (1) do nothing and suffer, or (2) utilize treatments that don't correct what's causing the problem and that have serious side effects. There has to be a better way that enhances our biochemical and biological nature. Rest assured, there is a solution. It lies in acknowledging the fact that all of our seemingly disparate hormonal symptoms all stem from the same root cause: disrupted endocrine function.

This is one of the most exciting findings in my research. When I first put together the FLO protocol, described in *WomanCode*, I was excited to discover that most hormonal symptoms stem from the same root causes. In nature, as explained by Einstein and Mandelbrot, things are often elegant and straightforward despite seeming complex. Women's menstrual disturbances may appear to be complex, but they mostly all come down to the ways in which the endocrine system has been interrupted. The FLO protocol I created is designed to address the underlying endocrine dysfunction that results in all those symptoms. If you have a diagnosed menstrual issue, there are three critical steps in the FLO protocol that must come *before* you start syncing with your cycle:

1. Stabilize your blood sugar.
2. Nurture your adrenals.
3. Support the organs of elimination.

Addressing these in this order is the key to restoring balance to your endocrine system. Stabilizing your blood sugar is critical because unstable blood sugar wreaks havoc on your hormonal health. Your brain and body need glucose to function, but many of us consume too much refined sugar, which disrupts our endocrine function. Eating carbohydrates triggers the body's insulin response, but too much glucose and too much insulin send your blood sugar levels soaring, followed by a big crash. The spikes disrupt ovulation, reducing the production of progesterone, and can lead to estrogen dominance, which you now know is behind many common period problems. Nurturing your adrenals helps to balance cortisol levels—another key hormone that, out of balance, can disrupt your cycle—and helps protect your body against stress. And supporting the body's pathways of elimination—the skin, liver, large intestine, and lymphatic system—helps your body eliminate excess estrogen.

Because we're left in the dark about how our bodies work, we don't see the interconnectedness of each symptom, and we believe that every period problem requires some individualized, targeted treatment. That is not the case. I want you to stop thinking of your period problems as a collection of random symptoms that you need to address one by one, and start thinking of them as signs of a systemic endocrine imbalance. When you see things this way, the path to hormonal health becomes clearer. It becomes obvious that taking a pill without changing anything else can never heal your hormones. Remember, your endocrine system is made up of several glands and organs. How can one medication address your thyroid, hypothalamus, adrenals, ovaries, and so on? It's not logical. There's only one way to address such a complex, interconnected system within the body, and that's by supporting your endocrine system as a whole. In this section, you'll discover the cleanup work you need to do to balance your hormones before you can begin syncing with your cycle.

Step 1: Check Your Fifth Vital Sign—
A Personalized, Monthly Hormone Test

I'm all for high-tech self-optimization trackers. In addition, the body has so much biofeedback available to provide you with real-time health information if you know how to evaluate it. Your period is an excellent hormonal self-evaluation tool. It's like getting lab work every month that gives you an immediate heads-up about any hormonal imbalances. The key to taking advantage of what your period is trying to tell you? You've got to look. Yes, before you double-wrap that tampon or pad in toilet paper and toss it in the trash, give it a good once-over. Getting familiar with your flow can provide invaluable clues to your overall health. As I mentioned earlier, your period health is so critical a vital sign as temperature and blood pressure that the American College of Obstetricians and Gynecologists have decreed it a fifth vital sign. Think of it as your own personal monthly hormonal checkup.

After working with thousands of women, I've identified five period types, which I call V-Sign™ Types. Check the descriptions that follow to find your type, and take the quick assessment at www.FLOliving.com/what-is-your -v-sign to learn more about what you need to do to get back on track. Whatever type you are, remember that changing your diet and supplements can modify a troublesome period within a cycle or two.

Red V-Sign Type: If you see cranberry or cherry red when you change your tampon or pad and the blood is clot-free, it's an indication that your hormone levels are balanced. Celebrate your good hormonal health this cycle!

Purple V-Sign Type: When you look at your period blood, is it a deep purple-blue color with clots and clumps? This is a sign that your estrogen levels are too high in proportion to progesterone, which can cause the uterine lining to be thicker than normal. This results in heavier periods and more severe PMS symptoms, including stronger cramps, bigger mood swings, and depression. Excess estrogen can lead to common period problems, such as fibroids, cysts, or endometriosis. When high estrogen levels remain unchecked, it can increase the risk of certain medical conditions, including thyroid dysfunction and breast or ovarian cancer.

Brown V-Sign Type: Without enough progesterone, the uterus doesn't shed completely, and the leftover lining oxidizes and turns brown. If you're trying to conceive, low progesterone makes it harder to maintain a pregnancy during the first trimester. Does your period blood resemble prune juice? Seeing a brownish color on Day 1 or on the last couple days of your period indicates your progesterone levels may be too low, which increases your chances of longer cycles or skipping cycles. Women with this type of bleeding may experience mood swings, anxiety, depression, trouble concentrating, sleep disturbances, headaches or migraines, and low libido.

If you're trying to conceive, be aware that low progesterone makes it harder to carry a pregnancy through the first trimester. Many of the women I see with low progesterone also experience hot flashes and other symptoms usually associated with perimenopause, even if they're still in their twenties or early thirties. Over time, your uterine lining may build up abnormally, leading to a condition called endometrial hyperplasia, which can lead to uterine cancer in some cases.

Pink V-Sign Type: If your blood is pale pink in color on the first and last few days of your period, it's a sign that your estrogen levels are too low. When your body doesn't pump out enough of this hormone, your uterine lining doesn't build up the way it should with each cycle. Shorter periods are a common side effect of low estrogen levels. Insufficient estrogen can also put you on the fast track to aging and is associated with osteoporosis and heart issues later in life. Low estrogen is one of the hallmarks of perimenopause and menopause and is associated with loss of skin elasticity, vaginal dryness, low sex drive, hair thinning, anxiety and depression, and difficulty conceiving. Younger women with low estrogen levels may experience these same symptoms even if they are years away from perimenopause.

Missing/Irregular V-Sign Type: Is your period erratic and unpredictable? Is it a toss-up if you'll see purple, brown, pink, or red blood when it finally does show up? These are signs that something is off-kilter. If you go months without getting your period, it's a major red flag that your hormones are out of whack. Do you get your period more than once every month? Does it only last one or two days? Do you have spotting between periods? If so, your period is too short, which can be caused by low estrogen levels or thyroid dysfunction. If you have a short cycle, it's a good idea to

BIOHACKING TOOL KIT   PART 1

have your gynecologist check your hormone levels. On the flip side, if you go more than thirty-five days between periods, your cycle is too long. This may be an indicator that your body isn't producing adequate amounts of FSH and LH to trigger ovulation, or that progesterone levels are too low to prompt the uterus to shed its lining. Long cycles may also be due to adrenal or pituitary issues, so be sure to make an appointment with your health care provider to get to the root cause. If your cycle goes MIA for more than sixty days, it could be due to one or more of the issues described above. Another reason your period may have gone on vacation is you may not have enough body fat for a healthy cycle. A period that's gone missing can be a sign of medical conditions, such as PCOS, amenorrhea, or adrenal hyperplasia, so don't hesitate to see your doctor for a diagnosis. If your cycle gets shorter or longer or becomes unpredictable, it may also be a sign that you're entering perimenopause, depending on your age. Check in with your gynecologist for a hormone workup.

PERIODS: WHAT IS "NORMAL," ANYWAY?

Cycle length: Your cycle should last twenty-eight to thirty-two days—anywhere in between is fine as long as it is regular and consistent *for you*.

Color: Your bleed should be the color of deep red cranberry juice or dark cherry juice from start to finish.

Flow length: Ideally, your period should last four to seven days.

Flow consistency: You should have a strong flow without any clots, and it shouldn't be inconveniently heavy or have you feeling like you're bleeding through menstrual care products every hour.

Physical sensations: You should be able to feel your uterus in action with some slight sensations or warm feelings, but you shouldn't experience any kind of pain that would make you reach for drugs or hot water bottles.

Analyze Your Results

After you've completed your personal audit, take stock of your situation. If you only have mild or even severe PMS—bloating, acne, cramps—but everything else with your period is relatively normal, go ahead and start syncing with your cycle; doing so will help alleviate those symptoms. If, however, your period is missing or you have been diagnosed with a menstrual condition like PCOS or endometriosis, then you need to do a little more groundwork by following the steps in the rest of this chapter. If you're postpartum or breastfeeding and are wondering if you can sync with your second clock, see chapter 9 for specifics on these particular life stages.

Step 2: Adopt a Biohacking Mindset

"Everybody gets cramps." "PMS is normal." "You're destined to suffer from your period." As you now know, these menstrual myths are BS. The biggest falsehood associated with your monthly cycle is that once you have period problems, you're stuck with them. This particular myth, which is so deeply ingrained in our society, is fundamentally disempowering and perpetuates a course of inaction when it comes to your hormonal health. This myth makes your cycle seem so mysterious, so unpredictable, and so unmanageable that there is nothing you can do about your period problems. So you do nothing. And guess what? Your period problems get worse, so you assume the myths were correct. So not only do you feel that you have to continue suffering from your monthly woes, but you also put your biological systems at risk, which can lead to serious long-term health issues. In addition, you don't get to take advantage of any of the magic that happens when your hormones are balanced and you're in sync with your cycle. You miss out on the revved-up energy, happier moods, and cognitive clarity that come with a finely tuned cyclical life.

It doesn't have to be this way. You don't have to suffer with PMS, PCOS, uterine fibroids, endometriosis, or any other hormonal issue for the rest of your life. Natalia had been dealing with endometriosis for five years. There were times the pain was so intense she couldn't even walk. She tried birth control pills as suggested by her doctor, but they didn't help. When she got off the pill and started supporting her hormonal health with foods and supplements and eventually by syncing with her cycle, things changed. After six months, her endometriosis pains vanished almost completely—once in a while when she's ovulating she feels some minor cramping, which she rates as a one or two on a scale of one to ten. She says 95 percent of the time she's acne-free, bloating-free, PMS-free, refreshed, and energized. And when she does feel these symptoms, even a little bit, she immediately knows what caused them and can take action to address them. That's the beauty of the Cycle Syncing Method™. As you've seen, it can keep symptoms in remission. But it's up to you to be your own hormonal advocate. I learned this lesson the hard way. When I first got my PCOS diagnosis, I couldn't believe that medicine had nothing to cure my condition. But that was the push I needed to become the Biohacker-in-Chief of my own body. Now it's your turn.

Step 3: Remove Endocrine Disruptors

It's not easy these days for hormones. Our modern environment is filled with chemicals, pesticides, pharmaceuticals, and artificial lighting that make it hard to keep our hormones happy and humming. On a daily basis, we're exposed to hundreds of chemicals found in the air, water, soil, food, and consumer products that interfere with the production, secretion, transport, metabolism, binding action, or elimination of the body's natural hormones. These endocrine disruptors often mimic naturally occurring hormones—including estrogen, thyroid, and androgens—which confuses the biological endocrine system and can lead to imbalances. Disruptors may bind to receptors within cells, which prevents the natural hormones from being able to do so, and effectively interrupts the typical messaging and

BIOHACKING TOOL KIT   PART 1

signaling that is supposed to occur between the hormone and its intended destination. These dirty disruptors can also trip up the way the liver metabolizes and eliminates hormones. Ultimately, these disruptors can wreak havoc with our hormones and negatively impact our biological systems, setting us up for physical and mental health issues.

Sadly, these infiltrators are everywhere. You come in contact with them in household cleaners, skincare products, cosmetics, personal care products, pharmaceuticals, plastics, and food. An independent research group, Women's Voices for the Earth, discovered that twenty of the most popular household cleaning products contain reproductive toxins, such as toluene and phthalates, as well as a hormone-disrupting synthetic musk, among other toxins. Research shows many of these toxins are bio-accumulative and can disrupt hormonal balance.

Exposure to endocrine disruptors has been linked to a laundry list of conditions, including estrogen dominance, early puberty, and infertility, as well as increased risk for breast and thyroid cancers. With so many environmental toxins affecting our endocrine system, we can't be passive and expect our hormonal cycle to sing in harmony. And we can't count on our government to do it for us. The European Union has banned more than 1,300 chemicals from being used in cosmetics, according to the Campaign for Safe Cosmetics. How many has the US banned? About thirty, says Credo Beauty, which has created a Dirty List of ingredients linked to health or environmental issues. It's up to us to take charge of our own health.

Now it's time to take stock of your exposure to potential disruptors. Check any of the following that apply to you:

1. Do you eat nonorganic foods?
2. Do you eat meat that isn't antibiotic-free and hormone-free, or do you eat farmed fish?
3. Do you drink water from plastic bottles?
4. Do you use chemical-laden household cleaning products and detergents?
5. Do you use drugstore cosmetics and skincare products?

6. Do you use hair care products that aren't all natural?

7. Do you use standard nail polish?

If you checked several of these questions, you could be stacking the deck against your hormones. Fortunately, positive changes can happen quickly. According to a study in a 2014 issue of *Environmental Research*, switching your diet from conventionally produced foods to organic foods reduces urinary output of pesticides by nearly 90 percent—*in just seven days!* This reveals how quickly you can begin to turn things around if you make a concerted effort to eat in a way that supports your hormones.

Step 4: Use Food to Fight Your Symptoms

Whether you have a serious or mild menstrual condition, the foods you eat can minimize your symptoms and help balance your hormones. If you have any of the following conditions or symptoms, take strength in knowing that you can eat your way to improving these conditions. Here are the best and worst foods for your condition.

Fibroids

Have you been told you have uterine fibroids? Research shows that most women will develop these benign tumors in their lifetime. These noncancerous growths develop in the wall of the uterus and can be as small as a pea or so large that the fibroid makes the uterus swell as if you were six or seven months pregnant. Some women have fibroids but aren't aware of them because the women have no symptoms. Other women, however, get hit with a storm of symptoms, including heavy bleeding, periods that last more than seven days, painful periods, spotting between periods, pain during intercourse, lower back pain, frequent urination, and reproductive problems. The medical community has yet to identify what causes some women to develop fibroids, but researchers point to hormones as a factor. Fibroids tend to grow when levels of estrogen are high. They usually stop growing and shrink in size after menopause, when estrogen levels typically decrease. Because of this link to estrogen, it's important to support your body so it can effectively flush out any excess estrogen.

FLO-approved biohack: Eat more flaxseeds. They act as a natural type of selective estrogen receptor modulators (SERMs), substances that impact estrogen's effect in the body. SERMs may block estrogen sensitivity in the uterus, and some studies have found them to be beneficial for women with fibroids. These tasty seeds are also high in fiber, omega-3 fatty acids, and lignans, which help flush excess estrogen out of the body and prevent absorption of excess estrogen. Add *unprocessed*, organic fermented soy in the form of tempeh and miso to your diet for its anti-estrogenic effect on the uterus. Beans—especially kidney beans, lentils, and mung beans—provide healthy fiber and protein. And because they have a low glycemic index, beans can reduce inflammation, which researchers are increasingly looking at as another factor that can cause fibroid growth. High-fiber whole grains, such as oats and brown rice, also crank up how quickly your body processes and eliminates excess estrogen. Eat pears and apples, which contain a flavonoid named phloretin that inhibits tumor growth.

Worst foods for fibroids: Avoid all processed soy products, such as soy cheese, soy meat, and other meat and dairy replacements. Skip processed red meats, and ditch white starchy foods, including bread, pasta, and noodles. It's also best to eliminate alcohol and caffeine, which can overtax your liver and reduce its ability to clear excess estrogen from the body.

Fibroid biohacking guide: www.FLOliving.com/fibroids-guide.

Endometriosis

Endometriosis is a painful condition in which the tissue that lines the inside of the uterus—the endometrium—grows outside the uterus. This tissue is sensitive to fluctuating estrogen levels throughout the cycle as well as to the prostaglandins that contribute to either uterine contractions or uterine relaxation. This endometrial tissue can adhere to other tissues like the intestines and bladder or even within the abdominal cavity and can create spasms that affect digestion and elimination and can cause pain. At its foundation, endometriosis is a combination of an autoimmune-like hormonal disorder with symptoms that are triggered by chemical stress and excess estrogen.

FLO-approved biohack: Eat anti-inflammatory foods, including leafy greens, broccoli, salmon, bone broth, blueberries, and flaxseeds. To reduce pain, increase your intake of foods high in magnesium, such as almonds, avocados, sunflower seeds, pumpkin seeds, spinach, and black beans.

Worst foods for endometriosis: Say good-bye to dairy, alcohol, gluten, pesticide-laden foods, and red meat.

Endometriosis biohacking guide: www.FLOliving.com/endo-guide.

PCOS

Polycystic ovarian syndrome (PCOS) is a hormonal health condition that affects an estimated 10 million women. I was one of them, but consider myself "in remission" from this issue, which is often—but not always—associated with cysts on the ovaries. There are several types of PCOS, but women with the condition tend to have higher levels of androgens, such as testosterone, which can lead to hirsutism (excess hair), thinning hair, acne, and irregular periods. This condition is also associated with lower progesterone levels, which further contribute to irregular periods. And as my gynecologist told me when I was finally diagnosed with PCOS, it set me up for insulin resistance and increased risk for serious health consequences, including diabetes, heart disease, obesity, metabolic syndrome, infertility, miscarriage, liver inflammation, and endometrial cancer.

FLO-approved biohack: Consume high-fiber foods like beans and lentils, cruciferous veggies, sweet potatoes, and almonds to combat insulin resistance, and remember it's always a good idea to cook cruciferous veggies (broccoli, kale, Brussels sprouts, cabbage, and collard greens), because they contain goitrogens that suppress thyroid function, contributing to PCOS.

Worst foods for PCOS: Steer clear of caffeine, sugar, dairy, red meat, artificial sweeteners, soy products, cooking oils (canola, sunflower, and vegetable oils), and margarine.

PCOS biohacking guide: www.FLOliving.com/pcos-guide.

Cramps

Are cramps keeping you on the sidelines? You're not alone. I meet so many women who tell me they spend several days a month curled up on the couch or in bed waiting for the pain to subside. I was one of them, too. I suffered from debilitating cramps that rivaled labor contractions and would practically knock me out. Of course, I needed to know *why* this was happening. Turns out, there are two causes for cramps—one chemical, one functional. Hormone-like substances called prostaglandins, which are involved with pain and inflammation, stimulate the uterine muscles to contract. Prostaglandins also play a part in the vomiting, diarrhea, and headaches that might come with your cycle. There are three types of prostaglandins: PgE1, PgE2, and PgE3. The culprit that causes uterine contractions and pain is PgE2. The more PgE2 you make, the more intense your cramps. PgE1 and PgE3 are antispasmodic in nature, relaxing the uterine muscles, which makes them natural painkillers. On the functional side, pain can be caused by any of the following conditions: endometriosis, fibroids, infections, use of an intrauterine device (IUD), ovarian cysts, narrow cervix, or a retroverted (tipped) uterus.

FLO-approved biohack: When cramps hit, don't automatically reach for the ibuprofen. Try a few almonds or hazelnuts instead—they're good sources of vitamin E, which has been shown to reduce period pain. And eat leafy greens like collard greens for the magnesium, which reduces the prostaglandins that cause cramps. To help prevent cramps, take vitamin E and magnesium for a few days before your period and for a few days after it starts. On a long-term basis, you need to increase PgE1 and PgE3. Eating the right fats will help you do it. For example, linoleic acid—found in foods like salmon, sardines, flaxseeds, pumpkin seeds, sunflower seeds, and sesame seeds—can help, so be sure to eat these foods on a regular basis.

Worst foods for cramps: Dairy and saturated animal fats increase PgE2, so limit them as much as possible, or ideally cut them out of your diet. Omit canola oil and other refined oils high in omega-6 because they increase the production of cramp-causing PgE2.

Bloating

Do you know the most common causes of bloating? Check out these three culprits that may be making it hard to zip up your jeans.

- A compromised microbiome: When you have an overgrowth of bad bacteria in your gut, which is known as dysbiosis, it can lead to inflammation. An inflamed gut can lead to—no surprise here— bloating. As you've seen in this book, the microbiome is made up of trillions of microbes that play a role in processing and flushing hormones out of the body. In particular, it's the bacterial colony known as the estrobolome that's involved in metabolizing estrogen, which is vital for keeping estrogen and progesterone levels balanced. When the estrobolome is out of whack, it can throw your hormones off balance and cause you to retain fluids.

- Chronic stress: As if you needed another reason to get out of perpetual productivity mode, chronic stress is linked to bloating. When your body produces excess amounts of the stress hormone cortisol, it causes you to retain sodium, which leads to water retention and uncomfortable swelling.

- Nutrient deficiencies: Not getting enough magnesium could be one of the reasons you feel bloated. Magnesium helps relax the muscles and eases constipation.

FLO-approved biohack: Support your microbiome with probiotics and take a magnesium supplement, or try my Anti-Bloatini juice recipe. Drink it every day of the week before your luteal phase to prevent bloat and other PMS symptoms.

Anti-Bloatini

2 beets, 2 carrots, 4 celery stalks, 1 lemon

Juice everything, and serve immediately.

Worst foods for bloating: Caffeine, salty foods, and dairy. Cut them out, especially before your period.

Acne

Do you tend to get a big zit during your period? Do little bumps appear on other parts of your face during the other times of your cycle? Or are you plagued with cystic acne as I was? Acne can be demoralizing, robbing you of your confidence. I hear from women every day who want help to get rid of acne and blemishes. Dermatologists will prescribe acne medication, and gynecologists will prescribe birth control pills. But acne is caused by excess estrogen, the improper metabolization of this hormone, gut dysfunction, and micronutrient deficiencies—yes, the same causes of any hormonal problem. Acne medication that treats your face won't get rid of the root cause, so those zits will keep coming back. In addition, the side effects of acne medications can include depression and liver and gut issues. Instead of medicating, you can simply track your cycle and hormone levels. Acne can be triggered during ovulation or when you're moving from the ovulation phase to the premenstrual phase. Acne can also appear when your hormonal patterns change as you age from your twenties to your forties.

FLO-approved biohack: Eat lots of leafy greens (my fave breakout buster is cilantro) and root veggies to up your vitamin A intake. Vitamin A is fat-soluble, so be sure to eat your greens with healthy fats, such as olive oil or avocado. Add more zinc to your diet by eating whole grains,

BIOHACKING TOOL KIT   PART 1

sunflower seeds, and tree nuts. Consume more essential fatty acids by adding flaxseeds to your meals, and take fish oil and evening primrose oil supplements.

Worst foods for hormonal acne: Dairy, soy, peanuts, vegetable oils (canola, sunflower, and safflower), caffeine, and gluten.

Breast Tenderness

In the days leading up to your period, do your breasts feel sore and painful? If so, you're one of legions of women who experience this common PMS symptom. Premenstrual breast tenderness, which is known as cyclical mastalgia, can be a sign that you have excess estrogen circulating in your body. When you have estrogen dominance, it leads to swelling of the breast ducts. If your breasts feel lumpy before your period, it could be a sign of fibrocystic breast disease and might merit a trip to the gynecologist.

FLO-approved biohack: Load up on foods that are high in vitamin E, including almonds, sunflower seeds, spinach, chard, kale, avocado, mango, and kiwis. Vitamin E is a powerful antioxidant that calms the inflammation that causes breast tenderness. Consider taking an essential fatty acid called evening primrose oil, which acts as an anti-inflammatory agent.

Worst foods for breast tenderness: Kick all forms of caffeine to the curb—including coffee, black tea, and green tea—and dump dairy.

PMS biohacking guide: www.FLOliving.com/pms-guide.

Step 5: Replenish Your Micronutrients

Endocrine disruptors, synthetic birth control, and stress—these all negatively impact your hormonal health. Sugar, dairy, and gluten—staples in so many women's diets—can mess with your microbiome and prevent your body from adequately absorbing nutrients. Cappuccinos, chai lattes, and energy drinks—which many women rely on to power through their day—

deplete micronutrients. And don't forget all that dieting, overexercising, and rampant stress that further drain our reserves. Mix them all together, and you've got one nasty cocktail for micronutrient depletion and endocrine dysfunction. Because we've been brought up without a fundamental working knowledge of our biochemistry or how to live in sync with our cycle, we try diets and engage in exercise routines and self-care that actually deplete the body of the very micronutrients the endocrine system needs to create hormonal balance. So our hormones go off-kilter, causing us to turn to yet another diet, fitness fad, or self-care ritual that only compounds the problem. It's a vicious cycle.

If you're like the vast majority of American women, you probably haven't been nourishing your monthly cycle. You may not be eating foods that provide enough of the micronutrients your body needs to optimize endocrine function throughout your cycle. Or you may be consuming nutrient-dense foods, but your body can't absorb enough of the goodness they contain due to gut dysbiosis. Whatever the reason, the result is the same—a lack of sufficient micronutrients to keep your hormones happy. The risk for vitamin deficiencies is significantly higher in women compared with men, and can you guess who is at highest risk for deficiency? Women ages nineteen to fifty and pregnant or breastfeeding women—in other words, women of reproductive age—are most likely to be missing out on micronutrients that are vital to hormonal health. Vitamin deficiencies put you at a greater disadvantage, keep you in hormonal dysfunction, and prevent you from accessing the gifts of your feminine biology.

In addition to eating nutrient-dense foods, you may want to add certain key supplements to the protocol. Science shows us that using specific supplements can support the body in achieving and maintaining hormonal balance. In a 2017 *Nutrients* study, people who didn't use any dietary supplements had a 40 percent risk of a vitamin deficiency, compared with just a 14 percent risk for those taking multivitamin and multimineral supplements. Don't fall into the trap of thinking that supplements can take the place of a healthy, phase-specific eating plan—*nutritious food always comes first!* And don't expect one single supplement to solve all your symptoms or to provide all the micronutrient support you need. After years of practice and research, I have identified the nonnegotiable micronutrients that your endocrine system needs to balance your hormones. Think of these micronutrients as a sort of "insurance policy" against that harmful cocktail that is wreaking havoc with your endocrine system. Learn more about these micronutrients here, and find the formulations at www.FLOliving.com/supplements.

B Vitamins

B vitamins are critical for hormonal health, in addition to playing an integral role in your energy, moods, skin, and stress response. Vitamin B6 is essential for the development of the corpus luteum, which is formed when a follicle releases an egg. The corpus luteum secretes progesterone and plays a vital role in conception and maintaining a pregnancy. B vitamins are also essential for your skin, helping your cells regenerate and renew. B6 prevents skin inflammation and overproduction of sebum, the oil your skin produces that can create acne issues. Vitamin B5, also known as pantothenic acid, promotes healthy functioning of the adrenal glands, which are responsible for pumping out the stress hormone cortisol. A 2008 study showed that supplementing with B5 helps stimulate adrenal cells, which in turn helps regulate your stress response. This is one reason some people refer to B5 as the "anti-stress vitamin."

When B vitamin levels are low: Low levels of B6 can translate to low levels of progesterone, which can trigger PMS symptoms during the luteal phase and increase the risk of miscarriage. Hormonal acne and adrenal fatigue are also associated with insufficient levels of B vitamins.

B vitamin disruptors: Many everyday things—stress, overexercising, alcohol, lack of sleep, and the pill—deplete B6 and subsequently, progesterone. Research has made it clear that oral contraceptives impair microbiome health, which prevents proper absorption of vitamins and can lead to depletion.

Magnesium

Magnesium is magic for your hormones. It's essential for hormone creation, and also contributes to cortisol regulation, thyroid function, blood sugar balance, and sleep. As if that weren't enough, magnesium also has a powerful anti-inflammatory effect. This micronutrient is essential for pituitary health and helps ensure that we produce optimal amounts of hormones like FSH (follicular stimulating), LH (luteinizing), and TSH (thyroid stimulating) for healthy endocrine function. Magnesium encourages relaxation, calms the nervous system, and promotes better sleep. Magnesium also helps regulate your body's stress-response system and prevents excess cortisol production. When your stress hormones are under control, the way is paved for progesterone, estrogen, testosterone, FSH, and LH levels to reach a happy balance as well. Magnesium helps keep insulin production in check, which reduces sugar cravings. Fewer cravings means less consumption of things like cookies and cupcakes, which translates to fewer blood sugar spikes and crashes. Keeping blood sugar stable is absolutely vital when it comes to healing hormonal issues, such as PCOS. Thanks to these benefits, magnesium can help heal PMS, PCOS, adrenal fatigue, menopausal symptoms, and all other health problems related to the hormone cycle.

When magnesium levels are low: Unfortunately, you could be lacking in this all-important mineral. In all my years working with women to balance their hormones, I haven't met a single woman who didn't need to boost her magnesium levels. People who don't get enough magnesium are more likely to have elevated levels of inflammation, which is associated with endometriosis and the painful cramps that come with it, breast tenderness, and acne. Other problems associated with low levels of magnesium include irregular ovulation, thyroid issues, excessive cortisol production, insulin or diabetes, and trouble sleeping.

Magnesium disruptors: Many things can deplete levels, but some of the most common are chronic stress, caffeine consumption, and high sugar intake.

BIOHACKING TOOL KIT   PART 1

Omega-3 Fatty Acids

Mountains of evidence point to omega-3 fatty acids as potent soothers of menstrual-related symptoms, mood boosters, stress busters, anti-inflammation agents, and skin rejuvenators. They can help ease symptoms related to PCOS, PMS, uterine fibroids, breast tenderness, and acne. In fact, when it comes to pain relief for menstrual cramps, taking omega-3 fatty acid supplements, most commonly in the form of fish oil but also found in vegan sources, is more effective than popping ibuprofen, according to a 2001 study by Iranian scientists. Omega-3 goes a long way in reducing perceived stress levels, and many studies have shown that supplementation with omega-3 may help ease depression.

When omega-3 levels are low: Low levels of omega-3 have been linked to many of the symptoms that come with hormonal imbalances, as well as fatigue, trouble sleeping, attention problems, dry skin, and achy joints. Low levels of omega-3 fatty acids have been associated with a higher incidence of depression and bipolar disorder.

Omega-3 disruptors: Eating a diet too high in omega-6 fatty acids, a type of essential fatty acid that is pro-inflammatory, can offset the anti-inflammatory benefits of omega-3. Foods high in omega-6 include vegetable oils (including sunflower, corn, and soybean), salad dressings, pizza, sausages, and potato chips.

Vitamin D3

Did you know the "sunshine vitamin" is actually a hormone? This micronutrient supports the health of many of your biological systems, including the brain, immune system, and nervous system. Vitamin D3 also regulates insulin levels, which helps stabilize blood sugar levels. It has also been linked to mood, dopamine production in the brain, and serotonin levels. Many women I meet are surprised to discover that vitamin D3 is also closely tied to fertility. For example, women with higher vitamin D3 levels are four times more likely to conceive via IVF than women with low levels, according to research in a 2012 issue of *Human Reproduction*. Bringing D3 levels up into the normal range can change your fertility story.

When vitamin D3 levels are low: A staggering 93 percent of women dealing with infertility have below-normal levels of vitamin D3, according to a 2008 study in *Fertility and Sterility*. This same study linked low levels of the micronutrient to an increased risk for PCOS. A low concentration of vitamin D3 is also known to cause estrogen dominance, which is the primary culprit behind many hormonal issues. Low levels have also been associated with an increased risk for depression.

Vitamin D3 disruptors: A lack of sunshine, a strict vegan diet, or avoiding dairy products may contribute to an insufficiency of vitamin D3.

Probiotics (Gut Bacteria)

I'm very pro-probiotics. These supplements contain billions of friendly bacteria intended to promote a healthier microbiome. A specific community of gut flora called the estrobolome produces an enzyme that supports the metabolizing of estrogen, essential for conception. Your gut is also an important part of the elimination system that is vital in ushering hormones, such as excess estrogen, out of the body.

When gut bacteria levels are low: If your microbiome is out of balance, it can put you on the path to estrogen dominance, weight gain, acne, diabetes, brain fog, cancer, acne, and rosacea.

Gut bacteria disruptors: If you take medications (including oral contraceptives), devour dairy, gobble up gluten, or eat foods covered in pesticides, you disrupt this hugely important bacterial balance. Imbalance in your microbiome compromises your ability to eliminate excess estrogen, which can significantly disrupt your reproductive ability.

Antioxidants to Promote Liver Function

Liver function is vital for healthy hormone levels. Antioxidants that support liver function include vitamin C, selenium, and alpha-lipoic acid.

BIOHACKING TOOL KIT   PART 1

When liver function is low: If your liver isn't doing its primary job of detoxification optimally, it could mean your body won't flush out excess estrogen adequately, making you vulnerable to estrogen dominance.

Liver function disruptors: Consuming large amounts of refined sugar or drinking too much alcohol can take a toll on your liver.

Hormone supplement guide: www.FLOliving.com/supplement-guide.

Step 6: Address the Emotional Causes of Your Symptoms

Did you know that our emotions, feelings, and the energy we hold can play a part in the development of reproductive health conditions? In *Women's Bodies, Women's Wisdom*, Dr. Christiane Northrup asserts that there's an emotional-psychological component to menstrual disorders. I have found this to be true with my clients and with myself. And although it's very important to look at the root causes of conditions from a functional nutrition and biological standpoint, and to go through all of the steps listed here to address those causes, it's just as important to make peace with some of the emotional issues that may be contributing to your menstrual problems. So far in this book, you've seen the biological and neurochemical underpinnings of hormonal dysfunction. You've grasped how trying to fit into a 24-hour world without taking your 28-day clock into account has put you at a serious disadvantage, and you've discovered how endocrine disruptors and synthetic birth control assault your body and damage your biological systems. Most important, you've seen how you can use food and lifestyle changes to put your period problems into remission and help you balance your hormones. Your emotions are the final piece to the hormonal dysfunction puzzle you may want to consider. Emotions are powerful, and they can cause real physical changes. You feel nervous, your hands get clammy. You feel scared, your heart starts to beat faster. You feel anxious, your stomach hurts. Research shows emotions can impact many of our biological systems—causing neurochemical changes, suppressing our immune system, and ramping up our stress response. It's not surprising that emotions may contribute to your period problems.

I find that emotions also need to be addressed for long-term hormonal recovery. What do I mean? For example, take a look at Sheri. She wanted help because she was experiencing continuous spotting. We had addressed her diet and lifestyle, but the spotting was still occurring. During one conversation she mentioned to me that the spotting had been happening since her father had passed away earlier that year. I suggested that Sheri's womb was holding her unprocessed grief, resulting in the symptoms, which were a literal weeping from the womb. Once she made that connection, she was able to release her emotions and address her grief, and this symptom pattern disappeared.

Think of your body having a "high heart" where your actual heart is, and a "low heart" where your pelvic basin is; the "low heart" holds on to your deepest emotions, the ones you may not even be aware of. These feelings will remain there until your "high heart" is ready to process them. A health condition like spotting can convey a message of the kinds of emotions being held in the reproductive organs. I see this in many women who are trying to live in perpetual productivity—being in never-ending go mode at work, in relationships, and in motherhood. When you push at work without rest, do what your partner wants but not what you need, and put your children always ahead of your own self-care, those unaddressed needs and feelings get stored in your pelvis. If you aren't creating space for yourself, your feelings, and your needs, period problems will be the price you pay for martyring yourself. Your cycle will shout it to the rooftops—*cramps! headaches! heavy bleeding! fibroids! breast tenderness!* Listen to your cycle. It's trying desperately to tell you something you need to hear. It's asking you to acknowledge these emotions. It's begging you to take care of yourself.

In my practice, I have found that certain hormonal conditions are speaking to you about specific emotional realities. Take ovarian cysts, for example—especially ones that are recurrent. They tend to represent unfulfilled creative expression. Maybe you feel stifled in your creativity at work, or maybe you don't have the energy to get your projects to blossom from the idea stage to fruition. This blocked creativity can manifest as ovarian cysts, which serve as a painful reminder that you must tap into the creative matrix. Look at endometriosis. The emotional connection here tends to relate to women who put all their energy toward caring for others while ignoring their own needs and desires. The uterus basically mirrors this behavior. Think of what the endometrium represents. This lush uterine lining provides a nurturing maternal cocoon for an embryo. When it grows outside the womb, it does so in an attempt to embrace and mother the woman who isn't mothering herself. These symptoms cannot be ignored, and they tell you that you can no longer ignore yourself.

I believe the best way forward is to bring these emotions out into the open, to talk about our traumas and the things we don't normally share openly—our individual experiences of miscarriage, postpartum depression, abortion, sexual abuse, rape, assault, and domestic violence, as well as the collective weight of sexism and misogyny. Releasing these emotions can mean we no longer hold them silently within ourselves, where they continue to do harm. I believe that understanding the emotional root of our hormonal issues can lead to more compassion for ourselves and for other women, and to an individual and collective recovery. Only through this understanding and recovery can we feel safe to come home to our bodies, and start living with our body's rhythms at the center of our lives.

To learn about the specific emotional root causes of your condition, download the guide at www.FLOliving.com/emotions-guide.

HOW TO GET IN THE FLO WHEN YOU HAVE SPECIAL CIRCUMSTANCES

Perhaps cancer treatments may have left you without a period. Or you may be a transgender woman who doesn't bleed. Or you have experienced premature ovarian failure or have adrenal hyperplasia or some other condition that is stopping your cycle. Adopting a cyclical practice can help you feel connected to the rhythm of the second clock. If you're not sure where to start, you have two options:

• Start this week as your follicular week and go from there.

• Look up the moon phases for the current month and chart your cycle according to its schedule: a full moon indicates the ovulatory phase, a waning moon represents the luteal phase, a new moon is the menstrual phase, and a waxing moon represents the follicular phase.

The idea is not that you'd do this with the intention of restoring your cycle. Instead it's a weekly practice that allows you to tap into a constantly shifting self-care practice and stay connected with creativity and productivity rhythms based on feminine energy. You can explore which aspects of the self-care practice give you the greatest boost physically and emotionally.

_____

What I hope you take away from this chapter is that whatever your particular challenge might be—endometriosis, fibroids, unresolved emotions—you have the power to change your hormones in a positive way by taking the steps outlined here. Understanding how to apply this practice to enhance your own body and health gives you a strong foundation to stand on. In part 3 of this book, you'll discover how to take the practice beyond your own personal well-being and make it work for you in your career, relationships, motherhood, and more.

What to Know If You're on Hormonal Birth Control

You quite literally are your hormones. And when you change your hormones—which is what hormonal contraceptives do—you change the version of yourself that your brain creates.
—Dr. Sarah Hill

The one endocrine disruptor that may do the most harm is the one we *purposely* choose to manipulate our hormones: synthetic birth control. If you've read my first book, *WomanCode*, or watched any of my Facebook live chats, you probably know my feelings on synthetic birth control. Let me be clear on my feelings: From a feminist point of view, I think every woman should have access to birth control anytime she wants. From a menstrual health point of view, period issues need better care, which birth control does not provide. One of my clients who took the pill for years to override a hormonal imbalance told me it felt like she was "using a Band-Aid to cover a deep wound that needed stitching." I couldn't have said it better myself. Synthetic birth control doesn't fix your hormones and it doesn't address any of the underlying root causes of hormonal imbalance. It simply masks the symptoms associated with conditions like estrogen dominance, PMS, PCOS, endometriosis, and fibroids. Gynecologists routinely prescribe synthetic birth control to treat or manage these conditions as if it were a magic pill. Unfortunately, there is no magic.

Here's how those synthetic hormones really work to hijack the four phases of your gorgeous cycle. Combinations of estrogen and progestin, a synthetic form of progesterone, conspire to interfere with your body's natural processes. They fool the brain so the hypothalamus never signals the pituitary gland to secrete luteinizing hormone (LH) or follicle-stimulating hormone (FSH), effectively preventing the follicles from swelling to mature the eggs they contain. The steady levels of synthetic hormones delivered by the pill thwart the natural midcycle surge in estrogen that typically kick-starts the release of an egg, so there is no ovulation. In the unlikely event an egg manages to be released in spite of all the synthetic hormones working against it, its chances of being fertilized are slim. That's because synthetic progestin thickens the mucus of the cervix, creating a sort of barrier that makes it harder for sperm to swim to an egg. In addition, unlike natural progesterone, which maintains the thickened lining of the uterus to make it inviting for a fertilized egg, progestin does the opposite, by thinning the uterine lining. If an egg is fertilized, the lining may be too thin for it to remain in the uterus, and it will be shed when bleeding occurs. Many forms of birth control pills try to mimic a natural monthly cycle with three weeks of pills containing the synthetic hormones and one week of placebos to make women feel as if they are still getting a period and therefore feel more comfortable taking the medication. During the placebo week, you typically experience some breakthrough bleeding. Don't be fooled: *This is not a real period!* Since there is no ovulation, you have no menstrual cycle.

This is a completely artificial pattern. Gone are the natural rise and fall of estrogen and progesterone. In its place is a static dose of synthetic hormones that basically keep you stuck long-term in a phaseless no-cycle land. Some of you might think, "Hey, that's great. I can be more productive and get more stuff done." Slow down, sister. This is not the case. Your estrogen levels are being suppressed, and you're getting a very low dose of progesterone that doesn't provide enough stimulation to the brain to fully mimic the luteal phase. So you don't have that fire to finish projects, and in fact, you're more likely to feel a little flat. You're basically stuck in a hormonal desert without access to the gifts of any of the four phases of your cycle, which means you won't have your inner creative matrix helping you bring your ideas and projects to life. Over time, the massive micronutrient depletion the pill causes will lead to a whole host of problems for your biological systems. This is a sure-fire way to burn out your adrenals, expose yourself to chronic stress and systemic inflammation, and increase your risk for autoimmune issues. Your body will pay the price. I see women every day who are dealing with the effects.

In my view, synthetic birth control has a huge opportunity cost. It distances you from your inner feminine power source and makes the HPO (hypothalamic pituitary ovarian) axis dormant. Synthetic birth control also comes with a host of nasty side effects (like shrinking your clitoris and ovaries), reduces your body's ability to absorb micronutrients, messes with your mate selection on a genetic level, and robs you of the opportunity to experience the magic that happens when you're in sync with your cycle.

I hear from women every day who are suffering from taking the pill or using another form of hormonal contraceptive. "I don't feel like myself," "I'm an emotional mess," "I'm so tired all the time," and "I feel depressed" are some of the more common complaints I hear. But these are only a few of the many side effects facing women on the pill, patch, ring, or hormonal IUD. Just look at the little information pamphlet that comes with your hormonal birth control prescription, and you'll see a very long list of potential birth control side effects. Women are not made aware of the health risks associated with the manipulation of their hormones through synthetic birth control methods. And although the pill in particular has seen many changes since it was first approved in 1960, many of the same potential side effects remain. You're probably well aware of the bloating, headaches, and weight gain, but did you know that the pill can also cause depression, shut down your sex drive long term, and decrease your fertility even after you stop taking it?

Did your gynecologist tell you about all these risks before writing a prescription for synthetic birth control? Probably not. If you're thinking about putting your daughter on the pill to mask her period problems, take a long hard look at these side effects and understand that with phase-specific foods and exercise, she can have regular periods without the consequences of hormonal birth control. And note that although many of these side effects and conditions look like individual problems, they may be signs of larger, systemic issues.

How the Pill Impacts Your Biological Systems

Increasingly, research is revealing how synthetic birth control can affect your (or your daughter's) biological systems.

Biological System 1: Brain. A 2014 review shows taking the pill is associated with changes in the brain's structure, neurochemistry, function, and mood modulation. Structural changes, which appear in brain regions associated with emotion, increase the longer you've been taking the pill, and some of them may not be reversible. Those little round pills can also mess with the intricate balance of your feel-good neurotransmitters—serotonin, dopamine, and GABA—which may contribute to mood swings, anxiety, or depression. Research from the University of Copenhagen suggested synthetic birth control could play a role in *causing* depression for some women. The researchers found that compared with women who weren't taking hormonal contraceptives, women taking birth control pills that contain both estrogen and progestin were 23 percent more likely to start using antidepressants for the first time. Even more alarming, women using progestin-only pills were 34 percent more likely to get a first prescription for antidepressants. Considering how many millions of women take hormonal birth control at some point in their lives, and the fact that women are taking it earlier with the younger age of menarche, it's critical for more research to be done to explore the effects of synthetic birth control on the brain.

Biological System 2: Immune system. Synthetic hormones have a profound effect on the immune system. A 2017 review of 352 studies found that using oral contraceptives with estrogen and pro-gestin is associated with a greater risk for autoimmune diseases, including multiple sclerosis, systemic lupus, and interstitial cystitis. Progesterone-only contraceptives are linked to progesterone der-matitis and, in one large developing world concurrent cohort study, are associated with increases in eczema, contact dermatitis, alopecia, acne, and related skin conditions.

Biological System 3: Metabolism. Are you one of those women who gains weight just thinking about taking the pill? I've met thou-sands of women who have experienced weight gain after starting the pill. The reasons why remain a mystery. Numerous studies have failed to show that hormonal birth control causes significant weight gain; however, the estrogen in contraceptives may cause you to feel less full after eating. According to Dr. Mary Pritchard, the low-dose estrogen in birth control increases the level of ghrelin, a hormone that increases appetite. This change can cause you to eat more, which is a sure-fire way to gain weight. Estrogen also leads to added fluid retention, which can add pounds. Taking the pill can also get in the way of your fitness goals. A 2009 study in the *FASEB Journal* found that women on the pill gain 60 percent *less* muscle mass than women who are not taking oral contraceptives. In a ten-week weight-training program, about half the participants were on the pill and the other half were not. By the end of the program, women who were on the pill had gained significantly less lean muscle tissue, had lower levels of hormones that build muscle, and had much higher levels of cortisol, which is known to break down muscle tissue. The pill is definitely not your workout buddy.

Biological System 4: Microbiome. The pill is your microbiome's worst enemy. It acts like an antibiotic in the gut, destroying the delicate microbiome balance. Bloating, constipation, nausea, irritable bowel syndrome, acne, eczema, headaches—these common birth control side effects may be signs of gut dysbiosis. The mechanism behind these issues could be interference by synthetic hormones with the ability of the hormone receptors throughout the digestive system to function normally. The science community is catching up to the link between hormonal contraceptives and gut health. A 2013 study found that women on oral contraceptives for more than five years are three times more likely to develop Crohn's disease.

Biological System 5: Stress response. Taking the pill may cause effects in the body that mimic chronic stress, increase levels of cortisol, and alter the HPA axis, according to a 2017 study in *Scientific Reports*. Bottom line: the pill can jack up your stress levels.

Having Options Is a Very Good Thing

When you look at all of these risks and the impacts on your endocrine system, it makes you wonder: Is it all worth it? Do you think men would be expected to endure these risks? Apparently not. Although research shows over 50 percent of men would be open to taking a hormonal contraceptive, and their female partners say they would trust them to take an oral "male pill," there still isn't a readily available product on the market. A 2016 study showed a male hormonal contraceptive injection was effective in preventing pregnancy, but the trial was cut short due to male participants not being willing to tolerate the side effects—mood swings, depression, acne, and suppressed fertility post-trial, among others. Researchers determined the risks outweighed the benefits and put a halt to the study. These are some of the exact same side effects women experience from taking hormonal birth control. They're also the kinds of complaints frequently dismissed or downplayed by doctors—an excellent example of gender bias.

Why are we expected to endure the effects of hormonal birth control, and why are we willing to subject ourselves to these risks, especially when we can get pregnant for only a maximum of seven days a month? Yes, you read that correctly. You're fertile only seven days a month—at most. This is due to the length of time sperm survives in the body (five days) and the egg is viable (two days). It's much harder to get pregnant than you're led to believe. It's not something you need to be fearful of every day of your life to the point where you need to take hormonal birth control on a daily basis. The ills of the pill have been concealed for too long, and it's time to make choices based on health, not fear.

Now, don't get me wrong—birth control is not all bad, and in fact, it's played a huge role in female empowerment. When the pill debuted in 1960, it was viewed as the great emancipator. It allowed women to finally take control of their bodies and enjoy newfound sexual freedom, and it was a key part of the women's movement. I'm not ungrateful. I completely agree that women must have access to birth control, and we must have the right to make our own choices regarding our bodies. However, having helped so many women use a food and supplement protocol to restore hormonal balance, I think it's important for you to know that there are other options for fixing your period and preventing pregnancy that don't force you to shut down your hormonal system.

Millennials are taking the lead here. A 2018 survey of more than 2,000 young women by *Cosmopolitan* and Power to Decide, a national campaign to prevent unplanned pregnancies, found that more than 70 percent of them said they had stopped taking the pill or had thought about quitting in the past three years. I talk with young women every day who are doing yoga, juicing, drinking adaptogenic lattes, and eating organic produce, and now they're beginning to wonder how synthetic hormones align with their overall values and lifestyle.

Women of *all* ages need to understand that with synthetic birth control, you're giving up access to this powerful cyclical process in your body. What I would love to see in our society is women getting full disclosure about

these medications, learning about natural means of support, and then making the decision they feel is right for them. Whenever I share all of the information here with a client and then ask her if she would have elected to take
this medication to treat her hormonal imbalance if she had known then
what she knows now, the answer is always a resounding no. I've met with
thousands of women who, once they understand the reality of the trade-off,
decide they want to go off the pill. I always let them know it's important to
transition off the pill safely. More details on how to transition off the pill
without crazy side effects appear later in this chapter.

Usually, when a woman makes the decision to come off hormonal contraceptives, the next question I hear is, "If I go off the pill, how am I going
to prevent pregnancy?" Here are some options.

Nonhormonal Birth Control Options

- **Condoms:** When used correctly and consistently, condoms are about
  98 percent effective at preventing pregnancy—about the same as
  the pill's 99 percent success rate when used perfectly. In addition,
  condoms prevent sexually transmitted diseases (STDs), such as human
  papillomavirus (HPV), as well as bacterial and viral infections.
- **Diaphragm:** A diaphragm is a small, flexible cup that is inserted into
  the vagina. It prevents pregnancy by covering the cervix so sperm are
  blocked from reaching an egg. When used correctly, diaphragms are
  94 percent effective. A one-size-fits-all diaphragm called Caya recently
  hit the US market. It's available by prescription only but doesn't require
  a doctor to do a fitting.
- **Cervical cap:** Similar to a diaphragm but smaller, a cervical cap is a
  small cup shaped like a sailor's cap that covers the cervix to prevent
  pregnancy. Cervical caps, such as FemCap, are 71 to 86 percent effective
  and work best when used with spermicide.
- **Copper IUD:** This tiny device is inserted into the uterus and is more
  than 99 percent effective at preventing pregnancy for up to twelve

years. The copper IUD allows you to continue ovulating, but it causes an inflammatory response in the uterus that prevents sperm from reaching the egg and fertilizing it and may interfere with implantation. Note—this form can increase copper levels in the body and increase the severity of cramps.

- **Intrauterine ball (IUBTM):** Considered the next-generation IUD, this string of copper pearls is inserted into the uterus to prevent pregnancy for up to five years. Like the copper IUD, it doesn't prevent ovulation, but it prevents egg fertilization and is more than 99 percent effective. The unique shape also makes it less likely to perforate the uterus, which is a major advantage.

- **Sponge:** This small, squishy sponge contains spermicide and is inserted into the vagina to cover the cervix. When used perfectly each time you have sex, it's 91 percent effective at preventing pregnancy. You can use this along with a condom during your fertile window for extra pregnancy prevention.

- **Fertility awareness methods (FAMs):** Being aware of where you are in your cycle week to week can help you track ovulation and pinpoint your fertile window to prevent pregnancy. There are three ways to do so. You can track your basal body temperature (BBT) with a device like Daysy or Lady-Comp, observe changes in your cervical fluid (it should look like uncooked egg whites), or chart your cycle using a calendar or the MyFLO app. Then avoid sex completely during your fertile time, or use condoms plus a spermicide to be extra safe. Individually, these methods are about 76 to 88 percent effective, but when all three are used together, the prevention rate increases.

- **Wild carrot seed (also known as Queen Anne's Lace):** This ancient herbal remedy has been used for centuries by women to prevent the implantation of a fertilized egg into the uterine wall. You can take wild carrot seed if you have sex when you're fertile and the condom breaks—*these things do happen!* For more information on studies and dosage, visit famed herbalist Robin Rose Bennet's website.

Can I Sync with My Cycle If I'm on the Pill?

The short answer is no . . . and yes. You'll do it in a slightly different way from a woman who isn't taking the pill. Because the pill and other synthetic contraceptives shut down your hormonal system, you lose your cyclical nature. Gone is the follicular phase. No more ovulating. The low doses of estrogen and progesterone put you in a phaseless cycle but without any of the benefits. And the bleed you get during the placebo week isn't a real period. Even though you don't experience the natural ebb and flow of your hormones while on the pill, that doesn't mean you can't try this cyclical program. Although you're missing out on all the gifts of your natural cycle, you can still reap benefits from consuming nutrient-dense foods, engaging in a variety of exercises, and scheduling your life with right-timing in mind.

Here's how you do it:

• Map out on a calendar when you finish the last day of your period.
• Consider the following day the first day of your follicular phase. Follow the follicular phase guidelines for seven days.
• The next day is your ovulatory phase. Follow the ovulatory phase guidelines for four days.
• The next day is your luteal phase. Follow the luteal phase guidelines for twelve days.
• The next day is your menstrual phase. Follow the menstrual phase guidelines for five days.
• Begin with the follicular phase again.

Experiment and see how you feel, but don't expect to experience the creativity, energy, productivity, or intuition that comes with each phase when you're not on the pill. My hope is that you will want to have access to all the physical and neurochemical opportunities that occur when your hormones and biological systems are operating at optimal levels, so you would make the decision to transition off the pill, and work with your physician to do so. And if you do decide to transition off, starting this process will help you transition more successfully.

You Can Quit the Pill (or any Hormonal Contraceptive) Without Crazy Side Effects

Think back to why you started taking the pill. Was it just to prevent pregnancy? Was it to regulate an irregular cycle? Was it to "treat" symptoms of hormonal imbalance—severe PMS, heavy cramps, migraines? As you understand now, the pill doesn't actually correct the root causes of any hormonal condition, so be aware that when you come off these synthetic hormones, all those unpleasant symptoms will come back, and often times with a vengeance. Post–birth control syndrome is real and can wreak short-term havoc and create long-term problems if the transition isn't handled properly. I hate to break it to you, but even if you didn't have any issues prior to going on the pill for pregnancy prevention, quitting can cause hormonal upheaval and bring on symptoms you never had before. It's so unfair. To avoid this, follow the steps outlined in the Biohacking Tool Kit—remove endocrine disruptors, use foods to fight your symptoms, replenish your micronutrients, and track your symptoms. Follow these steps for two months while you're still on the pill, and then you can improve your chance of transitioning without experiencing an intense relapse of your symptoms. Stopping abruptly is never the way, and I highly recommend that you let your gynecologist know about your plans so you can be monitored by your physician as you make the transition. Taking this approach can make the changeover much gentler. When you begin to experience what it feels like to have balanced hormones that allow you to access your natural gifts, you may decide that you want to continue on this path. It's really up to you.

This is how Shawna did it. She originally started using hormonal contraceptives—a vaginal ring that's inserted once a month—in part to take care of terrible acne. It seemed to flare up at all the wrong times and made her feel self-conscious at work and on the dating scene. Her acne had cleared up while on birth control, and the first time she came off it, she said her face "exploded." So she went right back on it. The next time she made the decision to stop hormonal birth control, she was nervous about the acne coming back. This time she started syncing with her cycle a few months before her big quit day, and after she stopped her skin stayed completely clear. She couldn't believe it. Now she says she wishes she had started this practice seven years earlier instead of hiding and medicating the problem using birth control.

Get more support about synthetic birth control at www.FLOliving.com /birth-control-rehab.

FOUR STEPS TO GET IN THE FLO

To recap how you can begin to get in the FLO, these are the four simple steps to follow:

1. Audit your period.
2. If you have hormonal problems, read the Biohacking Tool Kit section and follow the directions in it.
3. Keep it simple when easing into syncing with your cycle by adding more phase-specific foods and activities as you progress:
   • Week 1: Choose vegetables recommended for this phase.
   • Week 2: Add the other phase-specific foods into your meals.
   • Week 3: Use the recommended cooking methods for each phase.
   • Week 4: Add in some phase-specific workouts.
4. In the following weeks, continue building on the progress you're making by including more elements of the program.

PART 3

GETTING YOUR LIFE IN THE FLO

Don't think about making women fit the world—think about making the world fit women.

—GLORIA STEINEM

CHAPTER 7

Sustainable Success at Work

I believe when you put women in any equation,
the equation gets better.
—SHELLEY ZALIS

Now that you've seen how to weave the concept of syncing with your cycle into your personal life and time management, how do you apply the concept in the workplace? How do you incorporate your second clock into our corporate culture, which has been operating on a single clock for centuries? First, think about how you've been faring so far by ignoring your second clock and trying to fit in to that single-clock culture. Have you ever noticed that you feel completely different at work from week to week? Some weeks you're excited about going to networking events and giving presentations, but other weeks you'd rather hole up in your office and organize your invoices for your expense reports. If you're like most women, you probably work in an environment that doesn't honor your infradian rhythm and doesn't give you the freedom to manage your projects in a way that works with your innate rhythm. You're just supposed to do whatever is asked of you whenever it's asked. And just as our cultural conditioning has us believing that we are supposed to suffer with period problems, it also has us convinced that we are supposed to suffer in every other area of our lives, especially work. So you put your head down, dig in, and get the job done—buying in to the perpetual productivity notion that the only way to succeed is to work harder, put in longer hours, and sacrifice your personal life and self-care for the sake of the job.

Whether you're just beginning your career and still trying to figure out what you want to do with your life, climbing the corporate ladder, running your own business as I do, or dealing with the roller-coaster freelance life, you're probably feeling stretched to the limit. You might be taking on extra projects at the office in the hope of getting a promotion. You might have a side hustle in addition to your regular gig to pad your portfolio and hopefully land a better job. You might be spending nights and weekends on a passion project that could be your big break. But if you're sacrificing your well-being as a result of all the extra work, you won't be able to perform your best. When you don't have the bandwidth to devote to each of those projects, you can wind up making mistakes or turning in subpar work. Even worse, you could wear down your immune system, get sick, and have to take a short leave of absence. I've seen many women get so frustrated by the frenzy of nonstop productivity at work that they eventually think there's something wrong with the company, and they find a new job or switch careers only to get caught up in the same relentless pace again.

The truth is, our hormonal changes throughout the month play a role in our communication, creativity, energy, and productivity at work. Everything you do that focuses on managing your time rather than your energy and that isn't in sync with your cycle phases increases stress, dampens your energy, and slows your progress, making you feel pressured and unfulfilled in your job. But what if I told you it doesn't have to be this way? You don't have to ignore your second clock at work or get stuck in nonstop productivity mode. In this chapter, you'll discover how to tap into your monthly cycle in the work environment so you can optimize your work flow, unlock your creative process, and feel energized about your career.

That's what happened to Allie. This entrepreneur used to travel a lot for work. Whenever she was at home or on the road, she did what she'd always done—started the day with an intense workout, drank a smoothie followed by a big mug of coffee, and then worked all hours of the day, and attended dinners and networking events most nights. At home she would squeeze in time with her boyfriend, too. All of this in between cross-country or international flights—nothing had a rhythm; it was just go, go, go, no matter what time zone or cycle phase she was in. Inevitably, her period problems and symptoms got worse. She was looking for a way to feel good and live her dreams, and it was becoming clear that she wasn't getting away with taking shortcuts with her health or her projects.

When she started tuning in to her cyclical energy, everything changed. "Now I make sure I'm not just wiping myself out in the beginning of the day with intense workouts in the morning without enough sleep and just powering through," she says. "Instead, it's making me more productive at work because it's ensuring that I'm not burning the candle at both ends, which was really my experience before. I'm so thankful I'm feeling like I cracked the code on myself and knowing what's appropriate for me."

Reset the Corporate Clock

If you think it sounds like I'm advocating for some special, unusual accommodation for our infradian pattern, keep in mind that accommodating the male single clock hormonal pattern is the status quo. In fact, corporate culture is set up to optimize performance for male biological rhythms. Check out the typical workday described here.

Typical Workday on the 24-Hour Clock

Morning: Testosterone and cortisol are at their highest, which makes men efficient at getting stuff done—holding meetings and powering through projects.

Late afternoon: Testosterone is waning, making men more sensitive to their estrogen, which sparks a desire in men to connect through socializing, such as going to happy hour with clients or coworkers.

Evening: Testosterone is at its lowest, which makes men want to crawl into their man cave and power down for the day.

I'm not recommending that we do something radical here; I'm simply suggesting we acknowledge and make space for both realities so everyone can thrive equally. Historically, women have had to disconnect from our biochemical nature to fit in. How can we forget the women in the 1960s and 1970s who worked hard to earn a seat at the male table by downplaying their female-ness? We saw this suppression reflected in the fashion trends of the 1980s—have you seen pictures of those "power suits"?—and even in the shifting of our own beliefs that our biology is a liability that must be overcome in the pursuit of success. They did the absolute best they could do to gain access in an unfair environment. It's because of their sacrifices that we can envision even more for ourselves now. The fact is that corporate culture acknowledges only one biological rhythm, and ours deserves to be included now.

Would working in tune with our infradian clock somehow set us back? I would argue that this is an important next step in the evolution of a corporate culture that began and developed without envisioning a day when women might be part of the landscape. Women often feel forced to leave the workplace because it continues to refuse to acknowledge our different but equal needs—think maternity care, sustainable hours, and wellness programming. The disconnect with our cycle is taking a toll. In fact, a growing number of women are leaving the workforce altogether. Since 1999, when female employment peaked at 77 percent, it has declined to less than 74 percent among women of reproductive age—about twenty-five to fifty-four, according to a 2017 New York Times article. About one in five women are opting for part-time work for noneconomic reasons—things like childcare, family obligations, and health issues—compared with about one in ten men, according to 2016 data from the US Bureau of Labor Statistics. Women are also turning away from corporate jobs in favor of entrepreneurship, starting new businesses at a rate higher than men. In a 2018 report from SCORE that drew on data from more than 20,000 small business owners, 47 percent of women said they had launched a new business within the past year compared with 44 percent of men. A desire for flexibility in their professional and personal lives ranked among the top reasons cited for choosing to start a business. "Creating balance and control over my own schedule was paramount for me as a mom to two young kids," said one of the study respondents.

Quitting or starting your own business aren't the only options. The more we take up space instead of trying to fit into the existing cultural norm, the more we create policy, and the more we normalize our biorhythmic differences, the sooner we can reimagine a work experience that not only accepts our biological reality, but that also creates a more sustainable human work environment as we race toward a future where AI and "always on" will challenge us even further. We've sought to eradicate gender bias with sexual harassment policies, hiring laws, and more, and we should push further here. But we can't wait for the corporate world or government agencies to do it for us. We have to be the change we wish to see. When you embrace this paradigm it will impact not only your own effectiveness from a personal professional standpoint, but also that of your team and your business, creating momentum to both reach your goals sustainably and change the culture.

Put Your Cycle to Work for You

How can you harness your cyclical nature to get into the flow and be your most productive and powerful self? First, remember you're not the same week to week, so stop expecting to work that way. Second, discard the cultural conditioning that has led us to believe that our hormones have a negative impact on our capabilities at work. Although our hormones can affect the way we think, feel, and relate to others, and influence what we're naturally interested in and stimulated by, there is not one single day or week when women are not just as capable as men in every work-related capacity. Yes, we are creatures of our chemistry, just like men are, but our cycle doesn't dictate that we have to lose a week each month to PMS and your period. It just means that by noticing these shifts and scheduling your days to work *with* your hormones, you can make your hormones work *for you* to help you sustain your energy, creativity, and productivity regardless of the demands on your schedule. Work smarter, not harder, by playing to your dominant interests based on your cycle phases. Here are the job-related strengths you possess during the four phases of your cycle, and how you can be a total boss during each one.

PHASE 1: PREPARE
Follicular Phase: 7–10 Days
Cyclical Strengths: Creativity and Planning

As estrogen rises during the follicular phase, it boosts the brain's working memory capability—the ability to handle complex processing tasks, according to research in *Frontiers in Science*. That's why you should schedule your most mentally challenging assignments for this week since estrogen's effect on your brain improves your ability to solve problems, strategize, and plan. Hormonal levels during this phase also spark creativity, making this the ideal time to focus your energy on new projects at work, starting a new business, or going after new clients. Engage in brainstorming sessions with your coworkers to take advantage of the boost in your cognitive creativity.

PHASE 2: OPEN UP
Ovulatory Phase: 3–4 Days
Cyclical Strengths: Communication and Collaboration

Surging estrogen during the ovulatory phase increases synaptic connections, which can boost mental sharpness, creativity, and communication skills, according to a study in the *Journal of Comparative Neurology*. Connecting with others is at the heart of this phase. This is the time to have important conversations with your team, your boss, or your clients. If you are able to schedule key conversations during the ovulatory phase, your heightened communication skills will allow you to convey your thoughts and opinions more clearly, as well as to be more receptive to those of others. If you're planning to ask for a promotion or a raise, or give that big presentation, do it during your ovulatory phase. Harness your communication powers to work on your marketing and advertising messaging, write a month's worth of blogs for your social media pages, or post a video of yourself giving a talk. Your physical energy is at one of its highest points during your ovulatory phase. Emotionally, you feel outgoing, upbeat, and revitalized. Tap into this energy by slotting lunches, client meetings, and after-work networking for this time.

PHASE 3: WORK
Luteal Phase: 10–14 Days
Cyclical Strengths: Completion, Nurturing, and Tending

As the corpus luteum expands and then is reabsorbed, your energy begins to focus and turn inward. You'll notice that you have the desire to get things done, making the luteal phase an ideal time to take care of work tasks. The particular ratio of estrogen to progesterone in this phase makes you notice things around you that you didn't see before. As a result, your brain begins to prioritize detail-driven responsibilities you may have ignored all month, such as putting together your quarterly report, finalizing contracts, or editing marketing content. You'll also have a natural desire to wrap up projects and bring things to completion. On the social side, try slowing down your networking and outside meetings during your luteal phase, so you won't feel needlessly exhausted and so you have time to do what feels most pleasurable to you this phase—which is getting your work done.

PHASE 4: REST
Menstrual Phase: 3–7 Days
Cyclical Strengths: Evaluation, Analysis, and Intuition

Analysis and evaluation are dominant desires now. During your menstrual phase, the communication between the right and left hemispheres of your brain is more powerful than at any other time. This communication enables you to judiciously evaluate how you're doing in your career or with a project and, if necessary, to begin identifying and making course corrections that will reposition you in the direction you want to be heading. Ask yourself how you performed in the previous month. Did you feel energetic and happy about your work, or overwhelmed and underappreciated? Are you working on the kinds of projects that excite you, or are you feeling uninspired at work? Is your career headed in the right direction and, if not, what are some steps you can take to veer it toward your overall goals? Use this time of the month to reassess your career goals. Do you still want the same things as last month or last year, or have you developed a new interest in following another path? Because of the way your hemispheres are firing back and forth during your period, you're also most likely to receive clear intuitive-gut messages during this phase. Check in. Listen to those subtle messages. Are they telling you a proposed project at work is a nonstarter? Are they indicating that one of two potential hires is the right one for the job? Are they screaming that your job is going nowhere, and it's time to start looking for a new gig? Pay attention! Use your female-centered planner to jot down what your gut is telling you each month. You may find that after a few months go by, your intuition during this phase is reinforcing certain thoughts you've had in general—whether those thoughts are about chang-ing jobs, changing careers, venturing out on your own as an entrepreneur, or knowing that you're already in the best place for you. Many women feel restless or dissatisfied during their period. Are those feelings caused by low levels of hormones during this phase, or is this your gut's way of telling you to make some changes in your life? When you optimize your hormonal pat-terns with the phase-based practices you're learning about, you'll be able to clearly understand what you need rather than feeling uncertain. Sometimes you need more rest; other times you need a bigger change. By decreasing the lag time in understanding and addressing your needs, you gain time to start living your best life sooner rather than later. And by tuning in and trusting your instincts, you can then take action in the next set of phases to work toward your vision.

For Katja, who owns a growing company, planning business initiatives and projects around her cycle keeps her fueled with energy and excitement for her work. "I use the Cycle Syncing Method™ to run my company to my best ability by not letting myself get run down," she says. "By organizing things based on priority level and my cycle phase, it makes it easier to keep things running smoothly." She says planning according to her cycle keeps her in a creative groove, seeing projects come to life and building her business in an intentional and purposeful way rather than simply reacting to the latest crisis.

The Cycle Syncing Method™: Work FLO

FOLLICULAR Duration: 7–10 Days Creativity	OVULATORY Duration: 3–4 Days Communication	LUTEAL Duration: 10–14 Days Administrative Tasks	MENSTRUAL Duration: 3–7 Days Evaluation and Intuition
Start new projects.	Have important conversations.	Handle administrative tasks.	Evaluate the past month.
Brainstorm with coworkers.	Ask for a raise or a promotion.	Organize desk/office/paperwork.	Review your monthly planner and notice patterns.
Tackle challenging mental tasks.	Go on job interviews.	Devote time to deep work.	Ask yourself if you like the projects you're working on.
Problem solve.	Write blogs and craft marketing copy.	Review documents, contracts, and financial reports.	Ask yourself if your career is heading in the right direction.
Seek out new clients.	Post on social media.	File expense account reports.	Analyze project data and reports.
Research new ideas.	Attend networking events.	Order supplies.	Reassess your career goals.
Make plans for the month ahead.	Negotiate deals.	Wrap up projects.	Listen to your gut instincts.
Make decisions.	Give talks and keynotes.	Help your team meet deadlines.	Take frequent breaks.
Dream big.	Go to happy hour with clients or colleagues.	Organize computer files.	Take a personal day (if possible).

Planning your work schedule around your cycle sounds great, but what if you have to do something that is out of sync with your cycle phase because of a project deadline? First, remember that you can do *anything* in any phase—you're infinitely creative, communicative, collaborative, and more—but there is a natural ebb and flow to these energies. Working with your cyclical strengths infuses you with more energy, so you have more time to focus on the things you want to do and have energy to spare to handle those time-sensitive projects. So it's fine to do tasks that are out of sync with your cycle, but they will create a slightly bigger energy drain on your system. Just practice what you learned in chapter 6 about boosting your self-care on those days to compensate for this energy drain.

Do You Have to Tell Everyone at Work About Your Hormones?

How exactly do you incorporate a cyclical practice at work? Do you have to be in sync with all your female colleagues in order to get anything done? Does it mean you have to let all your coworkers know where you are in your cycle at all times? Do you have to put up a menstrual chart on your office door that says, "I'm in the ABC phase. My strengths this week are XYZ." *No!* Engaging your second clock at work can be a silent, internal process. Men certainly don't go around telling their coworkers in the morning that their testosterone levels are peaking so it's time to have a meeting, do they? Of course not. To give you an idea of what engaging your infradian clock looks like, let me show you how it works at my company, FLO Living. I typically like to schedule strategic planning meetings when I'm in my follicular phase and ready to embark on new ideas. I might excitedly introduce five new projects, definitely biting off more than we can chew in a month. My marketing director might be in her menstrual phase—a time for evaluation and course correction—and will diplomatically let me know that the last time we took on five new projects at one time it wasn't very efficient. So we may narrow it down to one or two new initiatives. Our operations manager might be in her luteal phase—ideal for detail-oriented tasks—and will enthusiastically map out a list of necessary duties by department to make the new projects a success. And our social media manager might be in the ovulatory phase—when you're a communications star—and will share her vision for the best ways to share the new project with our wonderful community on social media. Because we're all in different phases of our cycle, we each bring different and necessary aspects to the meeting. It's actually better if our cycles *are not* synced up. This way, we get more diverse viewpoints. If we were all in the follicular phase at the same time, we might rally around all five new project ideas without pausing to consider that it might be too much to take on at once and not get down to the brass tacks of how to make them happen. In a follicular foray, the result might be lots of great ideas without the follow-up to bring them to fruition. I schedule meetings with people when it works for my cycle phases, and they do the same; we all benefit from not being in the same phase and move forward more efficiently—a truly unique way to collaborate.

The big takeaway here is that you don't have to worry where your female colleagues are in their cycles, and you don't have to tell anyone what phase you're in. Just support your own cycle and bring the best of your phase into meetings, brainstorming sessions, and your daily workflow. When each individual increases her own awareness of her biological rhythms, collectively leveraging that awareness will create a much more efficient process for everyone.

HONOR YOUR BUSINESS AND
PROJECT CYCLES, TOO

If you're a "solopreneur," business owner, or C-level exec, you'll notice that businesses and projects are cyclical, too. Like all things in nature, they follow the creation matrix—initiation, growth, completion, rest.

Many companies go through periods of rapid expansion, then con-traction. You might have high-revenue seasons followed by lower-income phases. With your projects, you may go through phases when you are building and launching new products, and phases when you evaluate performance and focus on new customer acquisition rather than product innovation. Working with these phases helps keep your projects and your business focused and moving forward. Most suc-cessful businesses do not do many things at the same time. Instead, they focus on one initiative for a month or a quarter and then move on to the next big idea. The fastest way to fail in business or with a project is to multitask, overextend your resources, and fall short of your goals. Just as it is on a personal level when you sync with your own cycle, you can gain so much insight on a business level from letting projects have space and time to evolve and go through their growth cycles.

Redefine What Success Means for You

In spite of the concrete findings in favor of right-timing, it can still be diffi-cult to resist the cultural conditioning that says you should work constantly to reach your career goals. Even after so many years of living in sync with my cycle and engaging my feminine energy, I can still get sucked back into that male paradigm and perpetual productivity mindset. For example, when we were working on the launch of the MyFLO app, I overextended myself. I was super excited about bringing this idea to life, because *WomanCode* read-ers had been asking for it for years, and because it makes it so much easier for women all over the world to adopt the Cycle Syncing Method™. I was so immersed in prepping for the launch with my team and powering through my to-do list that I went too long between meals, started feeling the effects of blood sugar ups and downs, and overworked my stress response system. I ended up getting a nasty cold, which forced me to return to the basics of the practice. I'm grateful my body shares her feedback on what I might be doing that isn't in my best interest.

I went back to syncing my food and exercise with my cycle and using my planner—the three key tools I use to get myself back on track fast. Thanks to this biohacking triage, I bounced back pretty quickly with renewed focus and energy. We shifted some of the launch strategy. I delegated more to my team. To make sure it didn't happen again, I made notes in my planner to remind myself to eat so I wouldn't fall into that starve-crash-burnout pattern again, and reprioritized my self-care, especially during times of intense stress. Now a successful launch or project means the whole experience is positive and spacious for me and my team.

You may occasionally find yourself getting sucked back into the old patterns we've been conditioned to follow. If this happens, don't be too hard on yourself. Listen to your body, biohack like a boss, and go back to working *with* your cycle so it will start working *for* you again. Your body provides the ultimate inner blueprint to your career success, as well as your success in every other area of your life. But it's important to remember success doesn't necessarily mean perpetually chasing goal after goal, sprinting up the corporate ladder, or sacrificing your personal life for your work. Anything that costs you your health, relationships, or happiness isn't really success. Just as you shouldn't be forced to suffer with period problems due to hormonal imbalances, you shouldn't have to suffer or make yourself sick to get ahead in the workplace. Fine-tune your own picture of career success. What does it look like to you? What is the most sustainable path for you? What would make you most happy? When you have a clear image of what career success is for you, make it happen and own it!

Six Steps for Cyclical Planning at Work

Now that you've seen the basics of how you can incorporate cyclical planning into a work environment that caters to the single clock, follow these six steps to keep building energy, stay in the flow, and maximize your creativity.

1. Do an end-of-month review. Set aside some time to look ahead at what's coming up with work deliverables.

2. Map out your cycle phases and slot projects in where you have the flexibility to do so.

3. Put in nonnegotiable deadlines wherever they fall in your cycle phases.

4. Remove some nonessential tasks from that phase and plan one self-care upgrade to compensate for the work that isn't in sync with your cycle.

5. Schedule all of your team meetings, and remind yourself to focus on bringing a point of view that is based on the strengths associated with that cycle phase to the conversation.

6. Encourage your coworkers to become aware of this as a team.

Lead like a Woman

Women are wired to lead in a unique way, and we can lead a change in the workplace by living and working in sync with our infradian clock. It's not just me saying this. Emerging research says so. A growing number of studies show it's a good idea to embrace your feminine energy in the workplace. In fact, tapping into your natural strengths is your secret strategy to achieving more with less effort. Being a woman in the workplace isn't a disadvantage; it's a huge benefit.

In 2014, leadership consultancy firm Zenger Folkman reviewed about sixteen thousand leaders, one-third of whom were women, to assess leadership effectiveness. In terms of overall leadership effectiveness, women outranked men 54.5 percent to 51.8 percent. When women and men were rated on sixteen leadership competencies—including taking initiative, displaying high integrity and honesty, practicing self-development, inspiring and motivating others, collaborating, and communicating powerfully—women scored higher than the men on twelve of them.

In their fascinating book *The Athena Doctrine*, bestselling authors and researchers John Gerzema and Michael D'Antonio set out to determine whether people are beginning to place greater value on female-centric traits and characteristics. The authors surveyed sixty-four thousand people in thirteen countries, and the results will blow your mind. Worldwide, 66 percent of people agree that the world would be a better place if men thought more like women. When it comes to leadership, typically female characteristics like collaboration and sharing credit are valued more than masculine traits like aggression and control. Other traits generally considered to be feminine—intuition, empathy, flexibility, and collaboration—were listed as desirable among leaders. And a majority of people cited traditionally feminine traits, including being creative, flexible, community-oriented, adaptable, giving, generous, cooperative, and nurturing, as essential to success. Overall, the authors discovered, "The countries with higher levels of feminine thinking and behavior also have higher per-capita GDP and higher reported quality of life." The *World Happiness Report 2018*, which ranked 156 countries across six factors, confirms these findings. The six factors used to gauge happiness include traditionally feminine traits, such as social support and generosity, as well as GDP, healthy life expectancy, freedom to make life choices, and freedom from corruption. The top five happiest countries, according to the report, are Finland, Norway, Denmark, Iceland, and Switzerland.

Still thinking you need to follow male patterns to succeed in your career? I'm going to let you in on something I've known intuitively for years: teams perform better when they include female members. Scientists proved it in 2010 when they administered intelligence tests to 699 people and then divided them into teams of two to five. Each team had to tackle a series of challenges, including brainstorming, problem solving, and decision-making—typical work stuff. The researchers gave each team a collective intelligence score based on their performance. Surprisingly, the teams with the highest individual IQ scores didn't get the top collective IQ scores. Teams with the most women on them notched the best collective IQ scores. It's compelling to imagine what additional benefits would arise from more women bringing their cyclical awareness, project management, and self-care into their work environment.

Who Runs the World? Women!

If we model a shift to a more sustainable career that nourishes and reenergizes us instead of draining us, we can inspire our coworkers to adopt a similar way of working. Women are powerful influencers, and I'm not just talking about on social media. Here in the United States, women are the nation's biggest consumers, and we drive the majority of buying decisions for our households. Statistics prove it. We control more than 50 percent of all personal wealth in the nation, and our purchasing power amounts to a staggering $5–$15 trillion annually. Returning to a work-life pattern that's in sync with our biochemistry's natural rhythms might be so influential it could shift our corporate and entrepreneurial culture to support this sustainable work model. Working based on both the 24-hour clock and the 28-day clock could ultimately drive up creativity and productivity, similar to the way Google's introduction of the campus office concept sparked companies to reevaluate office design, work culture, and corporate community. Syncing with our infradian clock may drive an even bigger conversation about how we can all live on this planet in a more sustainable way. Heal your hormones, do less, achieve more, enhance your personal happiness . . . save the planet. It's certainly worth a try.

The Future Is Female

Women are leading the charge to change the workplace in so many ways—demanding the end of sexual harassment and gender bias. Many companies have heard our demands and are making a commitment to gender equality, taking steps to narrow the wage gap, creating sexual harassment policies, and investing in corporate wellness programs to the tune of $8 billion a year. That investment can pay off. For every dollar companies spent on wellness programs, they see their absenteeism costs drop by $2.73 and medical costs fall by close to $3.27, according to a 2010 analysis in *Health Affairs*. These changes are promising, but there's one more piece that will move the needle—acknowledging a woman's infradian rhythm. In the space of being safe and free to work how we want, perhaps we can finally begin to include our reality in work culture.

In other countries, women's hormonal health is taken into consideration. For example, did you know that in some countries, such as India, South Korea, and Japan, women are allowed to take the day off for "menstrual leave" if they have painful periods? And that in the UK, women receive a full year of *paid* maternity leave? In the US, the Family and Medical Leave Act entitles women to only twelve weeks of *unpaid* leave. A growing number of major US firms, however, offer greater incentives to attract and retain female employees, especially at the management level. Google provides women with mentoring groups like Google Women in Engineering and Women@Google, gives new moms five months of paid maternity leave, and allows for flexible hours and work-from-home options. Global consulting firm Deloitte boasts women's leadership development programs, women mentors, and flexible scheduling. At health care company Johnson & Johnson, a women's leadership initiative aims to promote female employees from within the company and offers other female-friendly perks.

Corporate America is starting to wake up to the fact that we need to address women's needs in the workplace. I'm encouraged by the corporations that have invited me to share this message with their employees about how reenvisioning success and productivity through a female lens could unlock our competitive edge. Teams are simply engaging the Cycle Syncing Method™ themselves. It doesn't cost anything to implement or require any corporate policy changes. I was really thrilled to be the first woman to speak about female biohacking at the 2018 SXSW conference. Until I hit the stage before a packed audience, not a single presenter had ever broached the subject of how getting in tune with our 28-day clock is the key to women thriving in their bodies and in the workplace. This watershed moment made clear that corporations need to acknowledge our second clock and women need a new paradigm to define productivity and success in the workplace.

If you're a corporate leader, small business owner, or entrepreneur, pay attention to how this applies to your own workplace. Think about what you're offering and also what you're modeling for your employees. If you're running yourself ragged, your female employees will be compelled to do so, too, and they'll be more likely to fall victim to hormonal problems, health issues, mental fatigue, and burnout. Ultimately, these employees will be less satisfied and more inclined to jump ship. Considering that women make the workplace smarter, more effective, and more profitable, think about how important it is to respect their hormone reality. We know bioindividualism is the future in medicine: biohacking at work will drive individual and corporate growth. Biohacking for women at work will offer them a paradigm to define productivity and success on their own terms. We have to make the work environment work for us to include our needs around health, maternity leave, and motherhood. Here at FLO Living, we're operating at max efficiency and peak performance because the women who work here are in the zone and happier. A positive work environment fosters success—a win-win for everyone.

With all of this overwhelming evidence, it's clear that letting your feminine side shine can help you achieve sustainable career goals. Following the natural rhythms of your cycle and scheduling your days in tune with your internal biological clock gives you a competitive advantage. And by supporting the monthly hormonal changes that impact the way you think, make decisions, and create during each phase of your cycle, you will bring the best of yourself at all times to all that you do.

By learning to focus on doing one thing at the ideal time rather than trying to do everything at once, you will become more efficient, get into flow mode more often, and boost your overall performance. Dropping the pressure of constant productivity in favor of biohacking your creative process with food, exercise, and right-timing will allow you to do more of the work that matters to you, and do it better. And when you wrap up a job well done and take some time to reflect and learn from the experience, it's like hitting the reset button on your system. You end up feeling like you're doing less, and you come back reenergized and ready to go for the next big idea so you can achieve more and feel great about it. And this dynamic helps you build more energy for other areas of your life.

CHAPTER 8

Get More of What You Want in Sex and Relationships

If you want to be treasured, you have to treasure yourself first and then show someone how to treasure you.
—REGENA THOMASHAUER

Let's be real. If you're like many women—whether you're straight, gay, bisexual, or anywhere else on the sexuality spectrum—you probably aren't getting enough of what you want out of your sex life. Sure, you may tell your friends—and yourself—that your sex life is fine, but if you're being completely honest, it could be better. You aren't the only one. In a 2015 survey by Healthy Women, 60 percent of women admitted their sex life wasn't as good as it could be. That's because we aren't getting enough sex, and we aren't enjoying the sex we're having to the fullest. A 2017 study in *Archives of Sexual Behavior* found that Americans are having less sex than we did ten years ago; when the researchers controlled for age and time period, they discovered it's millennials and the iGen crowd who are having the least amount of sex compared with other generations. Even those born in the 1930s—*yes, your great-grandparents*—were having more sex than today's young adults. I hear about low libido and unfulfilling sex every day from the women who come to me for hormonal help.

Mariel is one of them. She had recently had a second child, and between the lifestyle adjustment, which was causing massive fatigue and some relationship tension, and her unresolved postpartum hormonal imbalance, her sex drive had flatlined. Remembering how things had been before the kids were born, she wanted to get that spark back for herself and her relationship. When she came to me in search of help for her period problems, she didn't fully appreciate how regaining hormonal balance would massively impact her sex drive. In addition, she gained the knowledge that her libido changes throughout her cycle. Now, she's confidently enjoying higher-quality orgasms on a more regular basis and feeling organic interest in sexual experiences with herself and her partner. Like Mariel, when you approach your sex life and relationships with your monthly cycle in mind, you can biohack your way to a heightened sex drive, more pleasurable sex, better orgasms, and a stronger relationship. Remember, however, that there are two people in a partnership, and it's important to know not only where you are in your cycle but also to know where your partner is with their circadian and hormonal patterns. This chapter gives you the six-part plan to get you to a more fulfilling sex life, with your hormones leading the way!

CALL ME BY MY NAME

If you take your sex and relationship cues from our general culture, you're probably used to having your sex organs discussed using euphemistic terms like "down there," "coochie," or "vajayjay." If we are confused about how exactly to reference our physiology, however, we won't feel confident about how to clearly communicate our desires to our partners. It's essential to talk about your body, and that's why I'm going to call your miraculous parts by their names—vagina, labia, clitoris, and so on. Only when we name and claim our bodies and hormonal reality will we be able to use them to get the pleasure we deserve.

Step 1: Engage the Four Stages of Arousal

Whatever you learned about the birds and the bees, I can guarantee it didn't do justice to the awe-inspiring reality of your biological and neuro-chemical sexual response. If most of what you expect about your sexual response is set against the standards of pornography or romantic movies, you probably think you should be able to go from zero to climax in no time. But that's just not how the female body operates. Getting turned on and reaching orgasm is a specific process that you can engage with reliable success once you know about it. For women, arousal involves four distinct stages: tumescence, orgasmic plateau, climax, and the refractory period. Understanding the mechanics of your sexual response is the first step toward biohacking the arousal process to prime your body for better orgasms and guaranteeing yourself consistent pleasure.

Stage 1: Tumescence

It's common knowledge that men get an erection as part of the sexual process, but did you know that women's sexual anatomy undergoes a similar process of engorgement called tumescence? This stage can begin the moment you feel the desire to have sex or within seconds of erotic stimulation. In some women, or during some phases of your cycle, it can take longer to start feeling aroused (how each phase of your cycle affects the arousal process is detailed later in the chapter). When arousal does kick in, your heart starts pumping faster, your breathing accelerates, and your blood pressure rises. Your brain's limbic system—the emotional center—sets off a chain reaction that leads to the release of a flood of neurochemicals that make you even more interested in sex than you already were. The release of the chemical nitric oxide increases blood flow to the genitals, causing the outer and inner labia to swell and become more responsive to pleasurable stimulation. Your clitoris—the seat of eight thousand nerve endings exclusively designed to generate the most pleasure for you—engorges as well, allowing maximum surface area for those nerve endings to fulfill their destiny. Vaginal lubrication is triggered, and the tissues of the vaginal canal engorge, making it expand and lengthen. The increase in blood flow may also cause the breasts to swell and the nipples to harden.

Stage 2: Orgasmic Plateau

As more stimulation takes place, your heart, breathing, and blood pressure continue to rise. The increase in blood flow may cause a flush that colors your face, chest, or abdomen. As if by magic, the increase in blood flow also intensifies the color of your labia, from its relaxed paler shade to a darker version of itself. In preparation for increased stimulation, the vaginal opening narrows while the part near the cervix expands, intensifying sensations of pleasure. Activity heightens in the brain's pleasure centers while the regions associated with anxiety take a break. The neurochemicals dopamine and epinephrine rise. Your clitoris becomes hypersensitive and retracts under the clitoral hood. As you near climax, your cerebellum sends signals to your muscles, causing them to tighten. You're almost there . . . *but wait!* So many of us are in such a rush to climax as quickly as possible that we miss out on the massive hormonal and health benefits of the orgasmic plateau phase. If you were to think of the climactic experience on a scale of one to ten, with climax being a ten, then your orgasmic plateau would be anywhere from a four to an eight. Spending more time here will generate more oxytocin and nitric oxide, which will flush cortisol, improve your period, your fertility, the regularity of ovulation, and your immune function. Oxytocin also makes you feel more connected to your partner. Together they can even lead to a bigger, more intense orgasm. So even though you may be tempted to rush to climax, do yourself and your body a favor by lingering in this phase by getting close to climax then backing away, repeating this edging process while staying between a four and an eight for as close to twenty minutes as possible, or more. Do this twice a week to reap all the benefits.

Stage 3: Climax

Climax is the most fleeting of the four stages, lasting mere seconds when the clitoris's eight thousand nerve endings—*that's twice as many nerve endings as the penis, FYI*—have had enough and need a break. Your brain's production of oxytocin, serotonin, and DHEA spikes, putting a hold on the release of the stress hormone cortisol and causing waves of pleasure to wash over you. Your muscles spasm, causing your vaginal walls to contract rhythmically. Your back may arch, and your hands and feet may clutch involuntarily. Some women may experience female ejaculation, which involves the secretion of vaginal fluid. (And contrary to a common myth, no, this fluid isn't urine.)

Stage 4: Refractory Period

As you bask in the glow of that oxytocin and nitric oxide rush after climax, your body returns to normal. Your heartbeat, blood flow, and breathing slow down; your sex organs return to their normal size and color; and your muscles relax. Your cervix, however, remains open for up to half an hour, a useful fact for couples trying to conceive, so sperm has time to find its way into the uterus. In men, the refractory period prevents them from being able to experience climax again for a while. But for women—*lucky us!*—we need only a brief resting period for those clitoral nerve endings to calm down and get set up for another ride through these four steps. In fact, many woman can experience multiple clitoral orgasms (although there are other types, the vast majority of women can achieve clitoral orgasms most easily). All that's needed for you to discover what's possible for your pleasure is to work these four stages and enjoy what each has to offer.

Step 2: Sync Your Orgasm with Your Cycle

The second part of biohacking your orgasms lies in syncing with the four phases of your cycle. The same way your monthly hormonal changes affect your energy levels, moods, cognitive powers, creativity, immune system, and other biological systems, they also impact how you experience the four stages of arousal, your interest in sex, and even the intensity of your orgasms. Your needs, emotions, energy, and desires fluctuate from week to week with the rise and fall of your hormones. If there are some days when you're not in the mood, you need more foreplay to feel hot and heavy, or it takes longer to climax, it's not because there's something wrong with you. No need to get in your head about it—it's just your biochemistry doing its normal thing. The more you know how it works, the less you'll be left unnecessarily wondering whether something is wrong with your sex drive. When this information finally sinks in, you'll realize you can stop blaming yourself, let go of the guilt, and get the love you deserve when you want it the most. You'll also gain a more thorough understanding that your partner's needs may fluctuate on a daily or monthly basis, so you can become more attuned to your partner's desires too. Throughout this next section, I'll describe healthy sex drive patterns throughout the cycle and give you pointers on how to support your body, relationship, and sexual pleasure in each of the four phases. Sex will never be the same again. If you read through this and realize your libido may be suffering from hormonal imbalances, then refer back to the Biohacking Tool Kit section to learn what you can do to regain your drive.

PHASE 1: PREPARE
Follicular Phase: 7–10 Days
Cyclical Focus: Novelty

Body focus: As your follicular phase begins, your sex hormones—estrogen, progesterone, and testosterone—are all lying low. Estrogen helps keep the vagina lubricated, and because it's in scarce supply now, your vagina may not be as wet as it is at other times of the month. This dryness is completely natural and doesn't mean there's anything wrong with you. In fact, the follicular phase is one of two dry phases you'll experience during your cycle. To optimize your orgasms during the dry phase, you should absolutely use a lubricant. Be sure to let your sexual partner know you're in a dry phase so they can reach for the lube for you.

Relationship focus: As you saw in chapter 3 when you learned about how your brain chemistry changes across the menstrual cycle, you're more receptive to novel experiences and filled with energy during the follicular phase, so get creative and try something new with your partner. Novel experiences bring you together, create lasting memories, and help you bond more closely. Take a cooking class together, visit a museum, hike a new trail, or take a weekend trip to a new city. In a long-term relationship, it's very important to keep things fresh and exciting by breaking out of your routine. The follicular phase provides an ideal opportunity—and reminder—to try new things on a monthly basis. Another bonus is that doing anything that amps up the brain's production of oxytocin and nitric oxide—like getting outside for a run together or trying something new—makes you feel closer to each other. It's a bonding mechanism that reminds you why you love this person and primes you for intimacy and sex.

Sex focus: This is the perfect time to keep it fresh by exploring innovative ways of pleasuring each other—experiment with new positions, give tantric massage techniques a try, or get into some role-playing. Linger in the orgasmic plateau phase so you can build up to a satisfying climax. The nitric oxide and oxytocin released during the orgasmic plateau and climax will strengthen your emotional bond.

PHASE 2: OPEN UP
Ovulatory Phase: 3–4 Days
Cyclical Focus: Receiving

Body focus: With estrogen and testosterone surging, your sex drive will be in overdrive. Because of these hormonal changes, your body produces up to twenty times more cervical fluid, making your vagina wetter than usual. This is one of the wet phases of your cycle and the time when your body is primed for receiving—receiving sperm for conception purposes, receiving attention from possible mates, and, most important, receiving maximal pleasure. Remember the concept of taking the egg approach from chapter 6? Think of yourself like the egg, waiting in the uterus. The egg does not chase the sperm; it sends out a signal to drive them into a frenzy, then waits to receive them. You should take a cue from the egg, and get what you want, just the way you want it.

Relationship focus: This is a great time for bonding and socializing with your significant other. When you hang out only with each other, it can lead to feelings of isolation and boredom, so use this time for dining out with other couples, hosting a dinner party at home, or going to other social gatherings. You'll feel more talkative and engaged, making this the ideal time to talk to your mate about your personal and couple goals, dreams, and fantasies. With my husband, I like to take this time to touch base on what we want from our future together and look ahead to see where we want to be in five, ten, or twenty years. This communication makes us feel closer to each other and strengthens our bond. If you're single, this is also an ideal time to go on first dates. Your increased communication skills make you more magnetic, and your soaring estrogen levels make you naturally more alluring during your fertile phase. In fact, a 2013 study in *Hormones and Behavior* found that both men and women find women's facial features and voices most attractive during the ovulatory phase.

Sex focus: One of the best things about the ovulatory phase is that you're naturally more orgasmic at this time of the month. And since your body is geared to draw more attention during this phase, the best practice is for you to focus on receiving. Take advantage of your super orgasmic powers, and encourage your partner to take the time to pleasure you just the way you like it. And don't feel guilty about it! We've been so conditioned to take care of everybody else and put our needs last that it may be hard for you to wrap your head around the concept of letting a sexual encounter be focused on your pleasure. Of course, you can reciprocate;

but make sure your needs are met first, then give. And since you're more verbally oriented during the ovulatory phase, don't hesitate to ask for what you want—"More to the left, slow down, faster, don't stop," and so on. If you have a hard time being on the receiving end of all that attention, use this as a way to become more self-aware about why it's difficult for you, and work through this difficulty in your sexual encounters. This process can help you become more comfortable receiving in other areas of your life, too.

PHASE 3: WORK
Luteal Phase: 10–14 Days
Cyclical Focus: Clarity

Body focus: The luteal phase is made up of two parts. During the first half of the luteal phase, you have robust levels of estrogen, progesterone, and testosterone, so you're well-lubricated—making this half a wet phase—and more readily in the mood for sexual activity. During the second half of the luteal phase, these hormones begin to decrease in concentration, and so does your lubrication—making this half a dry phase—and your interest in sex may be lessened.

Relationship focus: The first half of the luteal phase can feel like an extended ovulatory phase, so enjoy. As soon as estrogen recedes from your brain chemistry during the second half of the luteal phase, however, you'll be able to be more honest with yourself about anything that needs to be addressed in your relationship. Estrogen acts as a social lubricant and makes you more willing to overlook problems. If there's something that isn't working, you can bet it will bubble up to the surface during this phase. You simply won't be able to ignore the truth the way you can in the first half of your cycle, when you're bathed in high levels of estrogen and can let things slide. Our cultural conditioning dictates, however, that you shouldn't believe yourself in this phase, that you're just being "hormonal." In reality, your cycle has baked in the ideal time for you to prioritize your needs and address any issues that are bothering you. This phase is like a monthly checkup for the emotional health of your partnership and a major opportunity to move in the right direction and deepen your relationship. This isn't something that should be avoided or feared. If you're hormonally balanced, you'll be able to express your insights in a loving, constructive way. When hormones are imbalanced, however, you might find it harder to distinguish between PMS-related irritability and discontent with your partner or your relationship. Keep observing these feelings for a few cycles while you work on balancing your hormones. Either way, the truth of your feelings is your body's way of helping you have the relationship you deserve. If these feelings don't change after you balance your hormones, you might want to rethink your commitment to your mate. In fact, the easiest time for you to break up with someone would be during the second half of the luteal phase or during the menstrual phase. The luteal phase is also an ideal time to focus on domestic duties. It might not sound sexy, but to get the most pleasure out of your relationship all month long you do have to attend to the day-to-day stuff of life—budgeting, cleaning, and organizing. Doing it together gives you another chance to bond.

Sex focus: During the first half of the luteal phase, you may still be enjoying a strong sex drive. However, your sex drive is likely to start to wane during the second half of the luteal phase. This part of the phase is best suited to slower sex. See whether you respond better with lots of foreplay and lubricant.

USING YOUR CYCLE TO HELP WITH BREAKING UP

You can use your cycle to help you make decisions and take actions about relationships and commitments. I recommend going through many, many hormonal cycles with your life partner before you fully commit. Feeling yourself in relation to their energy as you shift through every phase is an excellent way to deepen your emotional intimacy with your partner and ensures you can live with them in every phase.

I remember noticing the value of cyclical awareness as it applied to relationships for the first time in one of my relationships. With every month, I was only at ease in the first half of my cycle—the follicular and ovulatory phases. Like clockwork, come the luteal and menstrual phases, I felt unsatisfied in my relationship. It was clear to me in the second half of the cycle what the issues were and why I wanted to end the relationship. But once ovulation started, I was more willing to overlook these issues. I had to go through a couple of cycles where I understood that the truth—with a capital T—of the situation was coming forward in my luteal and menstrual phases, and I needed to act on this precious information. So I timed the breakup during my luteal phase when I was strongest in my conviction—in my truth—and that made it so much easier.

Trust that as you live through many cycles with your partner, your body will offer you her feedback about a relationship. And if you do need to end it, use your hormonal advantage to do so.

PHASE 4: REST
Menstrual Phase: 3–7 Days
Cyclical Focus: Recharge

Body focus: As your hormone levels fall, your interest in lovemaking may dwindle, and you might even want physical distance from your mate. However, something else is at play here. Right before your bleed, your uterus increases slightly in volume. As a result, it's heavier on the pelvic floor, which can create pleasurable pressure on your whole genital structure. Even though your hormones aren't driving your desire for sex, the pressure of your uterus may stimulate the nerve endings in your G-spot, inner labia, and the clitoral legs (the paired "cura" that descend from the sides of the clitoris) and put you in the mood for sex. Many people assume that menstrual blood would act as a lubricant, but in fact it does not. The more friction you apply to it and the more air gets on it, the drier it becomes. It's similar to having blood on your skin; it dries out quickly. So contrary to popular belief, this is not a wet phase; it's a dry phase, and you'll need lube for maximal pleasure.

Relationship focus: You may want some alone time during the menstrual phase, and it can be very beneficial in helping you recharge and connect to yourself. Indulge in self-care practices that make you feel good, and enjoy some "me time"—read a good novel, watch a movie, journal, or have a phone chat with a friend. Spending quality time with yourself is always healthy and can boost your appreciation for your partner, whether you engage in sex during this phase or not.

Sex focus: In our culture, there's a stigma that says period sex is taboo. Many women think they should avoid sex and avert their partners from engaging during this time, because of the negative way we've been conditioned to perceive our menstrual blood. You may even have a history of dating people who are turned off by your bleed, typically because of a lack of correct information. Nature intends for you to be pleasured all month long. When your hormones are low, your uterus picks up the slack to stimulate you from within and build your interest in sex. It's up to you to explore and experiment with sex during your period. Some women find it hugely beneficial to relax the fascia that holds the uterus. Think of this as a sort of internal massage that can relax the action of the uterus and diminish cramps. Clitoral stimulation will release a flood of nitric oxide and oxytocin while flushing cortisol to help resolve any sort of menstrual discomfort. On both a physical and hormonal level, sex during your bleed definitely can be beneficial *if you want it*. Some women do prefer taking a break from sex during menstruation because of the natural dip in their sex drive. If you're concerned about your sheets, there are period sex blankets and other great products to get around that situation. Whichever way you feel—go-time or no-go—it's all good as long as you follow what your body and hormones are telling you to do, not cultural taboos.

The Cycle Syncing Method™: Love FLO

FOLLICULAR Novelty Duration: 7–10 Days	OVULATORY Receiving Duration: 3–4 Days	LUTEAL Clarity Duration: 10–14 Days	MENSTRUAL Recharge Duration: 3–7 Days
Take a trip somewhere new.	Enjoy dinner with friends.	Do domestic projects together.	Indulge in self-care.
Go to a show or museum.	Go to a party.	Evaluate your relationship.	Read a good book.
Try new sexual positions.	Talk with your mate about sex fantasies.	Cook together and stay in for date night.	Watch your favorite movie.
Get outside and do something physical together.	Discuss your relationship goals.	Ask what you can do to make the relationship better.	Ask for a foot massage from your partner.
Focus on foreplay and use lubricant.	Go on first dates.	Enjoy quickies in the first half of this phase.	Spend quality time with yourself.
Pay attention to the orgasmic plateau phase.	Have multiple orgasms.	Enjoy more foreplay in the second half of this phase.	Always use lubricant in this phase.

SOLO PLAY IS ESSENTIAL

No partner? No problem! And even if you do have a partner, it's essential for you to cultivate a self-pleasuring practice for two reasons: (1) it helps keep your hormones balanced, and (2) it increases your self-awareness of your sexual response, so that when you do engage in partnered sexual activity you're able to share your road map to pleasure with your partner so your needs will be met more consistently. Self-pleasure feels great, can alleviate PMS symptoms like cramps and moodiness, and is connected with improved body image and sexual functioning. Just keep your body's cyclical pattern in mind. Your needs and desires depend entirely on what's happening with your hormones, and knowing this information will empower you to access the right tools in your arsenal at the right time. Speaking of tools, if you want to maximize the benefits of alone time, skip the vibrator during wet phases. These sex toys are like taking an expressway to climax, and you miss out on many of the benefits of the orgasmic plateau phase.

Follicular phase: Use lube, try something new, and, if you want, experiment with toys to see what new stimulation you can create.

Ovulatory phase: Skip the vibrator and opt for your hand instead; linger in the orgasmic plateau phase.

Luteal phase: During the first half of this phase, ditch the vibrator and use your hand instead. Lube, and, if you like, the vibrator, are good for the second half of this phase. In both halves of this phase, set the mood for yourself—put on something that makes you feel good, take a bath, light a candle, and indulge all your senses.

Menstrual phase: If interested, use lube and turn on the vibrator. This can be a great cramp reliever.

Step 3: Nourish Your Libido and Orgasm

Did you know that certain foods and supplements can boost your sex life? Here are some of the best sex enhancers. Many of these are found in the FLO Balance Supplements (www.FLOliving.com/supplements).

B vitamins (found in foods like nuts, seeds, meat, poultry, fish, eggs, and dark leafy vegetables) help calm stress, which is one of the most common sex-drive killers. Specifically, during stressful times, B vitamins prevent dopamine and serotonin from breaking down, leaving adequate amounts of these feel-good neurochemicals so you feel energized instead of drained. When you aren't overwhelmed by stress, you're much more likely to be ready for sex.

Zinc (found in foods like meat, shellfish, legumes, and seeds) promotes healthy testosterone levels by blocking an enzyme called aromatase that converts this important hormone into estrogen. Unless your body has enough zinc, aromatase can transform too much testosterone into estrogen, lowering testosterone levels. And you know what happens then—your sex drive takes a nosedive. Decades of studies have found that zinc supplementation leads to an increase in testosterone levels in men. For example, a 2000 study in the *Journal of Exercise Physiology Online* found that men who took 30 milligrams of zinc on a daily basis experienced an uptick in their testosterone levels. Unfortunately, the researchers didn't include women in this study.

Magnesium (found in foods like almonds, avocados, dark leafy greens, and watermelon) reduces the amount of testosterone that binds to SHBG, allowing more of the hormone to remain in the bloodstream. Higher levels of the bioactive-free testosterone leads to more sexual desire. Magnesium also reduces symptoms of anxiety and depression, according to a 2017 study in *PLOS ONE*, which sets you up for enhanced enjoyment.

Omega-3 fatty acids (found in foods like salmon, walnuts, sardines, and flaxseeds) play a role in preventing hormonal imbalance and contribute to the release of the neurotransmitters dopamine, serotonin, GABA, and glutamate. Balanced hormones and healthy neurotransmitter function improve your health and mood in so many ways, they also make you more likely to give bedroom action the green light. A 2014 study also points to a link between omega-3 fatty acid consumption and nitric oxide, a gas produced naturally by the body that promotes better blood flow. More blood circulating to your lady parts causes them to swell during the sexual arousal stage, leading to bigger and better orgasms.

Probiotics (found in foods like sauerkraut, tempeh, and kombucha) may not have a direct effect on your sex hormones or reproductive organs, but probiotics *do* impact your overall gut health, which is linked to moods and mental health. You're already well aware of how much your moods impact your sex drive. A 2017 study in the *Annals of General Psychiatry* linked psychiatric disorders like depression to imbalanced gut bacteria. Other research, including a 2005 study in *Medical Hypotheses*, suggests probiotics have the potential to restore microbiome balance.

PHEROMONES

Pheromones are scented airborne molecules humans secrete that can be powerful aphrodisiacs or strong repellents. You may not be consciously aware that a person's scent is turning you on or off; you just know intuitively that you're wildly attracted to, or totally not into, that person who's chatting you up at the bar. A 2013 look at pheromones and their effects on women's sexuality in *Facts, Views & Vision in ObGyn* suggests the molecules play a positive role in our moods and sexual response as well as in mate selection, proving even further that our biology often drives our behavior. You can even biohack your male partner's pheromones to boost your sex drive during the luteal phase of your cycle, when your interest in lovemaking fades. Here's how I do it. During the luteal phase I prepare dishes for my husband with celery because it's packed with male steroids called androstenene and androstenol that cause him to pump out more of his intoxicating pheromones. The more of these sexy scented molecules he secretes, the more attractive he becomes. And the more likely I am to get in the mood. It's a win-win.

Adaptogens—including maca powder, ashwagandha, reishi mushroom, and holy basil—are natural substances that can support your sex drive when you are under stress or when you are perimenopausal or postpartum. Check the resources section for more on adaptogens.

MAKE A SUPER SEX-DRIVE SALAD

Here's a recipe that's chock-full of the micronutrients just listed that are libido enhancers for both sexes. Enjoy!

Super Sex-Drive Salad

6 slices watermelon	2 stalks celery
1 bunch asparagus	2 tablespoons olive oil
¼ cup raw pumpkin seeds	2 tablespoons lemon juice
¼ cup raw walnuts	Sea salt or pink salt to taste

Cut asparagus into two-inch pieces and steam lightly, so they are still crunchy. Cut watermelon into matchsticks the size of the asparagus pieces. Use a spice grinder to grind the pumpkin seeds and walnuts. Toss into the salad. Break out your mandolin, shred some celery paper-thin, and sprinkle it on top of the salad. Drizzle with a little extra virgin olive oil and a pinch of sea salt and lemon juice.

Step 4: Loop Your Partner into Your Cycle

Wouldn't it be great if your partner were inherently tapped into your secret desires and needs and could give you what you needed sexually? It is great not to have to settle for less, and it's possible when you're tuned in to your cyclical needs. When you're able to educate your partner about not only where you are in your monthly cycle but also what that means for your physical, sexual, and relationship needs, your partner will find it so much easier to deliver what you want when you want it.

No matter how many years you've been together, you should never assume that your partner knows where you are in your cycle. It's up to you to let your partner know you're in a dry phase, for example. Whether you're in a female-male or same-sex relationship, you might say, "Let's keep the lube right next to the bed for easy access this week." And when your partner goes to get the lube, smile and give them some positive reinforcement. It helps to explain and give directions and clue your partner in to where you are in your cycle and what you'd like to make everything flow more smoothly. When your partner knows they're more likely to be able to give you what you need and create massive pleasure for you, it makes your partner feel empowered and creates a beautiful dynamic that increases emotional intimacy in addition to more satisfying sex.

I meet with many women who feel sexually shut down or emotionally disconnected from their partners because these women let too much go unsaid about what they need on a physical level. "Sometimes I want my partner to go slower when they go down on me." "Sometimes I need more foreplay." "I'd like to try some new positions that might stimulate my clitoris more during intercourse." These are just some of the things I hear from women. These women are left feeling unfulfilled, and I would bet their partners feel frustrated, too. Your partner can't guess what's going to turn you on each time. They might think that because you went wild over something they did last week you'll want that same thing again this week. And they don't understand why it doesn't have the same orgasm-producing effect week after week.

I've been with my husband for many years, and I still make sure he knows what phase I'm in and what kind of foreplay I need. He appreciates the information because it sets him up for success with me. When he makes me feel good, it makes him feel good, too. This practice of informing him of my hormonal and physiological reality has also gone beyond our sex lives. When I was pregnant and getting close to my delivery date, I prepared a four-page document for him about the four stages of labor, what he needed to know about them, and what he could do to maximize my comfort in each of them. Yes, I biohacked my labor and my husband was fully aware of what he was getting into when he married the woman who started the Period Club. And when the time came and I was dealing with my experience of labor, I didn't have to try to explain to him what was happening, nor did he feel clueless or helpless. I didn't have to say a word—and at the time I could not have articulated, for example, "Okay, honey, now I need you to apply counterpressure right above my hips to minimize pain." While your everyday sex life might not require a four-page document, when you understand your process and advocate for your needs, things can flow more naturally, especially in the bedroom.

If it feels overwhelming to keep track of your hormonal phase and notify your partner, you can simplify the process with one of the features in the MyFLO app, which alerts your partner when you enter a new phase of your menstrual cycle and gives them a heads-up about what's going on hormonally and physically. The app is just an additional way you can keep your partner in the loop for a smoother relationship. This can be a big benefit if you're one of the many women who struggle to tell your partner what you want and need sexually, or if you don't want to have to verbalize what you need during sex. Sometimes you just want to have one of those hot-and-heavy sessions where you and your partner are perfectly in sync and hitting all the right spots. The gift of looping your partner into your cyclical awareness beforehand is that you don't have to talk about it while you're in the middle of things. Your partner will already know what you need, so you can just get in the flow and enjoy the ride. You really *can* biohack your way to a better relationship!

It Takes Two

So much of what I'm sharing with you in this chapter focuses on what *you* can do to enhance your sex life and relationship. But achieving this kind of open, communicative, satisfying sex life and relationship isn't all on your shoulders. Just as you need to take responsibility to keep your hormones optimized and learn about your orgasmic process so you can enjoy all these benefits with your partner, you need to find a significant other who is invested in optimizing their own well-being and education, because the quality of their health and awareness will impact the quality of your relationship. You need a partner who will embrace this knowledge and actively participate in this new paradigm—someone who's willing to encourage you to live in sync with your cycle. Luckily, with wellness becoming more mainstream, it can be easier to find someone who is up for exploring and adopting a new relationship paradigm. If you haven't met your life partner yet, choose wisely! Imagine dating someone with cyclical awareness as the foundation of your relationship from the get-go. That awareness will make those important conversations and transitions down the road much smoother. When you're both healthy and hormonally balanced, it makes it so much easier to optimize your emotional and sexual life.

Step 5: Tune In to the Cycles of Long-Term Relationships

Okay, it's not all about sex: falling in love is one of the most blissful human experiences in the universe. When you meet your soulmate, you think the rush of attraction and lust will last forever. But true love goes through changes similar to all living things in nature. C. G. Jung, the influential twentieth-century Swiss psychiatrist and psychoanalyst, wrote extensively on something he called the inner marriage, an attempt to balance the feminine and masculine within ourselves. In his view, the drive to marry is merely an external manifestation of our desire for inner wholeness. Psychoanalyst Marion Woodman, who has authored numerous popular books exploring feminine consciousness, wrote in *The Maiden King* that both genders needed to incorporate elements of the other to be whole. This primal urge for oneness drives us to seek a partner in life for a long-term relationship. But making a relationship last can be hard work. The relationship must be reinvented at four critical inflection points during the life cycle as a whole. Just as knowing how to work with each of the four phases of your menstrual cycle is a huge advantage, so too is knowing that these four stages of a relationship are a normal and expected part of the journey. Having this knowledge in advance can help you navigate the process with increased awareness, compassion, and grace. By recognizing the interplay of your biochemistry and identity throughout them all, you can have a wonderful long-lasting relationship. You could even be one of those lucky, loving couples celebrating fifty years of togetherness. But if you fall headlong into these transitions without understanding the biological and neurochemical underpinnings that drive them, your relationship could be vulnerable at any one of the inflection points.

Stage 1: Romantic Courtship

The courtship stage is all about novelty and passion—which in a way makes it similar to the follicular and ovulatory phase of your cycle. In the early, blissful days of a relationship, you can't stop thinking about that special someone and can't keep your hands off each other. The infatuation is so strong, you think about each other constantly and want to spend every minute of every day with that special someone. You may feel intoxicated or completely out of control. And in a way, you are. When you're in the throes of romantic love, your biology works overtime to push you to mate. Helen Fisher, a scientist and the author of *Why We Love: The Nature and Chemistry of Romantic Love*, performed a study of college students who were madly in love. Fisher scanned the brains of the young lovers and discovered that showing them images of their sweetheart fired up certain brain regions and neurochemical circuits. Specifically, she found that the brain's reward system—involved in drive and motivation to seek out pleasurable things—lights up as well as areas that spew out dopamine. Dopamine increases the production of a host of other hormones and chemicals, including testosterone and norepinephrine. As you recall, your testosterone levels naturally rise during your ovulatory phase, which intensifies your sex drive and pushes you to seek out a mate. Norepinephrine acts as a stimulant that revs up your energy and heightens focused attention. The result? You feel more alive, think obsessively about your new love, and experience feelings of euphoria. These hormones communicate with your body, including your genitals and skin, so a simple touch from your lover can fire up the reward system and dopamine release, creating a powerful loop that drives you to fall more deeply in love. Be aware that some people can become overly infatuated with the rush of falling in love, so they have trouble getting beyond this stage of a relationship. This inherent vulnerability arises when the intense feelings subside, and such people then seek out a new partner so they can experience the love high again.

Stage 2: Domestic Bliss

The domestic bliss stage resembles the first half of the luteal phase of your cycle. As your relationship progresses, the adrenaline rush of new love wears off and transitions into a more comfortable commitment phase. The reward system and chemical cocktail that drove you to fall in love shift out of high gear and back to more sustainable levels. This can be a make-or-break moment for a relationship, because some people experience a sort of withdrawal from those heady chemicals or think it means they've fallen out of love. If you can make it through this period, the biological bonding chemicals oxytocin and vasopressin take over now. Researchers suggest oxytocin is such a powerful bonding mechanism it may promote fidelity. In a 2012 German study in the *Journal of Neuroscience*, researchers wanted to test whether giving men a dose of the "love hormone" oxytocin by nasal spray could entice them to go too far in a flirtatious encounter with an attractive woman. What they found was men who were in a committed monogamous relationship were more likely to keep their distance from the woman compared with single men or those who had received a placebo. In this phase of a relationship or marriage, you're washing dishes, changing diapers, and remodeling the bathroom, and those are just a few things on your seemingly endless to-do list. It's not sexy stuff. A key vulnerability of this phase emerges when couples let the stresses of child-rearing and work pull their focus from each other and stop putting in the effort to make each partner feel special. So how do you keep things fresh?

Syncing with your infradian clock is the answer. This can be a magical time when you're making the best of every phase of your cycle to keep things exciting for more fulfilling sex and a stronger relationship. You won't be feeling the stimulation of new love with a new person, but you can be continually learning something new about how your body functions and how your partner's body operates. I remember after I had our daughter, when my husband and I were just beginning to engage physically again. When I was in my luteal phase, I had to remind him that I needed more foreplay, because my biology wouldn't let me go from zero to sexy in sixty seconds flat the way he could. I had to let him know that we had to take it slow. I had him rub my shoulders for ten minutes, which helped me relax and primed my body for intimacy. And he realized that spending a little extra time on foreplay helped me switch out of mom-mode.

Keeping your sex life alive during this phase is critical to the success of your relationship. Sexual activity and orgasm cause the release of the "cuddle hormone" oxytocin, which strengthens feelings of intimacy, bonding, trust, and affection. Sex can also give you and your mate a happiness jolt thanks to the afterglow from a good romp. In 2017, the journal *Psychological Science* reported that newlywed couples experienced feelings of satisfaction up to forty-eight hours after sexual activity. The spouses who experienced the strongest sense of afterglow also reported the greatest happiness four to six months later.

Stage 3: Midlife Transition

The midlife transition is similar to the second half of the luteal phase, and provides a lot of clarity in a relationship. When you're in perimenopause, your values and interests shift. Jung calls this transition, from about forty on, the period when people become more interested in their relationship with their own soul. The potential is that you and your partner can wake up one day wanting very different things out of life. Several things are happening on a biological level that can make you question whether you're feeling fulfilled, or heading for Splitsville. If you're in a female-male relationship, understand that your partner may be experiencing his own version of "manopause," or may have erectile issues. As testosterone levels drop, men's sex drive can flounder. The result may be friction and a sexual disconnect. If you're in a same-sex relationship, your partner may be going through her own hormonal issues. If you haven't been nourishing your hormones throughout your reproductive years, you may have hormonal challenges now that are having negative effects on both vaginal lubrication and physical desire, making it harder for you to achieve orgasm.

You don't have to be blindsided by this situation. When you understand your biology and anticipate these changes, you and your other half can prepare for this new phase in your relationship. Your cycle actually provides you with the perfect practice model—the luteal phase. The hormonal levels during this time are similar to what you'll be experiencing in the second half of perimenopause. I make sure to let my husband know when I'm in my luteal phase as it's like a ten-day practice run for what's to come. It's a way for us to deepen our understanding of each other. During this transition, you're going to need a lot of patience and compassion for each other, and you'll have to be proactive to make sex more pleasurable. For example, use lube, increase foreplay, explore tantric practices, and focus more on the emotional connection and enjoyable physical sensations. You can also try biohacking to maintain a strong libido in midlife, such as doubling down on those B vitamins, omega-3s, magnesium, and zinc, or exploring safe and natural testosterone boosters or CBD oil. Knowledge is key to sailing through this transition.

Stage 4: Golden Years

The active work of career and child-rearing is done. Your time is your own. You may be pursuing travel, enjoying grandchildren, and exploring new hobbies. It can be a wonderful time. This is the stage when health issues could become more common, and you will need emotional resilience to navigate the changes aging can bring. However, since you're back to operating on a single clock, it's a chance for you to use the gifts of all the phases of your cyclical life to support your relationship. You can use all the lessons you've learned from your cyclical awareness and put them into action now. In essence, you'll be bringing all this wisdom with you into your golden years. Hormonal shifts in this stage lower your drive to take care of others and gives you the space to prioritize your own needs and interests. As you go through this transition, you'll have the opportunity to find new things that fill you with pleasure day to day so you will feel that you have some extra to give. Focusing on physical activities you can do together—as in the follicular phase of your cyclical years—is an excellent way to build oxytocin, strengthen your emotional connection, and maintain physical health. All of these are necessary to help you enjoy this time of your life together.

By preparing for this stage, you can shift more smoothly from your cyclical infradian clock back to a daily circadian rhythm. And when your partner is on board and aware of these hormonal changes, you can manage them hand in hand and enjoy your love throughout your golden years.

KEEP SEX SATISFYING THROUGHOUT YOUR LIFE STAGES

Your sexual needs and desires will fluctuate throughout your life cycle. Things that can negatively impact your sexual response include these:

• Hormonal birth control

• Pregnancy

• Postpartum

• Perimenopause transition

• Menopause

By syncing with your cycle, you can ease into these transitions with much more sensitivity to what is happening hormonally and physically, so you understand your needs. With more patience, compassion, and awareness of your biology and neurochemistry, you'll be able to continue getting maximal pleasure from your sex life throughout these life stages. You'll already be comfortable using lube when you need it, asking for what you want, and letting your partner know when your body needs more foreplay. Without this awareness, you can think you're experiencing some sexual dysfunction, or feel that something is wrong with your relationship. With a cyclical practice, you can avoid this confusion, feel great about yourself and your partner, and have a more satisfying sex life.

Step 6: Understand How Synthetic Birth Control Dampens Your Sex Drive

As I explained in the Biohacking Tool Kit section, the pill can cause you to fall for the wrong partner. It can also diminish your sex drive, shrink your clitoris, and make it harder to achieve orgasm. A 2010 German study in the *Journal of Sexual Medicine* found that in some women, the birth control pill stunts sex drive because of changes in a molecule called sex hormone-binding globulin (more on this below). When you're on the pill, you're basically in a no-phase zone. You have a low-dose combo of estrogen and progesterone that tricks your body into thinking implantation has occurred so you stop ovulating, and that means you miss out on the midcycle surge of testosterone. Higher levels of testosterone during your ovulatory phase make you interested in sex. Skipping that process in your cycle effectively suppresses your sex drive. Even worse, you may find that you're always dry vaginally and struggling to reach orgasm. You aren't imagining this. You're taking a medication that's hijacking your hormones and negatively impacting your sex life. Over the years in my practice, many women have sought out my help for their sex drive issues. Typically, these women have a history of using synthetic birth control. Here's how this medication interferes with your sexual function.

Your liver produces a molecule called sex hormone-binding globulin (SHBG) that's involved in transporting estrogen, testosterone, and dihydrotestosterone throughout your body. High levels of SHBG are associated with lower levels of testosterone. In a 2006 *Journal of Sexual Medicine* study involving 124 premenopausal women with sexual health complaints, researchers found that those taking synthetic birth control pills had SHBG levels four times higher than women who had never used hormonal contraceptives. Even after ditching hormonal oral contraceptives, SHBG levels remained elevated. The research suggests that long-term sexual, metabolic, and mental health consequences could result from continually elevated SHBG levels. In another study in a 2010 issue of the same journal, women taking hormonal contraception reported lower sex drive and arousal compared with women using nonhormonal birth control or no form of birth control at all.

What they feel is real. Birth control pills lower testosterone levels, dampening sexual desire. For some women who take synthetic birth control, their testosterone production and libido may never return to previous levels, even after discontinuing the pill, according to a 2006 study in *The Journal of Sexual Medicine*. If you're taking the pill, you may be experiencing a less-than-satisfying sex life due to the pill's effects on moods, testosterone production, estrogen levels, and SHBG. All of these effects can create a loss of interest, vaginal dryness, and difficulty achieving orgasm—a perfect recipe to sabotage your sex life.

Good Sex, Great Health

Why should you care about boosting your sex drive and having more fulfilling encounters? Aside from feeling amazing, a satisfying sex life has hormone-balancing superpowers and a host of other biological bonuses. A seminal 2007 report written by sex researchers and published by Planned Parenthood was one of the first to highlight the many health benefits of a happy sex life. Since then, researchers have continued to find that having regular orgasmic sex—whether it's with a partner or solo—supports your reproductive health, biological systems, and overall well-being in a myriad of ways.

Orgasm Can Balance Your Hormones

Sex is good for your reproductive health. Decades of science prove it. A series of studies has found that women who engage in sexual activity with a partner at least once a week have more regular cycles than those who are abstinent. In these studies, the first of which appeared in the journal *Psychoneuroendocrinology* in 1979, women who had sex at least once a week had cycles that averaged twenty-nine days with three days of bleeding. Women who had less frequent sexual encounters tended to have more extreme cycle lengths—either shorter than twenty-six days or longer than thirty-three days.

Having more orgasmic sexual encounters also improves your fertility. It isn't simply because there are more opportunities for sperm to fertilize an egg. Regular weekly orgasmic sexual encounters have a positive impact on basal body temperature (BBT), which promotes fertility. Your BBT is the temperature you have when you wake up first thing in the morning. Your BBT rises slightly during your most fertile days, giving you a sign that you're ovulating. Tracking BBT is a method I recommend for women who want help determining their fertile window. You simply take your temperature each morning before getting out of bed, and track when your temperature spikes. You can use a regular thermometer and paper charts or an app. In a 1985 study in *Physiology & Behavior*, women who were having weekly sex had the highest incidence of fertile-type BBT levels, getting into the baby-making range 90 percent of the time. Women who had sex sporadically achieved this level 55 percent of the time, while celibate women trailed, achieving this level only 44 percent of the time.

Having satisfying sex may also help alleviate two of the most common PMS problems—headaches and cramps. The next time you have either, you may want to skip the ibuprofen and just get some action. Many studies have found that sexual arousal, genital stimulation, and orgasm boost levels of endorphin and corticosteroids that have an analgesic effect. A 2013 study in *Cephalalgia* surveyed eight hundred migraine sufferers and two hundred cluster headache sufferers. Of those who engaged in sexual activity while having a headache, 60 percent reported improvement in migraine pain, and 37 percent said pain diminished from a cluster headache. And don't think you're the only one who is having sex or self-stimulating to curb cramps. In psychologist Carol Rinkleib Ellison's book *Women's Sexualities*, she reported that 9 percent of about 1,900 US women said they masturbated in the previous three months to relieve menstrual cramps.

There's also some evidence that the healing power of sex could go beyond everyday cramps. A 2002 study published in the journal *Gynecologic and Obstetric Investigation* suggested sexual activity could reduce the risk for endometriosis. Led by a researcher from Southern Connecticut State University, the study found that women who engaged in sexual activity and experienced orgasm during menstruation had a lower incidence of endometriosis. Considering I meet with so many women who are suffering from this painful condition, I would love to see additional research on this.

Sexual activity also promotes healthy estrogen levels to keep vaginal tissues supple and protect against heart disease and osteoporosis. And last but definitely not least, when you have healthy hormones, the radiance on the inside is reflected on the outside. Women having sex three times per week look ten years younger compared with those engaging in sexual activity only twice a week, according to psychologist David Weeks in his book, *Secrets of the Superyoung.*

Big Health Benefits of Orgasm on Your Five Biological Systems

Could the big O lower your risk for the big C and other major diseases? Some studies suggest sexual activity could lower a woman's risk for breast cancer. Research from a 1989 issue of the *Journal of Clinical Epidemiology* compared sexual activity among fifty-one childless French women who had been diagnosed with breast cancer within the three previous months and ninety-five healthy women. The researchers found a higher risk for breast cancer among women who had sex less than once a month.

Having sex gets your blood pumping and your heart beating faster, which could be good news for your ticker. A 2010 study found that men who had sex at least twice a week were at a 50 percent reduced risk for cardiovascular disease. Sadly, there is no comparable study looking at women's sexual behavior and risk for heart disease. However, in a 2016 study in the journal *Heart,* women diagnosed with coronary heart disease within the past four years were less likely to be sexually active than women without CHD.

By warding off disease, improving your hormonal health, and strengthening your biological systems, satisfying sex could be the secret to a longer life. In a study at Duke University that followed 252 women and men over twenty-five years, researchers looked for predictors of longevity. For women, the three most significant factors associated with greater longevity were good health, physical well-being, and past enjoyment—*not frequency*—of sexual activity. This is all the more reason why you should honor your cyclical nature in your sex life. When you're in sync with your cycle, you'll love your sexy time more and could live longer.

Orgasm and Your Biological Systems

Biological System 1: Brain. The big O is both a turn-on and a turn-off for your brain. What does that mean? Achieving orgasm activates a flood of mood-boosting neurochemicals—oxytocin (the bonding hormone linked to passion, intuition, and social skills), serotonin, and dopamine—that make you go "ahhh." But 2005 research from a team of scientists at Groningen University in the Netherlands shows that many regions of the brain switch off during female orgasm. Specifically, activity in the amygdala, hippocampus, and prefrontal cortex—areas involved in fear, anxiety, emotions, memory, and alertness—goes dark. For those few brief seconds, you can finally forget about your to-do list and all your worries and just enjoy the moment. Having sex on a regular basis could also make you smarter. A 2010 study in *PLOS ONE* found that having regular sex promotes neurogenesis in the hippocampus, an area associated with learning and memory. Numerous studies, including 2011 research in the journal *Nature*, have concluded that neurogenesis, which is the creation of new neurons, improves cognition. Orgasm also sparks the release of the hormone DHEA, which improves brain function, balances the immune system, helps maintain and repair tissue, and promotes healthy skin. Syncing with your cycle as your hormones and neurochemistry change each month helps you achieve orgasm on a more consistent basis so you can benefit from these positive impacts.

Biological System 2: Immune system. Who needs megadoses of vitamin C when sex boosts infection-fighting cells by up to 30 percent? Having frequent sex can help you stave off cold and flu bugs. A 2004 *Psychological Reports* study of 112 college students showed that those who had sexual intercourse once or twice a week had immunoglobulin A (IgA) levels higher than those who were abstinent or had sex less than once a week. A pair of studies in 2015 found a fascinating connection between sexual activity, the immune system, and the chances for conception. Researchers looked at thirty women—half who were sexually active and half who abstained from sex. The women who had regular sex saw changes in immune system activity that promoted conception, while those who were celibate showed no such changes. The two studies found that in sexually active women specific types of immune cells known as Type 1 helper T cells and IgA cells that fight foreign invaders are more abundant during the follicular phase of the cycle—helping to ward off infections, viral bugs, and bacterial invaders. During the luteal phase, however, there was a rise in the levels of Type 2 helper T cells and IgG cells, which help the body accept the sperm and fetus rather than viewing them as "invaders." In the women who weren't sexually active, this shift in immune system cells didn't take place.

Sexual activity also provides lymphatic massage, which is critical for a healthy immune system, and enhances the body's natural detoxification process. Lymphatic massage improves digestion and moods and helps prevent cancer.

Biological System 3: Metabolism. If you want to slim down, you may want to ramp up your bedroom activities. We all know that sex burns calories—well, okay, only about 69 calories for women—but did you know sex is also linked with a healthy BMI? A 2004 study in the *Journal of Sex & Marital Therapy* showed that frequent sexual activity—whether with your partner or solo—is associated with a smaller waist and hip circumference in both women and men. Remember that your metabolism changes from the first half of your cycle to the second half, so your sexual encounters may burn more or fewer calories depending on the time of the month.

Biological System 4: Microbiome. Having sex doesn't necessarily affect your microbiome, but your gut health can impact your desire for sex. An imbalanced microbiome is associated with mood disorders, sleep problems, and numerous health conditions, according to research in a 2015 issue of *Clinical Psychopharmacology and Neuroscience*. These issues all combine to sabotage your sex drive. On the other hand, a balanced microbiome contributes to healthy hormone and neurotransmitter production throughout your cycle. This leads to better moods, which are more likely to boost your sex drive.

Biological System 5: Stress response. It comes as no surprise that getting busy reduces stress. You can feel it when you have one of those toe-curling orgasms. Science credits the surge of oxytocin for this. What's more intriguing is that increased levels of this feel-good neurotransmitter can alter an individual's response to stress, according to a 2002 study in *Sexual and Relationship Therapy*. In her 2000 book, *Women's Sexualities*, psychologist Ellison interviewed 2,632 American women between the ages of twenty-three and ninety and found that 39 percent of those who masturbated reported doing so to relax.

The stress reduction action is so powerful, it can also help you sleep. Most of us think it's just men who have sex and then nod off soon after, but women also experience post-coital relaxation and better z's. The cocktail of neurohormones released during sexual activity induces relaxation to help you fall asleep, and an increase in the production of estrogen is associated with deeper REM cycles. If you're having trouble falling asleep, snuggle up to your partner or engage in solo play to help you get some shut-eye. In Ellison's work, 32 percent of women who said they masturbated in the previous three months did so to help them go to sleep. You can use your orgasms to biohack your sleep and relaxation throughout your cycle.

When you follow the steps in this chapter, you will discover a new positive relationship with your fluctuating sexual needs and desires, and you will no longer feel unnecessarily frustrated or confused. By understanding your biology, honoring your cycle and relationship stages, nourishing your sex hormones, and keeping your partner in the loop, your sex drive and sexual response will become more predictable, so you can start maximizing your enjoyment. Learning to work with your body's sexual cycle does more than just supercharge your sex life and give you more mind-blowing orgasms; it opens you up to another powerful way of energizing your biochemistry and fueling your creative nature that you can carry over into the other areas of your life.

CHAPTER 9

Making Motherhood Easier

I want them to see a mother who loves them
dearly, who invests in them, but who also invests
in herself. It's just as much about letting them
know as young women that it is okay to put
yourself a little higher on your priority list.
—Michelle Obama

I s there anything you wouldn't do for your child? Would you wake up
early to bake two dozen gluten-free cupcakes for your first-grader's
class bake sale? Would you help your middle-schooler complete a mind-
boggling STEM homework project after you've had a long day at work?
Drive your high school freshman fifty miles in hellish traffic for a volleyball
tournament? Of course you would! And if you couldn't, you'd be wracked
with mom guilt, feeling that you should have done more for your kids. We
all want to be the best moms and give our kids the best of everything. But
in addition, "popular mom" culture creates pressure to be perfect. Almost
every message we see in the media, on mommy blogs, or on social media
says we should be able to do everything for our kids without a hitch, look
flawless while doing it, and love every minute of it. As a result, we are
constantly feeling stressed and comparing ourselves to other moms. No

matter how much you do for your kids, you'll find images of some other mom who seems to be doing more—Instagram-worthy school projects, too-cute kiddie fashionistas, magazine-worthy school lunch bento boxes. Seeing these images makes you aspire to do more, but if you're trying to get it all done based on just the 24-hour clock, you will be left feeling exhausted and depleted.

Even though we're biologically made for motherhood, we need to acknowledge that the idea of the perfect mom is a myth. How are you supposed to be a sexy wife, kick-ass entrepreneur, mindful meditator, organic cook, fitness goddess, and doting mommy at all times? It's a lot. Trying to do it all week in and week out will put you on the expressway to exhaustion. And if you're dragging yourself to PTA meetings, soccer practices, and school plays while relying on your morning caramel latte to jolt you awake and your evening chardonnay to calm you down, you aren't doing yourself or your family any favors. Being stressed, sick, or zonked out from fatigue keeps you from being the best mom possible. In fact, it makes you more likely to lash out at your kids, be late *again* picking them up after piano practice, or be emotionally zoned out when you're supposed to be enjoying quality time. You are the heart and soul of the family unit. Your moods, energy, and words impact your children in long-lasting ways. This is the reason you need to rid yourself of the notion that you should sacrifice your health and well-being in order to do it all for your kids. Instead, you should live by those instructions you hear every time you fly: "Put your own oxygen mask on first." Practicing cycle-specific self-care is like putting on your oxygen mask. It won't give you more time in your day, but it will provide the foundation that gives you the optimized health and energy you need to be the best mom possible without the burnout. It also takes the pressure off from the never-ending to-do list and helps you prioritize, delegate, and set boundaries so things get done with less stress. Factoring in your infradian clock offers a more sustainable blueprint for motherhood, allowing you to draw on the unique gifts of each phase of your cycle so you can give your kids what they need when you're best able to offer it—no guilt required!

Wired for Motherhood

It isn't just society that drives us to go the extra mile for our kids. This drive is coded into our brain. Did you know that motherhood produces the most dramatic neurobiological changes in a woman's life? These structural and neurochemical changes, which encourage and support maternal caregiving and bonding, are far more profound than those that occur in puberty. We're all familiar with the awkward transition to adolescence, when our hormones are raging and our skin, body, and emotions act out accordingly. We treat adolescents with compassion and understanding during this time, because we know their whole way of thinking and viewing the world is changing and they're adjusting to their new hormonal reality. But the transition to motherhood? That remains largely a mystery. In a 2018 TED talk, reproductive psychiatrist Alexandra Sacks said, "There are entire textbooks written about the developmental arc of adolescence, and we don't even have a word to describe the transition to motherhood. We need one." *Matrescence* is the term she's encouraging us to adopt, and it deserves just as much attention as we give to puberty. After all, it's when you'll undergo the most sweeping neurobiological changes of your adult life—even more than what you can expect from menopause, which gets a lot more attention. Yes, we have lots of books, websites, and support groups that go into glorious detail about what you can expect your body to go through during pregnancy, birth, and postpartum, but most of them don't delve into the mind-altering, neurochemical aspect of this transition to motherhood (Angela Garbes's *Like a Mother* is a welcome exception). This lack of information leaves us ill-prepared for these dynamic changes, wondering why we no longer feel like ourselves, and too often assuming something is wrong with us. In *The Boston Globe's Globe Magazine*, journalist Chelsea Conaboy eloquently explored the radical transformation she experienced in her journey as a new mom, writing, "I feared that something deep within me—my disposition, my way of seeing the world, myself—had been altered. In truth, something very foundational had changed: my brain."

As scientific evidence on the changes in the maternal brain start to trickle in, it's becoming clearer that motherhood rewires our brain. That's what researchers concluded in a 2016 study in *Hormones and Behavior* that looked at the brains of new moms in the first, third, and fourth months postpartum. Several brain regions involved in important aspects of caregiving—maternal motivation and reward processing, sensory processing, empathy, and regulating emotions—increased in size throughout the study. Some of these brain changes may influence the anxiety and hypervigilance many new moms experience in the first few weeks postpartum, according to 2013 research in *Infant Mental Health Journal*. In this study, researchers suggested that this intense worrying tends to diminish after a few months.

Some of this rewiring, however, sticks around long after the early postpartum period. In a 2016 study in *Nature Neuroscience*, investigators used magnetic resonance imaging to look at the brains of women who were hoping to become pregnant. They conducted follow-up brain imaging tests after the women gave birth and compared those images with women who had not become pregnant. The brains of those who had given birth showed dramatic changes in gray matter volume that correlated to increased measures of maternal attachment, and these differences remained two years later in a subsequent follow-up. The differences were so clear that the researchers could easily distinguish which women had given birth based solely on the brain images.

Powerful neurochemicals also get in on the act to program us to bond with our babies and compel us to focus our attention on them like a laser. A 2014 study in *Scientific Reports* confirmed that oxytocin, the same compound that surges when you have an orgasm, is also released while you're breastfeeding, and fosters strong emotional bonding. Research has shown that for some women, simply hearing their baby cry initiates a let-down reflex that causes breast milk to start flowing. And groundbreaking research in a 2017 issue of *Proceedings of the National Academy of Sciences* found that dopamine, another mood-boosting brain chemical, is involved in the mother-child bonding process. All these things taking place in your brain serve an evolutionary purpose—making you ideally fit for the monumental job of keeping a tiny human alive. But when your brain is programmed to be overattentive, it can be easy to go overboard.

The Pursuit of Perfection

Are we doomed to think we aren't good enough as mothers? Are we programmed to strive to be better caregivers for the rest of our lives? Every bit of progress we make in the mom department is immediately followed by yet more yearning to improve. It's an endless pursuit of perfection, a lifetime of suffering. In her book *The Gifts of Imperfection*, Brené Brown writes, "Understanding the difference between healthy striving and perfectionism is critical to laying down the shield and picking up your life. Research shows that perfectionism hampers success. In fact, it's often the path to depression, anxiety, addiction, and life paralysis."

I understand the deep-seated desire to be the perfect mom, wife, friend, and career woman. I grew up with a productivity queen as a role model. My mom had a full-time job while also being a hands-on mom. Maybe being an immigrant spurred her to be in perpetual motion. She was indefatigable—whipping up hot meals three times a day, taking us to school and activities, and keeping the home perfectly clean and orderly. It's hard to fathom now, but I never ever ate at a restaurant until I moved out of our family home. When my mom wasn't at her job, she was bustling around the kitchen, doing laundry, taking me clothes shopping at the outlet, or getting crafty with some other project around the house. She was the most enterprising person I knew and was extremely creative in finding ways to stretch a dollar. She was so productive I never saw her sit down for more than the time it took to drink a cup of tea in the afternoon. Talk about living in perpetual productivity! But she was motivated to do all this because she had a deep desire to help her children realize their potential.

Like all moms of that generation, along with all the grandmothers and great-grandmothers who came before her, she was winging it in a society that was even more steeped in male-centered culture than we are today. Betty Friedan's 1963 landmark book, *The Feminine Mystique*, blew the cover off the plight of the stifled American housewife-mother, exploring the underlying cultural beliefs that forced women to conform to an idealized domestic role. The book depicted widespread dissatisfaction among unfulfilled women who were living zombie-like lives that prevented them from realizing their full potential. When women broke into corporate America, however, they felt stifled in a new way. On top of having to do it all at home, now they had do it all at work, reinforcing the belief that there was not enough time and that they had to suffer. With paying jobs during the day, largely invisible work at home, and the mental overload of managing all the details for both jobs, most moms then and now have been wound up tight. They don't have enough time, and they have no way to manage their energy, let alone factor in meaningful self-care. And worse, these moms feel guilty for not being the best, happiest, most "together" moms they want to be. We carry these wounds intergenerationally. We're still trying to figure out how to make all these roles fit together. There is a better way. Today, we are still healing from the wounds our female ancestors suffered. But we have an amazing opportunity to change our story and chart a new path for ourselves and our daughters.

I'm completely awed whenever I think of all the women who came before us who had to face hormonal health issues, a male-centered society, and the cult of perfection with absolutely no help. They must have felt so drained and depleted. I am so grateful to have found these insights into our biochemistry that we can now use to biohack like a mother. One of the most important lessons you can learn from listening to your inner biology is that you don't have to do everything all at once. This outdated concept of "doing it all in order to have it all" fed into the notion that we have to aspire to perfection. It's important to understand that syncing with your cycle isn't a method to help you get more organized so you can do all the things you think you should be doing. This cyclical practice is instead intended to help you get in tune with your inner wisdom and to make choices not just from your head but also from your center—your body, your heart, your hormones. Your biology will guide you to do what you want to do in a sustainable way, and helps you reorganize things you don't want to do, can't do, or need help doing. I would like to see us continue to evolve the narrative around motherhood to be more supported on all fronts, rather than that of self-sacrifice and burnout. If we truly want to honor our mothers and all the other women who came before us, what could be a better way than to create a new reality where we can be whole, integrated women living in tune with our biology?

Let Your Cyclical Nature Guide Your Mothering Style

I inherited my mom's perpetually active attitude, and I can easily fall back into this mode. I have a big appetite for life. I want to have a successful career and a strong relationship. I want to be a great mom who is fully engaged whenever I'm with my child. I want to be cooking homemade meals and keeping a beautiful home that looks as though it jumped off the pages of a magazine. And I want to have a fun social life. I want it all. But when I list all these desires out this way, I realize having all these expectations is a little crazy. How am I supposed to project-map all of this? How can I accomplish it all without draining my energy?

The cyclical way of living lets me practice the art of discernment. I do more of what's important to me as a mother—just at different times of the month. Letting your cycle provide a blueprint for a more effortless way to achieve your mom goals is the best way to prevent you from getting sucked back into the cult of perfection. Each phase of your cycle infuses you with unique talents and abilities that you can draw on to plan activities with your children, inform your parenting style, and tackle domestic tasks. Tapping into the natural strengths my cycle brings makes me a happier, more effective, and more fulfilled mom. When I map out activities and tasks in a phase-by-phase matrix, it makes my huge list of goals seem so much more achievable. By focusing on what I'm naturally best at each week, I end up getting to most of the items on my to-do list on a regular basis. Syncing with my cycle helps me feel that I can juggle more without dropping the ball.

But syncing your motherhood style with your cycle isn't just about optimizing your productivity in the domestic arena. It's also about having the energy and focus to be emotionally present with your children regardless of the activity. And there's another, even more pressing reason why right-timing is so important as a mom. As soon as my daughter was born, I quickly realized she wasn't going to be a little girl forever. It wouldn't be long before she entered her teenage years and then she'd be off to college. Acknowledging how special this childhood time is made me even more determined to make the most of it. Being disorganized or lacking the energy to be present with her would squander the magical phase of childhood. Discovering that my cycle provides a natural structure is like a gift that gives me more time with my daughter. And what mother doesn't want more time with her children?

This process is working for my client Jessie. This thirty-something pharmacist has found that syncing with her cycle does so much more than just alleviate period problems. "Before, I was pushing myself constantly and didn't realize that I was digging myself into a hormonal hole after multiple pregnancies. The Cycle Syncing Method™ has really given me the opportunity to get the most out of what I'm able to give to myself and to my family, and to my friends," she says. "It has also allowed me to manage the busyness of my life—three kids, a husband, a business, being an entrepreneur, being a pharmacist, and having friends. It's also given me the perspective of choosing more wisely, as well. I now have friends that only nurture me. There's no negative space. I don't have any room for any of that. And that's one big piece of this—it's allowed me to manage everything as well as say no and make a break from those things that were holding me back before."

THE MOTHER OF CREATION

Every woman, by virtue of being female and having access to the infradian clock, possesses the gift of being able to create something from nothing, to bring life from the fertile void. Whether you have children or not, you can apply maternal orientation to your own creative process. You can learn to be patient, compassionate, and nurturing with yourself the same way you would be with a child. The four phases of your cycle provide a guide for you to complete the creative cycle, and by tapping into your cyclical nature you can build your energy so you can bring your creative ideas and projects to fruition over and over again.

PROTECTING AND IMPROVING YOUR FERTILITY

If you aren't a mother yet, or you're currently trying to conceive, syncing with your cycle will protect and preserve your fertility for the long term. This method offers so many health and hormonal benefits, it can dramatically improve your reproductive ecosystem and improve your chances of conception. The earlier you begin living in sync with your cyclical nature, the easier time you'll have when you're ready to conceive. And the more aware you are of your life stages and matrescence, the smoother your transition to motherhood will be. A cyclical practice can also help boost progesterone if you have one of the 10 to 15 percent of pregnancies that end in miscarriage. With balanced hormones and foods that nourish your body, you will recover faster physically. On the emotional side, your cyclical practice will give you different ways to experience your grief and loss across several cycles as you heal your body and spirit.

Syncing Your Parenting with Each Phase

PHASE 1: PREPARE
Follicular Phase: 7–10 Days
Cyclical Focus: Curiosity

Activity focus: With supercharged energy during the follicular phase, you'll be primed to break out of your routine and try new experiences with your kids—visiting a new museum, taking a drive in the country, or going apple picking.

Parenting focus: Hormonal changes in the follicular phase lead you to be more cerebral and ramp up your curiosity, making this an ideal time to ask more questions when it comes to parenting. In this phase, it's also a good idea to break routines, take novel approaches with your kids, strategize with them, and find playful solutions if you come up against any resistance. For example, the other night, I let my three-year-old daughter know it was time to brush her teeth. I got out her toothbrush and was going to do it for her when she folded her arms across her chest and gave me an emphatic "No!" Instead of just pushing ahead with our usual routine, though, I paused and asked her why she didn't want to brush her teeth. I kept gently probing until she was able to express that she actually did want to brush her teeth; she just didn't want me to brush her teeth for her. It was one of those aha moments when I learned something new about her. So now we've graduated to letting her brush her own teeth, and she feels like a big girl doing it. Had I blindly stuck to the daily routine without inquiring about what was behind her refusal, I would have missed this new milestone, and we both would have felt frustrated. Instead, it was a win-win for both of us.

Domestic focus: The follicular phase is all about newness and bringing a fresh eye to things. Start planning home projects, think about what needs to be done this month, and loop your partner into the planning process. Is there something you've been meaning to do, such as painting a room or building a bookshelf? Lay out your plans to make it happen.

PHASE 2: OPEN UP
Ovulatory Phase: 3–4 Days
Cyclical Focus: Nurturing and Play

Activity focus: The best time to socialize during your monthly cycle is the ovulatory phase. Some ways to make the most of this phase are planning a family barbecue with all the young cousins, inviting kids over for a play date, visiting a family member, or planning an outing with other moms and their kids. In my latest ovulatory phase, I hosted a chess get-together for my daughter and her friends with an organization that uses storytelling to teach young kids how to play the game.

Parenting focus: In this phase, your estrogen's concentration level will boost your desire to nurture your kids and show them extra-focused love and affection. For example, during this phase you might want to go to a special meal for one-on-one time, help the kids with a project, or spontaneously make muffins with them. The ovulatory phase is the time when your verbal skills spike, so take advantage and use this time to talk to your kids. Do an emotional check-in and ask them how they're feeling and if there's anything they want to talk about. You'll also find it effortless to be a playful mom at this time, and you can resolve conflicts in a more physical, playful, lovey-dovey way. My latest game with my daughter is "mama jaguar and baby jaguar." If she's sitting on the couch and being difficult, I'll hop on the couch on all fours and start purring, growling, and nuzzling at her cheek in a fun way. She just starts laughing, then we cuddle, and before I know it whatever she was upset about has been forgotten.

Domestic focus: Your communication and social skills shine during this phase, so plan that parent-teacher conference, help your high schooler fill out those college applications, or have a family meeting when everyone is encouraged to share whatever's on their mind.

PHASE 3: WORK
Luteal Phase: 10–14 Days
Cyclical Focus: Collaboration

Activity focus: In the luteal phase, you're a superwoman when it comes to checking things off your to-do list. Use this time to include your kids in domestic chores. Ask them to help you fold laundry, chop the carrots, or pick up their room. They'll be building skills, and it will help you zoom through your list faster.

Parenting focus: As a parent, this is when I look at my task list and complete the items on that list. This is the time to give children the opportunity to learn to enjoy this process by helping them learn about sequencing, delayed gratification, skill building, follow-through, and completion. Now is also the best phase to let your kids practice working through issues on their own. With my daughter I might let her know it's time to wash her hands before dinner. If she doesn't follow through, I'll use love and logic questions with her. For example, "Do you want to go wash your hands by yourself, or do you want Mommy to wash them with you?" She usually thinks about it, and then she'll follow through on her own. What's amazing about this process is that she senses the underlying rhythm of my mothering phase, and she can tell when I've shifted into this different vibe. During my luteal phase, she'll be proactive and will proudly tell me, "Mom, I washed my hands before you asked me to!"

Domestic focus: During this phase, you'll feel a strong desire to get things in order. Honor that inner voice by getting organized and completing projects with the kids' help when appropriate. Once every quarter during the luteal phase, go through your children's closets and swap out those summer shorts for fall sweaters, or store the winter coats and break out the spring fashions. I like to do a deep cleaning once a month and ask my husband to pull out all the furniture so we can dust in places we can't reach the rest of the time. This is also when I tackle school administrative tasks, such as filling out forms or ordering supplies. I also go through the pantry and stock up on anything we need. If you're in the middle of a project—wallpapering, painting a room, or framing family photos to hang on the wall—now is the time to buckle down and see the project through. You—and the rest of your family—will feel so much better when you get it done.

PHASE 4: REST
Menstrual Phase: 3-7 Days
Cyclical Focus: Individuation

Activity focus: To be a happy mom, you need some alone time, and there's no better phase for that than during menstruation. Put your partner on bedtime duty with the kids and relax in the tub, read a page-turner, or tune in to something really juicy on TV. Giving your children some solo time is good for them, too. It encourages them to use their imagination and to entertain themselves. Being alone doesn't necessarily mean being apart from each other. For example, my daughter and I might be sitting together on the couch, and I'm reading my book while she's reading hers. We're still connected while doing our own thing. In fact, I think this is great practice for the oncoming pubescent years when she's going to have the itch to do things on her own—teaching us we can still be connected while pursuing separate interests. Plus, taking even the smallest break can make you miss your kids like crazy, so you are energized to come back renewed in the follicular phase.

Parenting focus: During this phase, I really like to lean on my partner and let him do more so that I can try to replenish myself. How do you do this if you're a single parent? Just try to give yourself one day of your bleed when you hire a babysitter if you can afford it, get your parents to come over, or leave your kids with your best friend for a night. Then you will have the opportunity to take a nap, go out to dinner by yourself, go to the movies, get a massage, or whatever will help refuel your resources.

Domestic focus: Your hormones align at this time to encourage analysis and evaluation. But in contrast with the ovulatory phase, when you ask questions and engage in conversation to explore issues, this process during the menstrual phase is about listening to your inner wisdom, your intuition. Do you have a weird feeling that something is going on with your kid at school? Has anything fallen off your radar with your self-care, relationship, finances, or friends? In the menstrual phase, your heightened intuition gives you the insights you need to catch things that need to be addressed. You're the CEO of your family, and it's important to evaluate all the things that go into making a happy, healthy home. This is also an ideal time to remind yourself of everything that's gone right in the previous month.

The Cycle Syncing Method™: Mom FLO

FOLLICULAR Curiosity Duration: 7–10 Days	OVULATORY Nurturing and Playfulness Duration: 3–4 Days	LUTEAL Collaboration Duration: 10–14 Days	MENSTRUAL Individuation Duration: 3–7 Days
Plan out the family calendar for the month ahead.	Attend family events.	Let kids help with chores.	Enjoy alone time.
Go somewhere new.	Arrange play dates.	Support your kids to practice problem solving.	Give your children solo time.
Ask questions to learn more about your children's needs.	Be playful with your kids.	Encourage your kids to practice follow-through on tasks.	Ask for help from a partner or friend.
Try a new activity as a family.	Get physical and have a dance party.	Handle school-related administrative tasks.	Up your self-care.
Plan meals for the month ahead.	Cultivate social community.	Tackle a domestic project.	Tune in to your children and feel how they are doing.
Make new recipes.	Have a family meeting.	Organize children's closets.	Evaluate family priorities.

Keep Your Life Stage in Mind

Your cyclical nature goes beyond your 28-day clock and also applies to the overarching seasonality of your feminine expression as you go through life. Think of the 28-day cycle as your own personal biological creation matrix that impacts your energy throughout your lifetime. From childhood to young adulthood, motherhood to "golden girl"—each of these life stages is tied to hormonal shifts in your body that impact the rhythms of your energy, vitality, and creativity. These hormonal shifts also affect neurotransmitters and shape the female brain, according to a 2015 review in *Frontiers in Neuroscience*. One of the best benefits of living with cyclical awareness is that it reduces stress by giving you permission to focus on the things that matter most to you. Similarly, keeping in mind where you are in terms of your life stage frees you up to embrace what's important to you at any particular stage. Cyclical awareness provides a guide to the seasonality of life and increases your understanding that there's a time to push hard in your career and a time to seek more balance, a time to develop forever friendships and a time to nest with your baby. The need to honor your life stage often becomes most evident during matrescence, when you may be struggling with your new identity as a mom. Ignoring the seasonal reality of your life can ramp up stress and guilt while putting your health at risk. There's no other time in your life when you're more likely to put others' needs first than when you become a mother. You may feel guilty about not doing enough for your kids, but on the other side you feel anxious that you aren't accomplishing enough in life, aren't being a good enough friend, and aren't giving your partner enough attention. This is the essential tension of motherhood.

Getting in tune with your seasonal life stage also ties in with the notion of right-timing and managing your energy. Right-timing applies not only to how you schedule your days, but also to where you focus your energy throughout your lifetime. Trusting your hormonal clock, and letting it guide you in shifting priorities, is very grounding and re-assuring. Your hormonal clock gives you permission to say no to the extra work projects or the night out with the girls. Of course you can try to find other ways to connect with friends. Just don't beat yourself up for not being "perfect" in every area of your life at all times. When things start feeling overwhelming, ask yourself: Where am I in my cy-cle? Where am I in my life stage? As spiritual teacher Ram Dass wrote in his seminal 1971 book of the same title, "Be here now." Honor your biology and let it guide you.

Going through the transitions from one life stage to the next can be challenging because they signal profound shifts in your identity. And no change is bigger and more culturally unsupported than going from sexual and carefree young woman to responsible, overstressed mother. This change can rock your foundation, especially if you haven't been taking care of yourself hormonally. The good news is it's never too late to start tuning in to your biological inner clocks.

Being aware of the changes that will come with each stage and preparing for them by nourishing your hormones can help ease these transitions. The women in your own family can give you a glimpse of what's to come. Jean Liedloff, an author who spent more than two years living in the South American jungle with an intergenerational tribe, wrote in *The Continuum Concept: In Search of Happiness Lost* that every person in their culture was able to learn from older indi-viduals while mentoring younger people. According to Liedloff, this provided for a smoother transition from one life stage to the next. Growing up in an intergenerational household that included your mom and grandma, for example, would have provided you with a model for what the different life stages look like. Back in 1950, about 21 percent of Americans lived with two or more adult generations in a single household, according to a Pew Research Center analysis of census data. That number plummeted to 12 percent in 1980, so most of you reading this book probably didn't grow up with multiple generations of women at home that you could emulate. The number of multigenerational households has gradually been inching its way back up, however, and reached a record 64 million people, or one in five Americans, in 2016. Being part of the "sandwich generation" living with your parents and your children definitely brings its own challenges, but it allows you—and your daughter, if you have one—to see that there's a right-timing aspect to a woman's life in addition to the monthly cycle. This awareness is especially helpful in motherhood, when you really need to honor all of your inner clocks. If you didn't have this intergenerational transmission of wisdom and you have uncertainty about what's to come, you can have anxiety about change in general—this is the same lack of preparation that leaves us feeling blindsided by or negatively about our puberty experience. Let's look to our biology to help give us confidence about how to navigate change successfully.

The Eight Hormonal Life Transitions

Childhood (Birth to About 12)

Body focus: During childhood, a girl's body, brain, and endocrine system undergo rapid development. The pituitary gland in the brain releases a growth hormone that causes kids to sprout taller. Thyroid hormone enables cells—especially those in the brain—to develop and function properly. The adrenal glands kick into action around middle childhood—a transition called adrenarche—and begin pumping out DHEA, which is critical for brain development, according to 2011 research in *Human Nature*. During childhood, girls are operating on a 24-hour biological clock the same way boys are.

Can I sync with my cycle during childhood? Since young girls are operating on a 24-hour biological clock, there is no need to cycle sync at this stage. However, a poor diet and exposure to endocrine disruptors in childhood could spell trouble when puberty hits. I recommend auditing your daughter's food intake and eliminating her exposure to endocrine disruptors starting as early as possible to lay the foundation for happier hormones.

Lifestyle focus: Everything is new and exciting during this stage. At first, life is all about mommy and daddy, but that changes in middle childhood when girls go to school and develop emotional, intellectual, and social skills and begin the process of individuation.

Puberty (About 12 to 21 Years Old)

Body focus: A girl's first period signals the wondrous beginning of her life as a cyclical creature in which she adds a monthly hormonal clock to her existing 24-hour clock. In the US, 90 percent of girls begin menstruating by age 13.75, with the median age for menarche at 12.4 years of age, according to 2003 research in *Pediatrics*. Fewer than 10 percent of girls have their first period before their eleventh birthday. Several factors may influence an earlier onset of puberty and menarche. Studies in the journals *Pediatrics and Pediatrics Research* show that a higher body mass index in girls may be related to budding breasts and the sprouting of pubic hair at a younger age. Other factors associated with an earlier age of menarche include exposure to endocrine disruptors, having a mom who smoked during pregnancy, growing up with one or more smokers in your household, and lower socioeconomic status. On the flip side, eating disorders, high levels of physical activity, and malnutrition have been associated with delayed menarche, according to a 2010 review in *Reproductive Biology and Endocrinology*.

When a girl first starts menstruating, it's not uncommon for the menstrual cycle to arrive in an irregular pattern. The median cycle length for adolescents is 32.2 days, but intervals ranging from twenty-one days to forty-five days are considered normal, according to the American College of Obstetricians and Gynecologists. It takes time for the hypothalamic-pituitary-ovulatory axis to build up enough of a hormonal concentration so a girl can ovulate and menstruate regularly. Within three years of menarche, 60 to 80 percent of girls will see their cycle length adjust to twenty-one to thirty-four days, which is similar to the patterns in adult women, according to 2003 research in *Human Reproductive Update*. The American College for Obstetricians and Gynecologists recommends teen girls monitor their menstrual cycles with the support of their health care practitioner. In the early stages, it can provide important information on health issues that need early diagnosis and understanding. If period problems arise during this stage, avoid suppressing the developing hormonal and cyclical processes with synthetic birth control. Refer to the Biohacking Tool Kit to help your teen nurture her hormones and save her years of suffering, time, and expense trying to get her cycle back on track.

Can I sync with my cycle during puberty? As a culture we're all too quick to assume that any issues with the menstrual cycle during this life stage need to be regulated with medication—namely, synthetic birth control pills. The birth control pill only masks reproductive health issues and delays proper treatment and care. Instead of jumping on the pill bandwagon, we need to do a better job of teaching girls and young women how diet and lifestyle changes can heal hormonal issues.

Lifestyle focus: This is a heady time for exploration, learning, new adventures, and discovering your identity. During this stage, teenage girls tend to shift their attention from their family to friends, who take on a much more important and influential role in their lives. Lifetime friendships are often forged during this stage.

Adult Menstrual Years (21 to 35 Years Old)

Body focus: During this life stage, the average menstrual cycle occurs every twenty-one to thirty-four days and lasts about two to seven days. This is the time to take action if the symptoms you had in puberty, such as cramps, PMS, or acne, didn't get addressed or don't resolve on their own, or if you begin developing new symptoms. Taking action isn't just about alleviating your symptoms so you can have easier periods; it's about preserving your fertility and setting yourself up to be able to unlock your hormonal advantage in every area of your life.

Can I sync with my cycle as an adult? As an adult, you have the opportunity to harness the potential of your feminine biochemistry by living in sync with your cycle.

Lifestyle focus: This is an exciting time of life when you'll likely be moving out on your own, getting your career off the ground, and diving in and out of passionate romances. You may have more exposure to alcohol and caffeine, both of which affect your hormones, so pay attention to their effect on you, and limit or eliminate them for optimal hormonal health.

Pregnancy (Age Varies)

Body focus: The female body is awe-inspiring when it comes to making tiny humans. Following implantation of a fertilized egg, your body's hormone production factory undergoes radical changes. About eight days after ovulation, your inner biological boss fires up production of human chorionic gonadotropin (hCG), which instructs your ovaries to halt the release of a mature egg each month. The primary job of hCG is to preserve the corpus luteum so it can dramatically ramp up the release of estrogen and progesterone in order to support pregnancy. In early pregnancy, your body produces hCG at a furious pace, peaking at about eight to ten weeks before lowering and leveling off for the final two trimesters. After hCG production tops out, the placenta takes over production of estrogen and pro- gesterone. Estrogen helps regulate other key hormones, supports the development and nourishment of the fetus, increases blood flow to the uterus, and contributes to the development of milk ducts. Un- fortunately, it's also to blame for the nausea many women experi- ence in the first trimester. Higher levels of progesterone suppress the maternal immune response so the mother's body won't reject the fetus as a "foreign invader." Higher levels of progesterone also maintains the placenta and buildup of endometrial lining, helps the uterus expand to support a growing fetus, and boosts your mood. This important hormone also plays a role in preventing miscarriages by stopping preterm uterine contractions. A 2017 study in *Fertility & Sterility* found that two-thirds of women who used a progester- one supplement prior to getting pregnant successfully delivered full-term babies even though they had previously suffered multiple miscarriages. If you're so exhausted you can't stay awake, you can blame it on this key hormone, because it tends to act like a sleeping pill. Your changing hormonal levels may also enlarge your breasts, darken the areolas, and increase breast sensitivity and tenderness. Fluid retention and swelling are common as a pregnancy progresses, as are a litany of other changes.

A lesser-known but magical short- and long-term gift of pregnancy is that fetal heart and brain cells are found in the maternal heart and brain permanently. The fetal heart cells help heal the maternal heart after it doubles in size during pregnancy, and they undoubtedly facil- itate emotional resonance between mother and child. The fetal brain cells give you that psychic link to your child so you can understand them before they are verbal and/or when they're not communicating as they get older—truly it's biology at its most poetic.

A number of other hormones get involved in the baby-making

process. Thyroid production increases to help with metabolism and the regulation of steroid hormones. Human placental lactogen (hPL) causes changes in your breasts to support breastfeeding and plays a role in your body's metabolism to provide adequate nourishment to the fetus. During labor, oxytocin stimulates the uterine contractions that push your new baby out of the womb. Your body intuitively knows what to do, but things can go haywire if you haven't addressed any existing hormonal imbalances. You can—and should—feel great during pregnancy, but it usually requires some preparation. If you're a hormonally sensitive person like me with my diagnosis of PCOS, it's even more important to prep for pregnancy, as you may be more susceptible to postpartum hormonal changes.

PLACENTA POWER

For far too many years, our culture has devalued the female body, its cyclical nature, and the birth process. Just look at the placenta, for example. This life-sustaining temporary organ, which nourishes the fetus during pregnancy, has traditionally been considered medical waste. Can you believe that? Many hospitals routinely dispose of it after birth like trash. This practice really irritates me because this amazing organ holds so much potential. Futurist tech innovators and other major influencers, including self-help guru Tony Robbins, are finally waking up to the placenta's immense power. Robbins raved in a 2018 Facebook post that he had received the transformative benefits of placental stem cell therapy, saying, "Stem cells saved my shoulder after struggling with excruciating pain from spinal stenosis and, more recently, a torn rotator cuff. Stem cell treatment is truly a next-level health innovation that can reverse the wear and tear we put on our bodies and prevent debilitating disease and injury from escalating further. This technological advancement will impact humanity in life-changing ways—it has the potential to transform and save MILLIONS of lives!" Robbins has teamed up with Dr. Peter Diamandis, cofounder of Human Longevity Inc. and one of *Fortune* magazine's World's 50 Greatest Leaders, to deliver placental stem cell therapy to consumers. Just as pharmaceutical companies pay consumers for their health data, women should be compensated for donating their placentas, and more women should get funding to do more research in this area. I can only hope this is just the first step in a major shift in thinking to view the female body as the ultimate, life-giving power source.

Can I sync with my cycle during pregnancy? No, absolutely not! However, I suggest you prep your body for pregnancy with phase-specific diet and lifestyle changes at least three months, but preferably a year, prior to trying to conceive. By fixing hormonal symptoms *before* that pregnancy test shows a positive result, you can increase your chances of a healthier, happier pregnancy.

Lifestyle focus: In the pregnancy phase, you're basically in an extended quasiluteal phase for forty weeks, which is why you have the desire to nest. You're literally nesting a human being, and then you'll nest your home. You'll be nesting everything. You'll get so turned on by getting things done—planning the baby shower, organizing the nursery, and filling the closet with baby clothes.

Postpartum (Age Varies)

Body focus: After your baby makes a grand entrance into the world, your hormone levels change dramatically, and you experience a rapid decline in estrogen levels, according to research in *Behavioural Brain Research*. Prolactin kicks in to stimulate your breasts to produce breast milk. Each time you breastfeed, your brain releases the powerful bonding hormone oxytocin, which strengthens your connection with your baby. Your first period post-delivery could arrive in six to eight weeks if you aren't breastfeeding. But if you are breastfeeding, your menstrual cycle may take some time to return. Among the women I work with, it takes an average of six months for the menstrual cycle to reestablish itself. Mine didn't come back for nine months. Research in a 2015 review in *CNS Spectrums* on the role of reproductive hormones in postpartum depression and anxiety suggests that some women who are "hormone sensitive" may be more at risk for developing this condition. In my experience with thousands of women, I've noted that the way you've been eating, exercising, and scheduling your life for the decade leading up to giving birth either helps protect you from developing postpartum mood issues or makes you more vulnerable to them. The way you nourish your body postpartum can make a difference, too.

Can I sync with my cycle postpartum? Do not cycle sync postpartum! Think of the first three months after giving birth as an extended menstrual phase. Focus your diet on warm cooked foods, including healthy fats, protein, and nutrient-dense fare. Think bone broth, liver paté, red meat, warm oatmeal, avocados, whole eggs, and coconut oil. This is not the time for salads, smoothies, or raw fruit—nothing cold! Forget trying to lose the baby weight by eating light. It won't work. You might think these hearty foods would make you pack on more pounds, but they helped me quickly lose sixty pounds of baby weight without trying. My post-baby eating plan also helped me avoid the mood swings that can arise from my hormone sensitivity. As soon as your period comes back and you are at least six months postpartum, you can then begin syncing with your cycle again.

Lifestyle focus: During this stage, your life can feel like it completely revolves around that tiny bundle of crying, eating, pooping joy. Try your best not to put pressure on yourself to attend to work, romance, and friendships perfectly while you're getting adjusted to being a mom.

Perimenopause Phase 1 (About 35 to 45 Years Old)

Body focus: The second clock unwinding process begins as early as your midthirties. Your body is still producing enough hormones to give you good energy, sex drive, skin tone, and muscle tone, but subtle changes are under way inside your ovaries. Ovarian reserve—the number of remaining follicles and eggs in your ovaries—may begin to dwindle. As your egg supply diminishes, cells within your ovaries secrete lower amounts of two key hormones—inhibin B and anti-Müllerian—which may cause occasional elevation of FSH levels during the follicular phase of your cycle, according to 2017 research in *JAMA*. With so many women over thirty-five having children, clearly how you care for your hormones greatly impacts your fertility during this stage. During this life stage, your cycle may still be arriving like clockwork every month, or it could begin to vary in length. In the later years of this phase, you could skip a period entirely.

Can I sync with my cycle in perimenopause phase 1? Yes! If you're already in the perimenopausal phase of your life and are just learning about the concept of living in sync with your cycle, you need to start doing it *now*! If you've been eating, exercising, and managing your energy according to your cycle, you may not experience any symptoms during this phase. If you've been neglecting or ignoring your female cyclical nature, however, your body will let you know it. You could be dealing with fertility problems, vaginal dryness, crepe-like or wrinkled skin, or bone-dry hair. This is your body's way of giving you a heads-up that underlying problems need to be addressed. Don't expect to solve your skin and hair issues at the spa or salon. The problem is more than skin-deep. It is critical to start biohacking your way to better-balanced hormones before you transition into the second phase of perimenopause, or you could be faced with unnecessarily intense symptoms. By taking charge of your health now with phase-specific foods and supplements, you can avoid many of the effects of premature hormonal aging and can reduce the likelihood of developing symptoms in the late phase of perimenopause. You can also slow down this process and delay menopause. A 2018 study in the *Journal of Epidemiology and Community Health* concluded that a diet high in fish and legumes delays the onset of menopause by more than three years, whereas eating refined rice and pasta results in an earlier end to your reproductive years. A high intake of vitamin B6 and zinc was also associated with a later age at menopause.

Lifestyle focus: By now you're hitting your stride in motherhood, career, and romance. When your hormones are optimized and you're honoring your cyclical nature, you can make it all work with less effort and feel more energized than ever. This can also be a time when you begin a journey back to the self. Psychologist Marion Woodman has written extensively about how women in midlife move away from focusing on external things and seeking external validation, and instead turn inward. Embrace this transition, and get to know yourself better.

Perimenopause Phase 2 (45 to 55 Years Old)

Body focus: As the infradian clock unwinds itself permanently, your hormone levels change even more dramatically. Over time, your body will make more and more FSH, and you will eventually stop having a 28-day cycle. By the time you reach perimenopause phase two, your ovarian reserve has shrunk, making pregnancy less likely but not out of the question. FSH levels rise, causing follicles to mature faster and shortening the follicular phase; luteal progesterone levels fall; estrogen production can remain steady or become erratic; and testosterone levels decline. These changes can all lead to more irregular cycles. Eventually, FSH levels rise to the point where you no longer ovulate. You may skip two or more cycles, going more than sixty days without a period. Your period may also increase or decrease in duration or be heavier or lighter in flow. This transition can be a relatively smooth one with your changing hormone levels remaining balanced in relation to each other *if* you've been syncing with your cycle. For women who haven't been practicing phase-specific self-care, however, hormones levels may fluctuate wildly and lead to a host of issues, including these:

• Hot flashes and night sweats
• Sleep problems
• Increased risk for fibroids and endometriosis
• PMS
• Weight gain
• Breast swelling and tenderness
• Fertility issues
• Forgetfulness
• Mood changes
• Concentration problems
• Headaches
• Loss of libido
• Vaginal dryness
• Urinary incontinence
• Decreased sexual response
• Lack of energy
• Fatigue
• Reduced motivation
• Changes in hair and pubic hair
• Increased susceptibility to urinary and vaginal infections
• Increased risk of osteoporosis

Can I sync with my cycle in perimenopause phase 2? You can use aspects of the Cycle Syncing Method™, but you have to allow for the timing to shift. You may need to spend longer times in various phases depending on what is happening hormonally and watch out for the desire to medicate this process away. Look at any perimenopausal symptoms as an opportunity to check in with yourself and see if you need to ramp up your self-care.

Lifestyle focus: If you have children, the day-to-day demands of motherhood gradually begin to ease up as they become more independent. Think of this as a time when you can put renewed focus on your relationship with your partner and your career. You may also find yourself reevaluating your life goals.

Postmenopause (55-Plus Years Old)

Body focus: Twelve months after your last period, you will join the estimated two million women per year who cross the threshold to postmenopause, according to the North American Menopause Society. If you're like most women, you'll make that transition around fifty-one, the average age for natural menopause in the US; however, as you saw earlier, your diet and lifestyle can either delay or accelerate onset. And as you've seen earlier in this book, the BioCycle Study has found that the longer PMS goes untreated, the greater the risk for cancer, heart disease, diabetes, and dementia in postmenopause. It's clear that your choices during your adult life and perimenopause journey will greatly impact your health and well-being postmenopause. In this phase, FSH has stabilized at its new, elevated levels, and estrogen, progesterone, and testosterone have locked into their lower levels for the long haul. As your hormones stop rising and falling in a rhythmic monthly pattern, your cyclical nature gives way to the return of the 24-hour biological clock you had in childhood. However, just because your second clock is no longer in the mix, it doesn't mean your female organs are useless. In fact, another reason to invest in your hormonal health while your second clock is still active is that you could increase the chance of keeping your uterus postmenopause. Did you know that about one-third of all women will have a hysterectomy by age sixty?

Or that research shows nearly all of them are unnecessary? When you were younger, your gynecologist wanted to give you birth control pills to override your hormonal system, and when you're older they say you don't need a uterus. It's the final piece in the trajectory of the thinking that says we need to medicate and suppress our natural biological process. But this surgery comes with problems for your long-term sexual and physical well-being. New research in 2019 has found that the uterus may play a surprising role in memory, and that having a hysterectomy has been linked to memory deficits. During this time of life, when supported, your hormones and brain circuitry are also rewiring themselves in ways that will open you up to a new life. I think Christiane Northrup says it best: "The woman in menopause, who is becoming the queen of herself, finds herself at a crossroads of life, torn between the old way she has always known and a new way she has just begun to dream of . . . imploring her to explore aspects of herself that have been dormant during her years of caring for others and focusing on their needs."

Can I sync with my cycle in postmenopause? Your body has returned to a 24-hour clock, so you don't need to live cyclically for health reasons and hormonal biohacking purposes, but if you enjoy it you may continue a cyclical practice. Some women like to stay connected to it by syncing with the lunar phases. The main focus here, however, is to consume nutrient-dense foods, proteins, and essential fatty acids because your body is no longer making as much in the way of hormones. You can continue eating the healthful foods listed in the Foods for Your Cycle chart in chapter 4, but you don't have to adhere to the phases. It's also important to exercise in ways that strengthen your body without increasing your risk for injury. And you can schedule your life at a more sustainable pace even though you're operating on a single clock. There is absolutely no reason to mourn the end of your cyclical life if you took advantage of your infradian clock while it was active. I feel women who express a sense of loss at this stage are coming to terms with a sub-conscious sadness about not living cyclically while they could. In fact, if you've been following a cyclical practice, you'll be accustomed to shifting from one phase to the next and from one life stage to the next, so you will embrace this new chapter with open arms.

Lifestyle focus: Look at this stage of your life as an opportunity to emphasize personal pursuits rather than taking care of others. More than half of American postmenopausal women report greater happiness and fulfillment compared with when they were in their twenties, thirties, or forties, according to research in the journal *Menopause*. Think of menopause as a time to draw on the wisdom of all the gifts of the cycle all at once.

MORE ON THE MOTHERHOOD LIFE STAGE

Whenever I'm overwhelmed or feeling guilty that I haven't seen my girl-friends in a while, thinking I should be spending more couple time with my husband, or contemplating responding to my work email on the weekend, I remind myself that I'm in the motherhood stage of my life and also in the early perimenopausal stage hormonally, and that reminder helps me put things into perspective. I give myself renewed permission to embrace the stage I'm in and not to put undue pressure on myself to do more. There are certain seasons of your life when you can hang out for hours and hours with your friends, rush off for romantic weekends with your lover, or spend major chunks of your free time working on your career, but not when you're actively raising small children. Your inner life clock tells you these things must be reprioritized in relation to baby. Research confirms what your inner clock says.

The magazine *Child* surveyed close to one thousand moms and dads to gauge how having children affected their friendships. The results show that women tend to drift away from their friends after having a child. Approximately 45 percent said they had fewer friends after becoming a mom, and they spent less time with them, down from fourteen hours per week before baby to only five hours per week. The way we connect with our gal pals changes too. Instead of lunches, cocktails, or shopping sprees, we shift to online chatting, email exchanges, or old-fashioned phone calls—and it's fulfilling in different ways.

Becoming a mom can cause a seismic shift in your romantic relationship, too. Is it any surprise? That tiny bundle of joy demands every second of your attention, prevents you from getting enough shut-eye, and just added 137 more things to your to-do list. It's hard to find time for yourself, let alone your partner. Decades of research point to a decline in marital bliss after transitioning to parenthood. A 2017 study in *Current Opinion in Psychology* concluded that the birth of a first child has a negative effect on the parents' relationship, whether you're an opposite-sex couple or a same-sex couple. And this isn't just a post-newlywed slump. In a 2008 study in the *Journal of Family Psychology*, researchers measured marital satisfaction among moms and women without children over a thirty-nine-month period. All of the women reported a decline in satisfaction, but the moms registered a much steeper drop—more than twice the decline that childless married women reported. When you use the strategies in chapter 8, you can buck this trend.

When it comes to working after baby, you can find yourself pulled in two directions. We all want to give 100 percent to our careers, but we also want to give 100 percent to our children. You don't have to be a math major to know this doesn't add up. Because we live in a culture of perpetual productivity, however, we're conditioned to think we must be available at all times to our clients, stay late to show we're working hard, and take on extra projects to prove our worthiness. When you add a baby—or a second or third baby—into that mix, there just isn't enough of you to go around. The biochemical pull to care for our children is so strong, and the culture of work is both so unsustainable and unsupportive of maternal needs, women often feel they must make a hard choice. In fact, more women are walking out of the workforce and back into the role of full-time mother. The percentage of women ages twenty-five to fifty-four in the workforce peaked in 1990 at 74 percent, but has since dropped to 69 percent, according to a 2014 article in the *New York Times*. The percentage of mothers who don't work outside the home skyrocketed to 29 percent—representing 10.4 million stay-at-home moms—in 2012, up from 23 percent in 1999, according to a Pew Research Center analysis. The *Harvard Business Review* analyzed a 2004 survey that looked at 2,443 highly qualified women—those with a professional degree, graduate degree, or an undergraduate degree with high honors—and found that 37 percent of them had chosen to leave the work force at some point. Among moms, the number jumped to 43 percent. As you might suspect, family responsibilities rank high on the list of reasons women are walking out of the workforce. According to a 2014 *New York Times/CBS News/Kaiser Family Foundation* poll of nonworking Americans between the ages of twenty-five and fifty-four, 61 percent of women cited family duties as a reason they weren't working. It's clear there is just not adequate flexibility and support on the corporate level for working moms. Many women who've quit working to be stay-at-home moms say they feel like failures. Why can't they "have it all" the way we've been told? Certainly, syncing with your cycle organizes and amplifies what you can accomplish over the course of a month, and it decreases the pressure you feel to accomplish everything in the span of a day. However, I would love to see more corporations helping women during the motherhood life stage by being open to these women creating working hours that are sustainable for family life. Redefining what success looks like in motherhood—achieving career goals, being available for your kids, and having time for self-care—is part of the biohacking needed in this life stage so you stop trying to just do more and instead decide to do more of what matters.

The Cycle Continues: When Your Daughter Begins Menstruating

If you have a daughter, the most important thing you can do as a mother is to model your cyclical nature for her. Raising her in a cyclical environment where she sees you living in harmony with your hormonal phases imprints this pattern in her so she will adopt it in her own life. Seeing you change your food, vary your workouts, and manage your energy according to your cycle will make this lifestyle seem like second nature to her as she matures. You might not realize it, but your daughter will notice the way you approach your life. I see this in my own daughter, and she's only four! One evening in my late luteal phase, I told her I'd been sitting all day at work and needed to move my body, but I didn't want to push it too hard. She watches me work out at home all the time, and she thought about it for a moment, then said, "What about that workout on the mat? That would be good." It was one of those beaming-with-pride moments for me, and I told her, "You're absolutely right. That's the perfect workout to do right now." So I did my thirty-minute mat Pilates workout, and she did the two-minute warm up with me.

Living a cyclical life is the foundation of the culture in my home. As I mentioned earlier, my daughter notices that things shift throughout the month, and she unconsciously observes shifts for each phase. By the time she hits puberty, she will take it for granted that she should live in a cyclical way. *Hallelujah!* I don't want her to have to try to wrap her head around this way of life in a cerebral way, as a concept I'm suggesting for her, but not doing myself. I would much rather have her tell me, *"Duh, Mom. Leave me alone. How else would I live my life?"* If that happens, I'll welcome the sass.

Unfortunately, this isn't the mainstream experience, yet. A client shared with me a conversation a few of her mom friends had with their daughters' pediatrician. The doctor suggested they put their daughters, who hadn't started menstruating yet, on Prozac so the moms wouldn't have to deal with the girls' "hormonal" behavior when they hit puberty, and also recommended that their daughters start taking the pill as soon as they started their first period. I feel we have to think extremely carefully about medicating girls whether they have any symptoms or not. My client said that these moms were also using the pill to handle their period problems and taking antidepressants to deal with their own mood issues, and they very likely thought that medicating their daughters early on would spare them whatever the moms themselves had gone through. The fact is, we all deserve so much better with our hormonal health care at every life stage. Depending on how old you were when you had your daughter, you may or may not still be menstruating when she hits puberty. There's beauty and wisdom to share in both of these scenarios. If you're both cycling, you can do a lot of role modeling for her during the process. She'll be discovering her identity, and at midlife you may be going through a rediscovery of yourself and your values. It's a big shift for both parties. You can help guide her through any turbulence, but remember that her brain is going through massive shifts, so be as emotionally nonreactive with her as you can. *Mothering and Daughtering* by Sil and Eliza Reynolds is a great resource. Model the self-care practices that will help her navigate all the life stage transitions throughout her lifetime. You can also include her on your own transitional life stage quest. If you enjoy wellness retreats and workshops, take your teenage daughter with you. Let her explore self-care practices like dance, yoga, meditation, journaling, or art so she can become invested in developing her relationship with herself and her inner world and identify with her biology as the source of her inner wisdom.

If you've already stopped cycling when your daughter enters her cyclical phase of life, you'll play more of a support role. Get in the kitchen with her so you can show her how this works. You may want to sync with the lunar phases to help you stay connected to the rhythms of nature and show your teenage daughter that it's important to bond with the world around her and care for it just as she's caring for her own body.

On a practical level, encourage her to use the MyFLO app, and have her send you alerts so you'll know which phase she's in. This way you will be able to be aware of the foods she needs and to help her practice being in tune with her phases so she can balance school and self-care accordingly. The alerts also help you as a mother to avoid taking things personally when your daughter gives you some abrasive energy or attitude. Simply acknowledge where she's at in her cycle and help her through it. Remember, you're midwifing her through the transition from a noncyclical being into a cyclical one. Be patient. Be kind. Be loving. Be supportive. The life-affirming guidance you provide during this time will lay the foundation for her to be a hormonally healthy woman with the ability to discern, balance, and prioritize her values, needs, and responsibilities, which will lead to lasting happiness and fulfillment. Think of how wonderful it would have been if you had been given this wisdom when you were transitioning to becoming a cyclical being. You could have avoided the path that led you to the pursuit of perfection, reclaimed your hormonal health, and enjoyed and taken full advantage of your infradian clock. She'll thank you for it . . . some day.

CHAPTER 10

Dynamic, Wise, and Free

A woman in harmony with her spirit is like a river flowing.
She goes where she will without pretense and arrives at her
destination prepared to be herself and only herself.

—MAYA ANGELOU

Think back to when you were a child—flying high on the swings, skipping down the street, and racing on your bike with your hair flying behind you. You barely thought about your body except to use it to help you do whatever you liked. Then one day your mom sat you down for the "period curse" talk, or you squirmed through a disappointing sex ed class like the one I had, and suddenly everything changed. You discovered what the world thought about your gender, that your body was a burden, and you were destined to suffer because of it. And this discovery broke your heart. It forced you to begin constructing a new set of beliefs about the body that had served you so well up until then, and to create a new inner dialogue to address this heartbreak. You started believing your body would betray you, so you disconnected from it. You learned to distrust your biology and its cyclical rhythm and tried to will it into submission to override its nature. And your body cried out with symptoms, trying to alert you to a fundamental issue you were missing. You tried to listen, but your doctor told you nothing could be done or encouraged you to mask the symptoms.

Meanwhile, the underlying hormonal imbalance remained, creating a vicious cycle and a self-fulfilling prophecy. As you've seen in this book, the foundational concept that your body is a burden couldn't be further from the scientifically evidenced, biological truth. In fact, the only true path to healing is through your feminine nature, through your body, and through integrating your infradian clock. I hope you feel validated as you have been reading, that your inner dialogue is affirming, "Yes, this is what I've been feeling," "I've had these instincts but didn't understand how they were connected," "We should have learned all this before," and "Yes, it makes sense to go with my own flow." Your inner voice and intuition have been calling you home. The Cycle Syncing Method™ is the bridge back to the body you loved, the body that made you feel like you could do anything. It's time to let the healing begin.

How Did We Get Here?

In workshops, I like to a share the story of how women ended up where we are today. Before the age of reason, when Descartes, Newton, and Galileo began exploring the "how" of things, we lived in an age of spirituality. During this time, all the activities in a person's life were connected to a sense of the sacred and the divine, and people lived their lives according to a natural order they observed in the world around them and believed supported the well-being of their soul and spiritual health. But this spiritual phase eventually gave rise to the age of reason as a necessary next step to understand the underlying mechanisms of things, to decode the mysteries that held sway in the age of spirituality. This new era sought to measure and delineate the world and everything in it, lending great power to linear time and specifically to the 24-hour clock. Only things that could be explained in this new model held value, and anything that couldn't be verified scientifically, including elements in the natural and emotional realm, was deemed unimportant. And anyone who focused on the natural was viewed as unthinking or unintelligent. People—*read "men"*—steeped in this new linear knowledge and way of reasoning assumed positions of power and prohibited women from educating and supporting other women. Eventually, this linear thinking fueled ideas of increased productivity. If you knew how things worked, you could outsmart the natural order and produce as much as you wanted, as fast as you wanted, whenever you wanted. Those in power realized they could remake the world in their image and for their benefit.

Of course, it followed suit that women's wisdom and cyclical energy were demoted. Midwifery, female-centric medical practices, and women's health concerns fell by the wayside, viewed as mysteries tied to natural laws that escaped reasoning. Although the age of reason introduced us to the beauty of science, it ignored women's biology and then vilified it because it couldn't be explained in this linear fashion. Women were viewed as sick and given diagnoses like hysteria—derived from the Greek word *hysterika*, meaning "uterus"—the alleged cause of our madness. And now, hundreds of years later, each and every woman's personal response to her hormones stems from that inaccuracy. This book marks the end of this long, painful, and unnecessary journey by uncovering the one missing piece of the scientific conversation the age of reason ignored: women have a second biological clock, and it is equally as valuable as the 24-hour clock. The 28-day clock can be measured; it is predictable; and it demands the same respect, attention, and priority as the 24-hour clock.

Moreover, in perfect lily-gilding fashion, this infradian clock is the physical embodiment of the sacred energy that once governed all of life. The 28-day clock reflects the inherent cyclical timing tied to creation. Women feel it on a visceral level. The word *ritual* derives from the Sanskrit word for menses, *rtu*. The earliest rituals were tied to women's cycles, to lunar and seasonal cycles. But we have been confronted with a cultural narrative that conditions us to deny and devalue our cyclical reality. We face this painful story with every representation of us, with every law governing us, with every story told about us. It's enough to drive any woman nuts and leaves us ungrounded and disconnected not only from a sense of self, but also from a connection to the sacred. This spiritual hunger to connect to ourselves and to embody cyclical timing in our lives explains why women make up the largest consumer base for personal growth, self-help, spiritual development, as well as wellness products and programs. From the beginning of our lives we're fed a tapeworm—a combination of misinformation and ignorance about our biology—that leaves us forever starving, striving to find something outside of ourselves to satisfy this hunger. We have been yearning for that elusive something throughout the centuries of our long oppression. And today, we continue seeking external things—the nicest house, the coolest wardrobe, a better figure, a prettier face, workshops, retreats—in an effort to feel connected to something bigger than ourselves. In fact, there's only one thing we need to restore our power, find our solid ground, and connect to our soul—the missing knowledge about our cyclical biology and the permission to follow our intuition through cyclical living.

Reclaiming Your Sovereignty

I needed to walk over the bridge of science to feel confident in taking on this great experiment in my own life. With so much water under the historical bridge, I wanted some security in stepping back into my own rhythm. It can feel a little daunting to swim against the current if you don't know that the current is already with you.

I find links connecting our female biology with nature all around me. For example, I was awestruck the first time I saw the Mandelbrot set and understood the way fractal geometry described perfectly the natural biological world I had fallen in love with in middle school. You don't have to be a math whiz to see the beauty in fractals. Studying the branches of a tree, the structure of bronchial tubes, or the architecture of the kidney—I was so impressed that all of organic life was based on the same self-replicating patterns. Though I'm no mathematician or physicist, it seems compelling that in our bodies we have this same fractal effect in our hormonal patterns, which influence every system in our body. We also have a quantum effect taking place. Along with the other fathers of quantum physics—Schrödinger, Bohr, and de Broglie—Einstein pushed us past Newtonian physics, past the traditional science that declared our universe was nothing more than an assembly of physical material. Quantum physics showed us that, in fact, nothing in this world is actually solid material, and everything is energy. In quantum mechanics, there's a wondrous effect in which particles can appear to be in two states at once. Our female biochemistry similarly allows us to access two different time patterns—the 24-hour and 28-day rhythms. Surely this combination of the fractal and quantum effects—found uniquely in the female body—is at the heart of the most powerful forces of nature in existence.

I've always been fascinated about how women were living before Euclidean geometry turned the focus to the man-made environment where everything was linear and Newtonian physics made everything finite. Scientists assumed everything in nature was chaotic and unpredictable and could not be described mathematically. They were wrong. Benoit Mandelbrot, an IBM researcher, figured it out in the 1970s. He understood that complexity doesn't mean chaos. Nature is genius, elegant, and efficient, just like you. I can only imagine what that pre-Euclidean life would have looked like—living closely in tune with the natural world, performing cyclical rituals, feeling more free. I wanted to find a way to create that life I imagined within our modern world, so I could live as an empowered and embodied woman. The cyclical pattern gave me a vision of how I could do that—and how any woman living anywhere could do it—without having to run away to the forest or give up technology. The past and how we might have lived in it centuries ago will always remain up for debate, but looking at ourselves through the lens of current science—seeing how our biology reflects the tides, the patterns of the moon, the rotation of a wheel—we no longer have to daydream about the past. We can simply stand in our own skin, emboldened by the forces of nature that power life within us and all around us. Ignoring the power of this biological process is just as limiting as the linear world was before allowing for nature to reveal itself. We simply must reject the conditioning we have received about these so-called hormonal limitations and embrace what we are—fractals of the cosmos, quantum beings, stardust made flesh—and shine a light on a new version of reality that does us and humanity justice.

Even though this new way of living involves connecting deeply with your biology, the science of your cycle doesn't mean your hormones rule your life. By acknowledging the simultaneous existence of your two clocks and syncing with your second clock, you're going beyond reductive materialist science (the notion that the brain creates consciousness) and biological determinism (the idea that you have no free will). You're not just the by-product of your body's hormonal mandate. With greater awareness, you can be tuned in to those hormones and bend them to your will for your benefit. If you were just a bag of biochemicals, you would have no ability to tweak your hormonal status—but as you've seen throughout this book, you have the power to heal your hormones and upgrade your well-being.

This is a beautiful opportunity for science and spirituality to converge and enhance our consciousness and self-awareness. So many forms of spirituality suggest we must transcend the body to connect to something bigger than ourselves. But what I've found personally is that for women, it is *through* the body that we come to this greater perspective and deeper conscious awareness. I'm not the first woman to try to show other women the way home to ourselves, to our feminine nature, to our connection to the divine. Jungian analyst Clarissa Pinkola Estés wrote one of the most seminal female empowerment books, *Women Who Run With the Wolves,* back in 1992. Marion Woodman and so many others have also shared the idea that reclaiming our inner wisdom is the key to fulfillment. I had the privilege of seeing Hilma af Klint's work at the Guggenheim Museum during its exhibition. Here was a woman during the suffragist movement of the early 1900s who was looking for validation of her intrinsic value in the midst of a society that marginalized women. She painted incredible representations of the intersection of the science of life and the geometry of the sacred to show that we are all truly equal. It was like getting a hug from a friend in the past, and it felt like no time had passed at all.

What I've gleaned from nearly twenty years of helping women balance their hormones and tap into the power of their feminine energy is that through healing the body we become whole. When you connect to this larger creative force of nature by going within your own body, syncing with your cycle becomes the physical daily practice that keeps you anchored from floating out into external distractions that are unfulfilling. You settle into a sense of greater self-awareness and realize that everything you're seeking is already within you. Nothing is missing; nothing is wrong. You are perfect in your ever-changing nature, just the way you are.

This understanding gives us an opportunity to reclaim our sovereignty, allowing us to recognize our true nature as powerful agents of change. And our ability to amplify this energy, by staying deeply connected to our biology, lets us focus on any aspect of our lives and create whatever change is needed—within ourselves, within our relationships, and within the world. By deeply investigating the *how* of our inner mechanics, we discover that we are not lesser, that we are not designed to be dominated, that our bodies are a gift that keeps the timing for a rhythm that is beneficial for all. Our perspective adds much-needed medicine to our unbalanced culture. And as we balance our hormones and get into harmony with our FLO, we can bring balance and harmony to the world around us.

Reimagining the Hero's Journey

Joseph Campbell outlined the concept of the hero's journey in his classic work *The Power of Myth*. Essentially, this journey involves an unlikely hero who receives the call to undertake an epic journey. He ventures out on a quest, makes progress, withstands setbacks, and ultimately achieves the goal, the grail, and/or the girl. It's about the conquest—doing something so you can get something—and this glorified tale has endured throughout the millennia.

Take a moment to consider how much the myth of the hero's journey has trickled down and seeped into your conscious and subconscious mind, dictating what you view as heroic, valuable, worthy, and laudable. In the telling and perpetuating of these stories, we're basically saying that the masculine energy of adventure, pursuit, and conquest is what society has been built on and what deserves to be valued.

Then notice that there are no stories in which a female hero is portrayed. That's why we struggle so much with our cyclical nature. We glorify the doing, and we're still very wary of the not doing.

A side effect of not having our stories told and represented is that we actually lack vocabulary to describe our reality.

Here's what I've experienced in the female version of the hero's journey. There is the call—but it's not for a grail or a goal; it's from the body or the heart, and it's a quest to come home to yourself. Then there is the journey within, into the unseen places of your psyche to access your wild, feminine nature and bring that to the light. Then there is the reclamation, which is the journey of the cycle—going through the phases to reclaim an appropriate balance of your masculine and feminine energy. Finally there is the rebirth.

You get to experience this every month. You get to go within to rest and incubate to make sure you have all that you need. And from that place of fullness, you can bring yourself out into the light. The deeper within you go, the farther you can launch forward when it is the time to do so in the first half of the cycle. You get to reinvent yourself every month. What an incredible gift.

The ordinary becomes extraordinary because you have this deeper self-awareness. Every little thing can become an opportunity for you to grow, learn more about yourself, and live more from a place of compassionate listening and compassionate responding.

It's Okay to Get Emotional

When I share this information in workshops, there is a palpable emotional process that takes place in the room. It's hard to describe, but it feels like the women in attendance go through several experiences. First, there's validation and excitement as the light flicks on and all the dots are connected. Then there's anger in recognizing what they have missed out on in their personal lives due to this misunderstanding. Then there's sadness at what can't be reclaimed. Ultimately, there's joy and elation that what they hoped for all along, what they dared to believe in quiet brief moments, is true—that they are worthy, powerful, equal, and capable leaders. This realization is emotional for them. It's emotional for me. And reading this book may be emotional for you, too.

WHAT YOU MIGHT FEEL

I talk with women on a daily basis who are confronted with very strong, conflicting emotions about this revelation.

- Martina, a thirty-four-year-old marketing executive, felt a tremendous amount of grief when she learned how syncing with her cyclical nature was the solution to her period problems and the path to greater happiness and fulfillment at work, in love, and as a mother. She felt like she had wasted twenty years of her life suffering needlessly from hormonal imbalance, and that her symptoms had contributed to the breakup of her marriage and her decision to take another career path. She mourned the life she could have had and *should* have had.

- Robin, a twenty-one-year-old student at an Ivy League university, was furious. She couldn't believe that in all her years as a student at the nation's finest schools, not one professor, not one counselor, not one school nurse had ever told her the truth about her biochemistry. Spurred to take action to ensure the spread of misinformation wouldn't continue to the next generation, Robin started her own version of a Period Club—*now there's a girl after my own heart!*—at her sorority and made each member vow to give any younger female siblings or cousins the *real* sex ed talk.

- Sarah, in her late thirties, felt the big difference for her was emotional. Before she'd always considered herself a quitter, but then she started to realize there are certain times of the month when she's really excited about trying new things and then there are other times when she really needs to just rest. She knows now that things that were really exciting before might not resonate right now, but if she just waits for the next phase, her excitement will come back. She also feels compassion for all the other women in her life—her mother, her friends, her grandmother—who put so much pressure on themselves to be perfect, and didn't know they could have lifted this weight off themselves if they had just connected with their cycles.

Waking up to the truth of who you are may place you on a roller coaster of emotions. Give yourself time to digest these insights, and start making changes slowly in your own life. Don't feel like you have to tackle these cultural wrongs on a societal level, leading the charge to change our sexual education system, institutional bias, or health care gaps. Start with yourself, and heal your hormones so you can feel better and live the best life you possibly can. My wish is for you to finally get off this hamster wheel of oppression—the one that has you running in circles trying to be perfect, pretty, thin, compliant, and docile; the one that values conformity. My wish is for women to bask in this corrected self-awareness, stand tall, throw off this yoke entirely, and walk together toward a new future. I can't fully envision what this future will bring, but my heart beats with joy at the thought of what we can create.

No Perfection Required

As we march forward into this new future, we need to make sure we don't simply take the same unhealthy approaches to productivity and apply them to this cyclical way of living. Don't think of syncing with your cycle as something you have to add to your to-do list in your quest for perfection. I understand that in our patriarchal environment, it's almost impossible to avoid being infected with the illness of perfectionism. As young girls, when we hit puberty, we're struck with myths about our bodies and faced with the challenge of figuring out how to survive the patriarchy. On a meta level, the way our society values women is tangled up in how perfect you are—perfect in looks, moods, performance, and everything else. A by-product of the intergenerational patriarchal wounding we have inherited, perfectionism is something we use as a survival response. It's how we unconsciously seek out safety and security. It's how we gain value from our peers and approval from our community. Mostly, it's the ticket to landing a man, which in our heteronormative society has long been viewed as the key to safety. The more perfect you are, the more successful the mate you can attract, and the better they'll be able to provide you with the economic and physical security you crave. This tired, old-school notion no longer has relevance today, because women can do it ourselves—provide for ourselves, gain economic independence, and install an alarm system for safety if we need to. So why do we still hold tight to this harmful story? It doesn't stand up. It doesn't hold water. It disintegrates in the light. Before you realize how faulty it is, however, this script screws up your relationship with your body. And unfortunately, this story can prevent you from gaining the benefits of engaging your cyclical clock. I see this far too often. In almost twenty years of working with clients one-on-one, I've never met a woman who hasn't had this psychopathology of perfectionism get in the way of a healthy relationship with her body. There are two sides to the perfectionism coin: procrastination and micromanagement.

- **Procrastination:** If you find yourself thinking, "I'm not going to start taking care of myself by syncing with my cycle yet because I can't follow the entire program the way I want to," you may be falling victim to the procrastination side of the perfectionism coin. When you know you can't give something your 100 percent effort, you may not bother trying at all. What's really a shame is that if you gave 50 percent of your utmost effort, or even 20 percent, you could still gain some benefit, but you're missing out on all that because you don't want to be judged for not doing enough. Sometimes the judges are outside of you—teachers, bosses, or coworkers—but more often your harshest critic is the one you see in the mirror. You don't want to let yourself down by not being perfect, so you don't even start.

- **Micromanagement:** If you're syncing with your cycle but micro-managing it with thoughts like, "Am I eating the right food today? Did I do the wrong exercise for this phase? Oh no, I planned my big presentation for the wrong phase!" you can drive yourself crazy. Eventually, this micromanagement adds to your stress, so you give up and assume it's too hard because you couldn't live up to your own expectations.

How can anyone survive in a mental ecosystem like this? It's so stressful and exhausting to be caught up in this dance of procrastination or micro-management. More important, how do you unhook yourself from the per-fectionist trap? Take it from me, a recovering perfectionist—you can do it. I use the phrase "recovering," because perfectionism is never really cured. You have to be vigilant each and every day to break free from the chains of perfectionism. I used to be a massive procrastinator, which is ironic con-sidering how much I do now on a daily basis. I'm a testament to breaking out of this trap. When I developed the Cycle Syncing Method™ to heal my hormonal issues, I began confronting the scripted thoughts in my brain at every turn. You don't have to be negative toward these thoughts. You just need to be objective and ask yourself, "Do I need this behavior to survive or feel safe?" "How is this thought serving me?" "Is it serving me to delay starting to sync with my second clock?" "Is it serving me to get so wrapped up in the minute details of this process that I miss out on the joy it's sup-posed to bring?" When you answer honestly, you may recognize that you're in perfectionist survival mode, which feels stressful. The Cycle Syncing Method™ is designed to help you break free from this pattern so you can thrive, not just survive.

The real genius of cyclical living is you don't have to do it perfectly. Yes, this book gives you charts to help you find foods, exercises, and planning tools to optimize your hormones, biological systems, and creativity, but following your instincts is your goal. Flexibility is baked into the method. I want you to do this program *intuitively*. That's a loaded word we've been conditioned to mistrust, but I mean it from a biochemical perspective: the right and left hemispheres of your brain cross-communicate about facts and feelings to inform you about your body's needs. This process also gives you access to a conscious awareness that transcends your body. You just *know* or *feel* what's right for you in the moment. If you're in your ovulatory phase, which generally calls for cooling foods, but you're exhausted from a tough work week and feel like you need a bowl of hot soup, go ahead and have the soup. That intuitive sense that you need something warm is coming from a wise, powerful, and conscious place. Listen to your self. Let this new cyclical practice be the bridge that connects you to your intuition, so you can respond dynamically to your body's needs. Trust yourself.

You can also give yourself permission to start syncing with your cycle by simply dipping your toe in the water and changing one thing, whether it's food, exercise, scheduling, or focusing on one specific phase. Wherever you start, celebrate and enjoy it, and build from there. I've been syncing with my cycle for almost two decades, and I keep learning and going deeper with my practice of living as an embodied woman. From your first baby steps it becomes an upward spiral of learning, appreciation, self-awareness, and growth. That's what I want you to have. If you're currently stuck in 24-hour clock perfection mode, just focus on unraveling your to-do list and stretching it into your second clock, the 28-day clock. You'll be less busy and will have more space to listen to your body, to tap into your intuition, and to respond with what's right for you. Syncing with your cycle should be fun for you, not stressful. It should be a joy for you to develop this kind of loving relationship with yourself and your body.

TELL YOUR INNER VOICE TO BE KIND!

Realizing that most of what you believe about yourself and your body has been based on misinformation is a real eye-opener. All of a sudden, you begin to see there is no truth in all those nasty things you have been telling yourself. The things you mistook for character flaws or imperfections are actually part of your strengths. And once you realize scientific evidence shows negative thinking can alter your genetic expression in a harmful way, while positive thoughts can enhance your DNA and genes, it becomes even more critical for you to reexamine your inner dialog. Instead of berating yourself for what you thought were personal failures, look for the biological root causes and attend to them. Here's a look at the conversations you should be having with yourself.

Old Inner Dialog	New Inner Dialog
I can't stick with a diet. I have no willpower.	When I switch hormonal phases, my metabolism changes and I have different caloric needs.
I'm a failure because sometimes I can't handle the stress at work.	In the second half of my cycle, my body heightens my stress response and releases more cortisol. I can practice targeted self-care to counteract this.
I always feel so anxious. I'm a weak person.	Maybe I have a hormonal imbalance that triggers certain neurotransmitters in my brain, or my body is lacking in omega-3 fatty acids.
I suck because I'm terrible at following through on things.	Maybe I'm just using the wrong clock and need to schedule things to work better with my body's natural rhythms.

A CHAIN OF COURAGE AND LOVE

Although the revelations in this book about your hormones and biological systems may be new to you, the notion that women are powerful biological creatures has deep roots. Books by other women have been the beacons of light for me on the path of self-remembering. I remember when I was in middle school reading about menstrual rites of Native American women in Carolyn Niethammer's book *Daughters of the Earth* and feeling a longing for something I couldn't name. *The Joy of Sex* changed my world view, as did *Woman: An Intimate Geography*, by Natalie Angier. A friend gave me Sharron Rose's book, *The Path of the Priestess*, which inspires women to get in touch with their powerful inner goddess energy, and gave me insight into a language I didn't even know existed. Then Eve Ensler published *The Vagina Monologues*. Christiane Northrup's *Women's Bodies, Women's Wisdom* validated our physical suffering. Most recently, Madeline Miller's *Circe* was the first fiction book I've read describing the hero's journey from a female's point of view. Each of these books read like a love note, encouraged me, validated me, nurtured me, brought me home to myself. These authors' courage in writing in historically unprecedented ways makes me believe change is not only possible, but inevitable. Authors like Miranda Gray (*The Optimized Woman*) and Alexandra Pope and Sjanie Hugo Wurlitzer (*Wild Power*), who share that the journey to enhancing our health, creativity, and spirituality lies in our menstrual cycle, are allied voices in the growing chorus of women seeking to get in touch with our cyclical side.

Is It Time for a Matriarchy?

Many of the women who have healed their period problems by syncing with their cycle ask me whether I think the next logical step in the feminist movement is the establishment of a matriarchal society to replace the oppressive patriarchy. Most of them look a little surprised when I tell them we've already had matriarchal societies. Archaeologist and anthropologist Dr. Marija Gimbutas described a goddess- and woman-centered culture from the Paleolithic era as far back as two million years ago, which was replaced by a patriarchy only about five thousand years ago. Based on her archaeological findings, she suggested the gynocentric culture was a peaceful one that revered the feminine nature and believed in economic parity. Doesn't that sound nice? Could it be true that women thousands of years ago enjoyed economic equality, while women in the US today still earn a paltry 82 cents for every dollar men make? The conversation about our matriarchal heritage doesn't get much attention, and in fact some dismiss or question the idea, as Cynthia Eller, a professor of religious studies, did in her book *The Myth of Matriarchal Prehistory.*

But don't give up on the idea of matriarchal ancestors too fast. Emerging research on genetics points to something bizarre that happened about five to seven thousand years ago. A 2015 study in *Genome Research* unearthed evidence that the population of reproducing men throughout Europe, Africa, and Asia took a dramatic nosedive. Researchers discovered a bottleneck in the Y chromosome, which is passed from father to son, causing the collapse of genetic diversity among males. What caused this mysterious drop-off? New research in a 2018 issue of *Nature Communications* claims the most likely scenario was war between patrilineal clans. Stone Age men were so vicious they were clubbing one another to death and decimating entire male lineages. This left behind a majority population of women— about seventeen women for every man. I think it's only logical to assume that while the men were off killing one another, the women must have been constructing cultures at home. I can imagine them creating a society steeped in female-centered values that catered to their biological reality.

I don't understand why some people find it so hard to believe we could have had a gynocentric prehistoric society. In fact, there are matriarchal cultures still in existence today. Just look at the Mosuo society in rural China. A beautiful 2012 documentary on PBS's *Frontline* called *The Women's Kingdom* explored this fascinating society's culture. The women there don't marry in the traditional sense. They practice what's called a "walking marriage" in which male suitors enter a woman's bedroom hoping to enjoy a "sweet night," and she holds the power to decide whether or not she wants him to stay for sex—no strings attached. After doing the deed, the man has to hit the road the following morning. A Mosuo woman can enjoy a walking marriage with more than one man if she wishes without any of the shame that American women sometimes feel about sex. In this way of life, lovers don't live under the same roof, and fathers aren't involved in raising their children. It's the mother and the mother's family who take charge of child-rearing, and it's the mother's name that is passed down to the children. In the all-important matrilineal family unit, relatives choose the most capable woman to be in charge of the household. For me, one of the most touching scenes in the documentary was watching a young girl talk about how proud she was to be female, saying, "I enjoy being a girl. Girls can do everything. Isn't that great?" *Yes, that is great!* And true!

After reading this book and understanding all the gifts your cyclical nature can offer you when your hormones are healthy and balanced, you might feel like banging the drum to overthrow our patriarchal society and replace it with a matriarchy. But we don't want a society where one biological clock dominates the other. In her essay "There Is No Hierarchy of Oppressions," feminist poet Audre Lorde wrote, "I have learned that oppression and the intolerance of difference come in all shapes and sizes and colors and sexualities; and that among those of us who share the goals of liberation and a workable future for our children, there can be no hierarchies of oppression." We need to envision a more inclusive future that honors our cyclical nature so we can optimize our physical, emotional, and social well-being while supporting inclusion, sustainability, and healing. You deserve to have truthful information about your body and its amazing gifts, and we all deserve a future that embraces our right to live according to our true nature.

Charting the Path Ahead

How will our feminine power evolve in the future? Now that we're aware of our infradian clock, we have an opportunity to spread that knowledge and expand on what we know. As you saw in chapter 1, women are woefully underrepresented in health research, and this is especially true of females of reproductive age. A 2014 report on sex-specific research from Brigham and Women's Hospital got it right: "Medical research that is either sex- or gender-neutral or skewed to male physiology puts women at risk for missed opportunities for prevention, incorrect diagnoses, misinformed treatments, sickness, and even death." It's time for researchers to stop assuming that findings from studies on men and postmenopausal women translate to menstruating women. In the past, scientists pointed to the potential risks to women of childbearing age and their future fetuses as reasons for excluding them from research studies. Scientists may have finally found a way around this roadblock. In a 2017 report in *Nature Communications*, researchers revealed they had succeeded in integrating cells from every organ involved in the menstrual cycle—ovaries, fallopian tubes, uterus, cervix—in a petri dish. This gives health researchers an easier, risk-free way to study women's cycles. For now, researchers are planning to use the system to study hormonal contraceptives and their effects on female biochemistry, and they also hope to look into the hormonal cycle's impact on the gastrointestinal tract and conditions like Crohn's disease and inflammatory bowel disease. This is a great start, but I can't help thinking of all the women-centered research we might be able to access thanks to this laboratory version of your cycle. I can't wait for researchers to take a deeper dive on the following:

- How nutrition impacts each phase of a woman's cycle
- How nutrition can ease symptoms of disease in women
- How fitness routines affect each phase of a woman's cycle
- How a cyclical fitness approach affects a woman's biochemistry
- How low-carb diets affect women's biochemistry and phases
- How vegetarian and vegan diets affect women's biochemistry and phases
- How intermittent fasting affects women's biochemistry and phases
- How a cyclical eating plan affects women's biochemistry and phases
- How women can best achieve autophagy (an anti-aging process that involves cleaning up damaged cells) in their reproductive years
- How women metabolize prescription drugs in each cycle phase
- How hormonal birth control given to teenage girls affects their mental health and future fertility

Thinking about everything we could learn about our biochemistry from this research makes me excited about our future and hopeful the day is coming when women won't ever again question our cyclical nature and won't dream of ignoring it or trying to mask it to fit into our male-patterned society. The more we know, the more we'll understand that biohacking our diets, exercise, and schedules with our monthly cycle is the only way to live that makes sense for women. And we need to make sure the biohacking world helps women understand they need to biohack for their own biological reality to reap the benefits of this practice.

It isn't just the medical field that needs to be more inclusive. The future of our work environments is also at stake. I was invited to speak on a panel about artificial intelligence (AI). What on earth was a hormonal health expert like me doing talking about AI, you ask? I'm the first to admit I'm not much of a techie, but I do want to make sure AI is developed with the female biochemical reality in mind. Did you know AI is largely based on male patterns? Or that developers may unconsciously be infusing it with gender biases? Or that AI could amplify existing gender inequality? Here's proof: Google's online advertising algorithm displays ads for high-paying C-suite jobs to more men than women, according to a 2015 study in *Proceedings on Privacy Enhancing Technologies*. This same study found that AI trained to process text determined that "man is to computer programmer as woman is to homemaker." And eye-opening research presented at the 2017 Conference on Empirical Methods in Natural Language Processing in Copenhagen, Denmark, found that image-recognition software ramped up sexist stereotypes. For example, looking up the word "cooking" in two popular stock image collections turned up 33 percent more pictures involving women than men. No surprise, right? When the researchers used machine learning to train the software, however, that percentage jumped to 68 percent. Machine learning magnified the existing bias! Can you imagine a world where machines reinforce sexism? We can't let that happen. Fortunately, this research team sought to reverse this unexpected trend and implemented a series of controls that effectively reduced the bias. That's the kind of AI development we want. Even more pressing is the need for more women in leadership roles in the creation of AI. In the AI and machine-learning arena, women make up as few as 18 percent of C-level executives, according to an analysis by TechEmergence. How can we expect a field that is more than 80 percent male-dominated to accurately reflect women's needs when creating algorithms, chatbots, and other forms of artificial intelligence that will fundamentally shape the future of the workplace and the world?

A Feminine Force of Nature

Once you start living in sync with your cyclical nature and according to your unique female biological rhythms, you'll unleash the superpower of your hormones. You'll minimize bothersome symptoms; boost your biological systems; enhance your long-term health; and gain access to greater creativity, more effortless productivity, deeper fulfillment, and greater self awareness. Do it for yourself, do it for your health, do it for your happiness. But remember, getting hormonally healthy isn't the ultimate goal; it's just the jumping-off point for a whole new life. In part 2 of this book you discovered how the Cycle Syncing Method™ can be applied to yourself to heal your hormones, improve your biological systems, and boost your overall well-being. In part 3 you saw how to build on your increased health, energy, and vitality to unleash your creativity at work, enhance your orgasms and relationships, and be a better mom without all the stress. Once all these areas of your life are firing on all cylinders, thanks to your new cyclical practice, you can begin to look outside yourself and see how you can be an agent of change in the world around you. With your new ability to continually increase your energy physically and emotionally, you can share your talents with the world and become a force of nature for good, which is what women are hardwired to do—to create out of the fertile void, to tend and befriend, and to lead like a woman.

So many women feel stuck and are looking for someone to tell them how to bring forth their creative talents. But as you now realize, you have an inner guidance mechanism that shows you the way and will lead you to give birth to your true self. Now that you are no longer in the dark about who you are, and you've freed up all of your extra inner energy from being on that hamster wheel of failed diets, failed workouts, and failed time management, what will you do with your one wild and precious life? Now that your head is no longer filled with that inner critical voice berating you for your alleged lack of willpower, self-control, and motivation, how can you harness your brainpower to take advantage of your unique talents? Who would you be if you weren't somebody who was always dealing with symptoms? How would you use your body to master your environment rather than working on your body as a never-ending project? What can you do to become a force of nature?

A Radical New Life

What you have learned in this book shouldn't feel like the next wellness trend or the next fad diet. The information here should feel like a radical departure from anything you have ever read, and it is. Syncing with your cycle brings you home to yourself. You no longer need to be critical of yourself, doubt yourself, or chase some idealized notion of static perfection. You can finally tune in to your body and listen to your natural rhythms so you can blossom in a dynamic, responsive, and compassionate way. With science on your side, you can have confidence to live the way that makes you feel good. You can go after all of your dreams and ambitions in a way that builds your energy, sustains your health, and decreases your stress. You can let go of being perfect and trying to be the same every day. There's nothing more beautiful or more powerful than a courageous, dynamic woman. Adopting this cyclical practice is a radical new way of thinking about your body and living your life that lets you celebrate being you. In revolutionizing your life, you will revolutionize the world. On your own time.

MEAL PLANS

Follicular Phase

Breakfast: Overnight Oats with Cashews, Goji Berries,
   and Cinnamon (page 330)
Lunch: Lentil Tomato Quinoa Pilaf (page 331)
Dinner: Chicken Veggie Buddha Bowl (page 331)

Ovulatory Phase

Breakfast: Sweet Green Protein Smoothie (page 333)
Lunch: Hearty Greens Salad with Salmon Toasts (page 333)
Dinner: Zoodles with Pumpkin Seed Pesto (page 335)

Luteal Phase

Breakfast: Avocado Tater-Toast (page 336)
Lunch: Turkey Tacos (with Vegetarian Option) (page 337)
Dinner: Chickpea Pasta with Garlic Kale (page 338)

Menstrual Phase

Breakfast: PBJ Bowl (page 339)
Lunch: Bento Salmon Soba Miso Lunch (page 339)
Dinner: Bunless Bison Burgers with the Works (page 341)

RECIPES

Follicular Phase

OVERNIGHT OATS WITH CASHEWS, GOJI BERRIES, AND CINNAMON

Serves 1

¼ cup organic steel-cut oats

¾ cup water or unsweetened almond milk

Small handful cashews

Small handful goji berries

Dash of ground cinnamon

Dash of sea salt

1 teaspoon apple cider vinegar

Combine all ingredients in a bowl and cover. Place in refrigerator and let soak overnight. In the morning, transfer to a pot and cook on medium heat until heated through.

LENTIL TOMATO QUINOA PILAF

Serves 2 or 3

1 cup quinoa

2 cups water

1 cup cooked lentils, canned or fresh

1 large tomato, chopped

Small handful fresh basil

Romaine lettuce (or greens of your choice)

Honey mustard dressing, organic

Cook quinoa in water according to package directions. Combine the quinoa, cooked or canned lentils, chopped tomato, and basil. In a separate bowl, toss the greens with honey mustard dressing. Divide the greens, top each serving with about ¾ cup of the quinoa mixture, and serve.

CHICKEN VEGGIE BUDDHA BOWL

Serves 2

2 boneless skinless organic chicken breasts

Coarse sea salt to taste

Freshly ground black pepper to taste

Fresh or dried thyme to taste

2 tablespoons extra virgin olive oil

4 carrots, peeled and sliced into ¼-inch rounds

1 cup of string beans, ends trimmed and cut into 1-inch pieces

1 head of broccoli, sliced into stems and florets

2 bunches baby bok choy

Black beans (optional)

For the dressing

¼ cup tahini paste

¼ cup olive oil

Juice from 2 lemons

2 teaspoons honey

Sea salt and pepper to taste

To poach the chicken: Fill a large skillet with about ½ inch of water. Bring to a boil over high heat. Add chicken, salt, and herbs, and let simmer. After 10 minutes, remove skillet from heat and cover. Let stand for about 15 minutes, turning chicken over halfway through, until the chicken is thoroughly cooked. Drain poaching liquid.

To steam the veggies: In a pot, layer carrots, then broccoli, then string beans, and bok choy on top. Add water to fill the pot to a level just below the broccoli. Sprinkle with salt. Steam for 15 minutes, or until broccoli is tender when tested with a fork.

For the dressing: Combine the ingredients in a food processor. Start with half the lemon juice, and add more as needed to your taste. Mix until well blended.

Arrange veggies in a large bowl, and add the black beans if you will be using them. Top with the sliced poached chicken, and drizzle with 2 to 3 tablespoons dressing.

Ovulatory Phase

SWEET GREEN PROTEIN SMOOTHIE

Serves 1

1 cup unsweetened almond milk

2 cups mixed baby greens

1 tablespoon chia seeds

1 tablespoon hemp seeds

1 tablespoon ground flaxseeds

1 date, pitted

1 tablespoon almond butter

¼ teaspoon vanilla extract

Combine all ingredients in a blender, and blend until smooth. Pour into a glass and enjoy.

HEARTY GREENS SALAD WITH SALMON TOASTS

Serves 2

For the salad

2 cups baby spinach

1 cup escarole, chopped

1 small fennel bulb, thinly sliced

¼ cup fresh parsley, chopped

For the dressing

½ cup extra virgin olive oil

½ lemon, juiced

1 tablespoon Dijon mustard

1 teaspoon honey

2 tablespoons fresh tarragon, chopped

1 clove garlic, minced

Coarse sea salt to taste

Freshly ground black pepper to taste

For the salmon and toasts

1 can wild salmon, drained

1 to 2 tablespoons Dijon mustard

Gluten-free or sprouted grain bread of your choice

Combine salad ingredients in a large bowl. Combine dressing ingredients in a mason jar, and shake until combined. Pour desired amount of dressing onto salad and toss well. Drain the can of salmon. In a small bowl, mix the salmon with Dijon mustard. Toast your bread, and then spread the salmon on it. Serve with salad and enjoy!

ZOODLES WITH PUMPKIN SEED PESTO

Serves 2

For the zoodles

> 3 zucchini, spiralized or julienned
>
> Sea salt to taste
>
> Olive oil for sautéing

For the pesto

> 1 garlic clove
>
> 2 cups fresh basil leaves (or use a combination of basil, spinach, and/or arugula)
>
> ½ cup raw pumpkin seeds
>
> ⅓ cup olive oil
>
> 1 lemon, juiced
>
> Salt to taste

For the protein

> **Your choice of grilled chicken or fish, or white beans**

Blend all the pesto ingredients in a food processor. In a large sauté pan, heat some olive oil and lightly sauté the zucchini noodles. Toss together the noodles and pesto. Add the protein of your choice on top, then serve.

Luteal Phase

AVOCADO TATER-TOAST

Serves 1

1 sweet potato, sliced lengthwise

½ avocado

2 eggs

Butter or coconut oil for frying

Juice of ½ lime or lemon

Turmeric to taste

Coarse sea salt to taste

Freshly ground black pepper to taste

Preheat oven to 350°. Place the sweet potato slices on a sheet pan, and bake them for 20 minutes. (Reserve the unused slices for a snack or another day's breakfast; they can easily be heated up in a pan.)

In a frying pan, heat the butter or oil, and prepare eggs over easy by frying them on both sides until the white is cooked through but the yolk is still runny. Sprinkle some turmeric, salt, and pepper onto the eggs while cooking.

Mash the meat of the avocado with the lime juice. Spread the mashed avocado on the warm sweet potato slices, season with sea salt and black pepper to taste, and serve with eggs on top.

TURKEY TACOS (WITH VEGETARIAN OPTION)

Serves 2

½ pound ground turkey or ½ head cauliflower

Salt and freshly ground pepper to taste

½ cup parsnip, cubed

1 teaspoon olive oil

1 teaspoon chili powder, or hot sauce or spice of your choice

½ cup cooked brown basmati rice

½ cup black beans

1 tablespoon shaved radish

4 small gluten-free corn tortillas

½ cup chopped tomatoes

Cilantro for garnish

½ lime, wedged

If you are using ground turkey, heat the oil in a pan. Season the ground turkey with salt and pepper, and sauté on medium heat until fully cooked. Set aside. If you are using cauliflower for the vegetarian option, roast the cauliflower with the parsnip in the next step.

Preheat the oven to 400°. Peel, cube, and toss the parsnip with olive oil, salt, and pepper. Place on a sheet pan and roast until tender, about 40 minutes or so. Set aside. If you are preparing a vegetarian recipe, break the cauli-flower into florets; toss with olive oil, salt, pepper, and chili powder or your favorite hot sauce or other spice; and roast at the same temperature and at the same time as the parsnip, until tender. Set aside.

Shave the radish with a grater or mandolin. Warm the tacos in a pan.

Assemble tacos with rice and beans on bottom, then add ground turkey or cauliflower and the rest of the toppings. Garnish with cilantro and a squeeze of fresh lime.

CHICKPEA PASTA WITH GARLIC KALE

Serves 2 or 3

1 box chickpea pasta (spirals or ziti shape)

1 head lacinato kale

Olive oil for sautéing

2 or 3 garlic cloves, peeled and finely chopped

Salt and pepper to taste

½ cup water

½ cup chopped raw walnuts

Bring a large pot of salted water to a boil, and then add chickpea pasta and cook for approximately 7 minutes or according to package directions. Drain and toss with olive oil.

While the pasta is boiling, wash and chop the kale. Heat the olive oil in a large saucepan, add the chopped garlic, and then quickly add the chopped kale. Stir until the kale is coated, add salt and pepper to taste, add ½ cup water, and cover the pan tightly. Steam-sauté until the greens are tender.

Combine the kale with the pasta, top with chopped walnuts, and serve.

Menstrual Phase

PBJ BOWL

Serves 1

Cream of buckwheat

1 tablespoon raisins

1 tablespoon sunflower seed butter or almond butter

Hemp seeds

1 teaspoon maple syrup

Cook the cream of buckwheat according to package directions. Mix the raisins in while hot. Drizzle sunflower seed or almond butter on top. Top with hemp seeds and maple syrup.

BENTO SALMON SOBA MISO LUNCH

Serves 2

2 4-ounce salmon fillets

Untoasted sesame oil to taste

Soy sauce to taste

1 8-ounce package buckwheat soba noodles

For the dressing

2 tablespoons low-sodium gluten-free tamari

¼ cup rice vinegar

1 tablespoon toasted sesame oil

For the soup

2 cups water

½ cup cubed tofu

2 scallions

2 tablespoons miso paste

1 nori sheet

Toasted sesame oil to taste

Grated daikon or pickled ginger (optional)

Preheat the oven to 350°. Toss the salmon in the untoasted sesame oil and soy sauce, place in a baking dish, and bake for 12 minutes.

While the salmon is in the oven, boil the soba noodles according to the package directions, rinse in cold water, and drain.

While the soba noodles are boiling, whisk together the dressing ingredients.

To make the soup: Bring 3 cups of water to a boil. Add the chopped tofu and sliced scallions, and continue cooking for 30 seconds. Remove from the heat and evenly distribute into two soup bowls. Stir 1 tablespoon miso paste into each bowl of soup. Tear the nori sheet into pieces, and add to each bowl. Drizzle with toasted sesame oil.

To assemble your bento, serve each diner the following:

A bowl of miso soup

A plate of cold soba noodles, with a dipping bowl of dressing on the side

A plate of hot miso-glazed salmon

Optional: grated daikon radish and pickled ginger

BUNLESS BISON BURGERS WITH THE WORKS

Serves 2

½ pound ground bison meat

1 tablespoon coconut oil

½ red onion, chopped

1 package shitake mushrooms

1 package of baby spinach

1 avocado

Form the bison meat into 2 patties and grill on a barbecue, or panfry for about 5 minutes on each side.

Heat a large saucepan to medium heat and add coconut oil. Sauté the chopped onions for 2 minutes, then add the mushrooms and sauté for another 2 to 3 minutes. Add the spinach and cook until it's wilted.

Add avocado slices to the burgers, and top with the spinach and mushrooms. If you feel you need some carbs, add a gluten-free bun. Enjoy!

GUIDES AND RESOURCES

I have created many helpful resources, guides, and e-books to help you as you get yourself in the FLO. You can find all of them below with links.

Biohacking Guides

Hormone Supplement Guide: www.FLOliving.com/supplement-guide

Fibroids: www.FLOliving.com/fibroids-guide

Endometriosis: www.FLOliving.com/endo-guide

PCOS: www.FLOliving.com/pcos-guide

PMS: www.FLOliving.com/pms-guide

Fertility: www.FLOliving.com/fertility-guide

Perimenopause: www.FLOliving.com/perimenopause-guide

Emotional Root Causes: www.FLOliving.com/emotions-guide

Birth Control Rehab: www.FLOliving.com/birth-control-rehab

Bonus *In the FLO* Content

See www.IntheFLObook.com/bonus for these guides:

Get In the FLO Now Quick-Start Program

Cyclical Self-Care Guide

Cyclical Skin-Care Guide

Adaptogen Guide

Access to the In the FLO Facebook group

More Support to Put into Action What You've Learned in This Book

Join me and our community of women in the revolutionary FLO 28: The Cycle Syncing™ Membership, an online group membership for women around the world to care for their bodies and find more flow in their lives. In FLO 28, you will be supported with everything you learned in this book. You'll have access to five key tools to help you optimize your biochemistry, leverage your neurochemistry, and live your best life: phase-specific recipes and workouts, the Cycle Syncing Method™ daily planner and guide, live monthly Q&A calls with Alisa, and a dedicated, private Facebook group for community support—as well as support from trained FLO Living counselors and Alisa.

For more information, go to www.cyclesyncingmembership.com. We hope to see you in the FLO 28 community soon!

Connect with Me to Stay in Your FLO!

Alisa Vitti online

www.alisavitti.com

Stop by and say hello!

Instagram: @floliving and @alisa.vitti

Facebook: www.facebook.com/floliving

Pinterest: www.pinterest.com/alisavitti/

YouTube: www.youtube.com/user/FLOlivingTV

Twitter: twitter.com/FLOliving

FLO Living

Discover the modern menstrual health care company at www.FLOliving.com.

FLO 28: The Cycle Syncing™ Membership

The revolutionary online program and community that supports women to live in their FLO. Sign up at www.cyclesyncingmembership.com.

MyFLO App

Download the only period tracker app that tells you what to do to be symptom free and helps you sync with your cycle at www.MyFLOtracker.com.

FLO Living's Programs, Books, and Recommended Supplements

You can find these all on www.FLOliving.com, home of the first modern menstrual health care company. We work with women all over the world who have any health issues from PMS to fertility to postpartum to perimenopause to address these symptoms naturally and safely using functional foods, supplements, and lifestyle changes.

Monthly FLO: The most widely used digital hormone recovery program worldwide, helping women put PCOS, endometriosis, fibroids, infertility, and period symptoms into remission naturally.

Balance Supplements: The bestselling female hormone biohacking supplements delivered to your door every other month. These five formulations provide essential micronutrient support that you need to balance your hormones.

One-on-One Support: Access our FLO coaches anytime to talk through questions and concerns and to get support and accountability to make lasting changes in your health and life.

ACKNOWLEDGMENTS

I am so appreciative of all the forces that conspired to make this book possible. So many people have encouraged me to believe in the audacity of this idea. Everything I've been able to create is in direct proportion to the love and support I've received.

My biggest thank-you goes out to my family. To my daughter, Ariana, who was very patient for such a little girl while I wrote this book, thank you for the gift of being your mother. Thanks for playing "office" and "author" with me. To my husband, Victor, thank you for believing in me and encouraging me on my journey. Thank you for being the most loving and supportive partner and devoted coparent and for being in the FLO with me.

To my mother, for your eternal love. Thank you for always encouraging me to go after my dreams and to follow my passion. To my father, thank you for always believing that I could do anything and for making the air I breathed as a little girl filled with your belief that women are powerful forces of nature. And to my mother and my paternal grandmother, for showing you that. And to my two brothers and their families, whom I love so much.

To Jelena Petrovic, thank you for being my sister. To Jess G., Lori F., Jackie C., Lauren S., and Meredith G., thank you for every conversation and your deep friendship.

To my incredible team at FLO Living, thank you for your work to help me modernize menstrual health care, and for helping women around the world know there is a place for them where they will be seen, heard, and supported.

I also want to thank all the fellow female entrepreneurs who have inspired me tremendously and supported me along the way.

I want to give a special shout-out to Nisha Moodley, the first woman to come to me and ask that I teach how I use my cycle to manage my time, my self-care, and my career. I appreciate you seeing me and holding space for me to workshop my ideas at her mastermind.

Danielle DuBoise and Whitney Tingle from Sakara Life—you have been incredible supporters from the way back. Michele Promaulayko, thank you for being a champion of the app and having me come teach the crew at *Cosmo*. Melisse Gelula, thanks to you for all your support since my first book, and for Well+Good making menstruation officially a wellness trend! And to Colleen Wachob at MindBodyGreen for giving me a space to share my message. To Claudia Chan and Dee Poku, for believing in the power of this concept and inviting me to share it in the sphere of women's leadership.

Thank you to Marika Frumes for being an amazing champion, to Hannah Bronfman for your support, and to Lee Tilghman for being an example of cyclical living to so many.

To Josh Zabar and the Summit community, for getting me and having me teach for the first time to both men and women. Thank you to the women at SXSW for inviting me to be the first female biohacker in the history of the conference.

JJ Virgin, thank you for your guidance and friendship. Your generosity and integrity are unparalleled.

To Stephanie Tade, who is the most extraordinary literary agent, thank you not only for getting this book concept, but also for all your work and emotional support in midwifing this book.

Hilary Swanson, my editor at HarperOne, it is a joy to work with you. Thank you for believing in the message of this book and helping me bring this book to life.

Thank you to Frances Sharpe for helping me pull all my content together, for your research support, for talking through my ideas, and for helping me refine this book. I loved each one of our conversations. I am so grateful for all of your help in making this book come to life.

To Judith Curr, thank you for being personally involved in this book's birth process.

To the team at HarperOne, thank you for the irresistible invitation to do a second book with you. And thanks to Melinda Mullin and Aly Mostel for taking such good care of me.

To the FLO Living community all around the world, thank you for believing in your body's amazing capacity to heal, for telling your stories of hormonal reclamation, and for spreading this message to the women in your life. Your appetite to learn more was the catalyst not only to create the MyFLO app but also to write this book. Thank you for inspiring me and for living in the FLO with me.

To my readers, thank you for trusting me, for your willingness to step into the new with me, for believing that you deserve a life that is easier, healthier, and more pleasurable on your own terms and in your own time. Together we can liberate ourselves, shift our cultural narrative to value our biology, and make sure the next generation of young girls know about their super powers from the start.

REFERENCES

In order to maximize the content within book-length constraints, I've selected key references here that provide the scientific evidence and basis for
this book. You can find the complete bibliography of references for free at
www.IntheFLObook.com/references.

Chapter 1: Ending Your Mys-education

Allickson J and Xiang C. Human adult stem cells from menstrual blood and endometrial
   tissue. *Journal of Zhejiang University Science B.* 2012;13(5):419–20. https://doi.org
   /10.1631/jzus.B1200062
American College of Obstetricians and Gynecologists, Committee on Adolescent Health Care.
   "Menstruation in Girls and Adolescents: Using the Menstrual Cycle as a Vital Sign."
   Committee Opinion Number 651. Dec. 2015. https://www.acog.org/Clinical-Guidance
   -and-Publications/Committee-Opinions/Committee-on-Adolescent-Health-Care
   /Menstruation-in-Girls-and-Adolescents-Using-the-Menstrual-Cycle-as-a-Vital-Sign
Bruinvels G, Burden RJ, McGregor AJ, et al. Sport, exercise and the menstrual cycle:
   Where is the research? *British Journal of Sports Medicine.* 2017;51:487–88. http://dx.doi
   .org/10.1136/bjsports-2016-096279
Buck S. "The Inventors of the Pill Decided Women Should Still Bleed Every Month." *Timeline.*
   May 3, 2017. https://timeline.com/birth-control-pill-history-marketing-e77ce609e749
Campaign to End Chronic Pain in Women. "Chronic Pain in Women: Neglect, Dismissal,
   and Discrimination." 2010. www.endwomenspain.org/Common/file?id=20
Costello JT, Bieuzen F, and Bleakley CM. Where are all the female participants in sports
   and exercise medicine research? *European Journal of Sport Science.* 2014;14(8):847–51.
   https://doi.org/10.1080/17461391.2014.911354
Dominguez-Bello MG, De Jesus-Laboy KM, Shen H, et al. Partial restoration of the
   microbiota of cesarean-born infants via vaginal microbial transfer. *Nature Medicine.*
   2016;22(3):250–53. https://doi.org/10.1038/nm.4039
Dusenbery M. *Doing Harm: The Truth About How Bad Medicine and Lazy Science Leave
   Women Dismissed, Misdiagnosed, and Sick.* New York: HarperOne, 2018.
Faro M, Sàez-Francás N, Castro-Marrero J, et al. Gender differences in chronic fatigue syndrome. *Reumatologia Clinica,* 2016;12(2):72–77. https://doi.org/10.1016/j.reuma.2015.05.007
Harlow SD and Ephross SA. Epidemiology of menstruation and its relevance to women's
   health. *Epidemiological Review.* 1995;17(2):265–86. https://www.ncbi.nlm.nih.gov/pubmed
   /8654511
Harvey RE, Coffman KE, and Miller VM. Women-specific factors to consider in risk,
   diagnosis and treatment of cardiovascular disease. *Women's Health.* 2015;11(2):239–57.
   https://doi.org/10.2217/whe.14.64

Liu KA and Dipietro Mager NA. Women's involvement in clinical trials: Historical perspective and future implications. *Pharmacy Practice*. 2016;14(1):708. https://doi .org/10:18549/PharmPract.2016.01.708

Mazure CM and Jones DP. Twenty years and still counting: Including women as participants and studying sex and gender in biomedical research. *BMC Women's Health*. 2015;15:94. https://doi.org/10.1186/s12905-015-0251-9

National Institutes of Health. "The BioCycle Study. A Longitudinal Study of Estrogen and Progesterone Effects on Biomarkers of Oxidative Stress and Antioxidant Status During the Menstrual Cycle." https://www.nichd.nih.gov/about/org/diphr/officebranch/eb /biocycle

Pinn VW. Sex and gender factors in medical studies: Implications for health and clinical practice. *JAMA*. 2003;289(4):397–400. https://doi.org/10.1001/jama.289.4.397

Women's health: Report of the Public Health Service Task Force on women's health issues. *Public Health Reports*. 1985;100(1):73–106. https://www.ncbi.nlm.nih.gov/pmc /articles/PMC1424718/?page=2

Xiao S, Coppeta JR, Rogers HB, et al. A microfluiditic culture model of the human reproductive tract and 28-day menstrual cycle. *Nature Communications*. 2017;8:14584. https://doi.org/10.1038/ncomms14584

Chapter 2: Break Free from the 24-Hour Clock

Baker FC and Driver HS. Circadian rhythms, sleep, and the menstrual cycle. *Sleep Medicine*. 2007;8(6):613–22. https://doi.org/10.1016/j.sleep.2006.09.011

Baron KG and Reid KJ. Circadian misalignment and health. *International Review of Psychiatry* 2014 Apr;26(2):139–54. https://doi.org/10.3109/09540261.2014.911149

Bellezza S, Paharia N, and Keinan A. Conspicuous consumption of time: When busyness and lack of leisure time become a status symbol. *Journal of Consumer Research*. 2017; 44(1):118–38. https://doi.org/10.1093/jcr/ucw076

Breus M. *The Power of When: Discover Your Chronotype and the Best Time to Eat Lunch, Ask for a Raise, Have Sex, Write a Novel, Take Your Meds, and More*. New York: Little, Brown, 2016.

Chang A-M, Aeschbach D, Duffy JF, et al. Evening use of light-emitting eReaders negatively affects sleep, circadian timing, and next-morning alertness. *PNAS*. 2015; 112(4)1232–37. https://doi.org/10.1073/pnas.1418490112

Csikszentmihalyi M. *Flow*. New York: Harper, 1990.

de Botton A. *Status Anxiety*. New York: Vintage Books, 2008.

Dietrich A. Neurocognitive mechanisms underlying the experience of flow. *Consciousness and Cognition*. 2004;13:746–61. https://doi.org/10.1016/j.concog.2004.07.002

Etkin J, Evangelidis I, and Aaker J. Pressed for time? Goal conflict shapes how time is perceived, spent, and valued. *Journal of Marketing Research*. 2015;52(3):394–406. https:// doi.org/10.1509/jmr.14.0130

Maslow A. *Motivation and Personality*, 3rd ed. New York: Longman, 1987.

National Institute of General Medicine Science. "Circadian Rhythms." https://www .nigms.nih.gov/education/pages/Factsheet_CircadianRhythms.aspx

Nicolaides NC, Charmandari E, Chrousos GP, et al. Circadian endocrine rhythms: The hypothalamic-pituitary-adrenal axis and its actions. *Annals of the New York Academy of Sciences*. 2014;1318:71–80. https://doi.org/10.1111/nyas.12464

NobelPrize.org. "The 2017 Nobel Prize in Physiology or Medicine." Press release, Oct. 2, 2017. https://www.nobelprize.org/nobel_prizes/medicine/laureates/2017/press.html

Saran S and Srikumar M. "AI has a Gender Problem. Here's What to Do About It." World Economic Forum, 2018. https://www.weforum.org/agenda/2018/04/ai-has-a-gender -problem-heres-what-to-do-about-it/

Schmidt C and Bao Y. Chronobiological research for cognitive science: A multifaceted view. *PsyCh Journal*. 2017;6(4)249–52. https://doi.org/10.1002/pchj.203

Schulte B. *Overwhelmed: Work, Love, and Play When No One Has the Time.* New York: Sarah Crichton Books, 2014.

Schwartz T and McCarthy C. "Manage Your Energy, Not Your Time." *Harvard Business Review.* Oct. 2007. https://hbr.org/2007/10/manage-your-energy-not-your-time

Semaan J. "The Hungry Ghost and Always Wanting More." Medium.com. Feb. 10, 2017. https://medium.com/@jessicasemaan/the-hungry-ghost-and-always-wanting-more-2bb397dbdc10

Sensi S, Pace Palitti V, and Guagnano MT. Chronobiology in endocrinology. *Annali dell'Istituto Superiore di Sanita.* 1993;29(4):613–31. https://www.ncbi.nlm.nih.gov/pubmed/7985925

Shechter A and Boivin DB. Sleep, hormones, and circadian rhythms throughout the menstrual cycle in healthy women and women with premenstrual dysphoric disorder. *International Journal of Endocrinology.* 2010;2010:259345. https://doi.org/10.1155/2010/259345

Winget CM, DeRoshia CW, and Holley DC. Circadian rhythms and athletic performance. *Medicine and Science in Sports Exercise.* 1985;17(5):498–516. https://www.ncbi.nlm.nih.gov/pubmed/3906341

Chapter 3: Beyond Your Period—Understanding Your Hormonal Advantages

Alvergne A and Tabor VH. Is female health cyclical? Evolutionary perspectives on menstruation. *Trends in Ecology & Evolution.* 2018;33(6):399–414. https://doi.org/10.1016/j.tree.2018.03.006

Amen DG. *Unleash the Power of the Female Brain.* New York: Harmony Books, 2013.

Amin Z, Canli T, and Epperson C. Effect of estrogen-serotonin interactions on mood and cognition. *Behavioral and Cognitive Neuroscience Reviews.* 2005;4(1):43–58. https://doi.org/10.1177/1534582305277152

Arciero PJ, Goran MI, and Poehlman ET. Resting metabolic rate is lower in women than in men. *Journal of Applied Physiology.* 1993;75(6):2514:20. https://doi.org/10.1152/jappl.1993.75.6.2514

Baker FC and Driver HS. Circadian rhythms, sleep, and the menstrual cycle. *Sleep Medicine.* 2007;8(6):613–22. https://doi.org/10.1016/j.sleep.2006.09.011

Baker JM, Al-Nakkash L, and Herbst-Kralovetz MM. Estrogen-gut microbiome axis: Physiological and clinical implications. *Maturitas.* 2017;103:45–53. https://doi.org/10.1016/j.maturitas.2017.06.025

Barsom SH, Mansfield PK, Koch PB, et al. Association between psychological stress and menstrual cycle characteristics in perimenopausal women. *Women's Health Issues.* 2004;14(6)235–41. https://doi.org/10.1016/j.whi.2004.07.006

Barth C, Villringer A, and Sacher J. Sex hormones affect neurotransmitters and shape the adult female brain during hormonal transition periods. *Frontiers in Neuroscience.* 2015;9:37. https://doi.org/10.3389/fnins.2015.00037

Barth C, Steele CJ, Mueller K, et al. In-vivo dynamics of the human hippocampus across the menstrual cycle. *Scientific Reports.* 2016;6:32833. https://doi.org/10.1038/srep32833

Borelli L. "Menstruation and the Female Brain: How Fluctuating Hormone Levels Impact Cognitive Function." Medical Daily. July 8, 2015. https://www.medicaldaily.com/menstruation-and-female-brain-how-fluctuating-hormone-levels-impact-cognitive-341788

Brizendine L. *The Female Brain.* New York: Harmony Books, 2006.

Cavill R, Eccleston C, Keogh E, et al. The effects of menstrual-related pain on attentional interference. *PAIN.* 2014;155(4):821–27. https://doi.org/10.1016/j.pain.2014.01.021

Chen KL and Madak-Erdogan Z. Estrogen and microbiota crosstalk: Should we pay attention? *Trends in Endocrinology and Metabolism.* 2016;27:752–55. https://doi.org/10.1016/j.tem.2016.08.001

Cornelis MC, El-Sohemy A, Kabagambe EK, et al. Coffee, CYP1A2 genotype, and risk of myocardial infarction. *JAMA.* 2006;295(10):1135–41. https://doi.org/10.1001/jama .295.10.1135

Davidsen L, Vistisen B, and Astrup A. Impact of the menstrual cycle on determinants of energy balance: A putative role in weight loss attempts. *International Journal of Obesity (London).* 2007;31:1777–85. https://doi.org/10.1038/sj.ijo.0803699

De Zambotti M, Nicholas CL, Colrain IM, et al. Autonomic regulation across phases of the menstrual cycle and sleep stages in women with premenstrual syndrome and healthy controls. *Psychoneuroendocrinology.* 2013;38(11):10.1016/j.psyneuen.2013.06.005. https://doi.org/10.1016/j.psyneuen.2013.06.005

Dye L and Blundell JE. Menstrual cycle and appetite control: Implications for weight regulation. *Human Reproduction.* 1997;12(6):1142–51. https://www.ncbi.nlm.nih.gov /pubmed/9221991

Fransen F, van Beek A, Borghuis T, et al. The impact of gut microbiota on gender-specific differences in immunity. *Frontiers in Immunology.* 2017:8:754. https://doi.org/10.3389 /fimmu.2017.00754

Gillies GE and McArthur S. Estrogen actions in the brain and the basis for differential action in men and women: A case for sex-specific medicines. *Pharmacological Reviews.* 2010;62(2):155–98. https://doi.org/10.1124/pr.109.002071

Goel N, Workman JL, Lee TT, et al. Sex differences in the HPA axis. *Comprehensive Physiology.* 2014;4(3):1121–55. https://doi.org/10.1002/cphy.c130054

Goldman, B. "Two Minds: The Cognitive Differences Between Men and Women." *Stanford Medicine.* Spring 2017, Sex, Gender and Medicine. https://stanmed.stanford .edu/2017spring/how-mens-and-womens-brains-are-different.html

Grigg-Spall H. *Sweetening the Pill or How We Got Hooked on Hormonal Birth Control.* Hants, UK: Zero Books, 2013.

Hamilton LD and Meston CM. Chronic stress and sexual function in women. *The Journal of Sexual Medicine.* 2013;10(10):2443–54. https://doi.org/10.1111/jsm.12249

Hinojosa-Laborde C, Chapa I, and Haywood JR. Gender differences in sympathetic nervous system regulation. *Clinical and Experimental Pharmacology and Physiology.* 1999: 26(2):122–26. https://doi.org/10.1046/j.1440–1681.1999.02995.x

Hulmi JJ, Isola V, Suonpää M, et al. The effects of intensive weight reduction on body composition in female fitness competitors. *Frontiers in Physiology.* 2017;7:689. https:// doi.org/10.3389/fphys.2016.00689

Klein SL and Flanagan KL. Sex differences in immune responses. *Nature Reviews Immunology.* 2016;16:626–38. https://doi.org/10.1038/nri.2016.90

Koebnick C, Strassner C, Hoffmann I, et al. Consequences of a long-term raw food diet on body weight and menstruation: Results of a questionnaire survey. *Annals of Nutrition & Metabolism.* 1999;43(2):69–79. https://doi.org/10.1159/000012770

Kwo PY, Ramchandani VA, and O'Connor S, et al. Gender differences in alcohol metabolism: Relationship to liver volume and effect of adjusting for body mass. *Gastroenterology.* 1998;115(6):1552–57. https://www.ncbi.nlm.nih.gov/pubmed/9834284

Lipton BH. *The Biology of Belief: Unleashing the Power of Consciousness, Matter & Miracles.* Carlsbad, CA: Hay House, 2005.

Lisofsky N, Mårtenssom J, Eckert A, et al. Hippocampal volume and functional connectivity changes during the female menstrual cycle. *NeuroImage.* 2015;118:154–62. https://doi.org/10.1016/j.neuroimage.2015.06.012

McCarthy, MM. Estrogen modulation of oxytocin and its relation to behavior. *Advances in Experimental Medicine and Biology.* 1995;395:235–45. https://www.ncbi.nlm.nih.gov /pubmed/8713972

McEwen BS, Gray JD, and Nasca C. Redefining neuroendocrinology: Stress, sex, and cognitive and emotional regulation. *The Journal of Endocrinology.* 2015;226(2):T67–T83. https://doi.org/10.1530/JOE-1-0121

National Institutes of Health. "The BioCycle Study. A Longitudinal Study of Estrogen and Progesterone Effects on Biomarkers of Oxidative Stress and Antioxidant Status During the Menstrual Cycle." June 2018. https://www.nichd.nih.gov/about/org /diphr/officebranch/eb/biocycle

Ngun TC, Ghahramani N, Sánchez FJ, et al. The genetics of sex differences in brain and behavior. *Frontiers in Neuroendocrinology.* 2011;32(2):227–46. https://doi.org/10.1016 /j.yfrne.2010.10.001

Oertelt-Prigione S. Immunology and the menstrual cycle. *Autoimmunity Reviews.* 2012;11(6):A486–92. https://doi.org/10.1016/j.autrev.2011.11.023

Roved J, Westerdahl H, and Hasselquist D. Sex differences in immune responses: Hormonal effects, antagonistic selection, and evolutionary consequences. *Hormones and Behavior.* 2017;88:95–105. https://doi.org/10.1016/j.yhbeh.2016.11.017

Shechter A and Boivin DB. Sleep, hormones, and circadian rhythms throughout the menstrual cycle in healthy women and women with premenstrual dysphoric disorder. *International Journal of Endocrinology.* 2010;2010:259345. https://doi.org/10.1155/2010/259345

Solomon SJ, Kurzer MS, and Calloway DH. Menstrual cycle and basal metabolic rate in women. *American Journal of Clinical Nutrition.* 1982;36(4):611–16. https://doi.org /10.1093/ajcn/36.4.611

Sundström Poromaa I and Gingnell M. Menstrual cycle influence on cognitive function and emotion processing—from a reproductive perspective. *Frontiers in Neuroscience.* 2014;8:380. https://doi.org/10.3389/fnins.2014.00380

Taylor SE, Klein LC, Lewis BP, et al. Biobehavioral responses to stress in females: Tend-and-befriend, not fight-or-flight. *Psychological Review.* 2000;107:411–29. https:// www.ncbi.nlm.nih.gov/pubmed/10941275

Tu C-H, Niddam DM, Chao H-T, et al. Brain morphological changes associated with cyclic menstrual pain. *PAIN.* 2010;150(3):462. https://doi.org/10.1016/j.pain.2010.05.026

Ullrich IH, Peters PJ, and Albrink MJ. Effect of low-carbohydrate diets high in either fat or protein on thyroid function, plasma insulin, glucose, and triglycerides in healthy young adults. *Journal of the American College of Nutrition.* 1985;4(4):451–59. https:// www.ncbi.nlm.nih.gov/pubmed/?term=3900181

Urbaniak C, Gloor GB, Brackstone M, et al. The microbiota of breast tissue and its association with breast cancer. *Applied and Environmental Microbiology.* 2016;82(16):5039–48. https://doi.org/10.1128/AEM.01235-16

Weaver L. *Rushing Woman's Syndrome: The Impact of a Never-Ending To-Do List and How to Stay Healthy in Today's Busy World.* London: Hay House, 2017.

Zagni E, Simoni L, and Colombo D. Sex and gender differences in central nervous system–related disorders. *Neuroscience Journal.* 2016;2016:2827090. https://doi.org /10.1155/2016/2827090

Zethraeus N, Kocoska-Maras L, Ellingsen T, et al. A randomized trial of the effect of estrogen and testosterone on economic behavior. *PNAS.* 2009;106(16)6535–38; https:// doi.org/10.1073/pnas.0812757106

Chapter 4: Never Diet Again

American Cancer Society. "Fibrosis and Simple Cysts of the Breast." https://www.cancer .org/cancer/breast-cancer/non-cancerous-breast-conditions/fibrosis-and-simple -cysts-in-the-breast.html

Baker JM, Al Nakkash L, and Herbst-Kralovetz MM. Estrogen–gut microbiome axis: Physiological and clinical implications. *Maturitas.* 2017;103:45–53. https://doi.org /10.1016/j.maturitas.2017.06.025

Beilharz JE, Maniam J, and Morris MJ. Diet-induced cognitive deficits: The role of fat and sugar, potential mechanisms, and nutritional interventions. *Nutrients.* 2015;7:6719–38. https://doi.org/10.3390/nu7085307

Bertone-Johnson ER, Hankinson SE, Bendich A, et al. Calcium and vitamin D intake and risk of incident premenstrual syndrome. *Archives of Internal Medicine.* 2005;165(11):1246–52. https://doi.org/10.1001/arcinte.165.11.1246

Bolúmar F, Olsen J, Rebagliato M, et al. Caffeine intake and delayed conception: A European multicenter study on infertility and subfecundity. European Study Group on Infertility Subfecundity. *American Journal of Epidemiology.* 1997;145(4):324–34. https://www.ncbi.nlm.nih.gov/pubmed/9054236

Buchhorn R. The impact of nutrition on the autonomic nervous system. *International Journal of Food and Nutritional Science.* 2016. https://www.ommegaonline.org/article-details/The-Impact-of-Nutrition-on-the-Autonomic-Nervous-System-/942

Carwile JL, Willett WC, Spiegelman D, et al. Sugar-sweetened beverage consumption and age at menarche in a prospective study of US girls. *Human Reproduction.* 2015;30(3):675–83. https://doi.org/10.1093/humrep/deu349

Chandra RK. Nutrition and the immune system from birth to old age. *European Journal of Clinical Nutrition.* 2002;56:S73–S76. https://doi.org/10.1038/sj.ejcn.1601492

Chavarro JE, Rich-Edwards JW, Rosner BA, et al. Diet and lifestyle in the prevention of ovulatory disorder infertility. *Obstetrics & Gynecology.* 2007;110(5):1050–58. https://doi.org/10.1097/01.AOG.0000287293.25465.e1

Chen M-N, Lin C-C, and Liu CF. Efficacy of phytoestrogens for menopausal symptoms: A meta-analysis and systematic review. *Climacteric.* 2015;18(2):260–69. https://doi.org/10.3109/13697137.2014.966241

Ghanbari Z, Haghollahi F, Shariat M, et al. Effects of calcium supplement therapy in women with premenstrual syndrome. *Taiwanese Journal of Obstetrics and Gynecology.* 2009;48(2):124–29. https://doi.org/10.1016/S1028-4559(09)60271-0

Gómez-Pinilla F. Brain foods: The effects of nutrients on brain function. *Nature Reviews Neuroscience;* 2008(9):568–78. https://doi.org/10.1038/nrn2421

Gottfried S. *The Hormone Reset Diet: Heal Your Metabolism to Lose Up to 15 Pounds in 21 Days.* New York: HarperOne, 2015.

Hall A. "Seed Cycling for Hormonal Balance." Herbal Academy. Apr. 20, 2014. https://theherbalacademy.com/seed-cycling-for-hormonal-balance/

Itoh H, Sashihara T, Hosono A, Kaminogawa S, and Uchida M. Lactobacillus gasseri OLL2809 inhibits development of ectopic endometrial cell in peritoneal cavity via activation of NK cells in a murine endometriosis model. *Cytotechnology.* 2011;63(2):205–10. https://doi.org/10.1007/s10616-0111-9343-z

Jahanian E, Nanaei HA, and Kor NM. The dietary fatty acids and their effects on reproductive performance of ruminants. *European Journal of Experimental Biology.* 2013;3(6):95–97. http://www.imedpub.com/articles/the-dietary-fatty-acids-and-their-effects-on-reproductiveperformance-of-ruminants.pdf

Koebnick C, Strassner C, Hoffman I, et al. Consequences of a long-term raw food diet on body weight and menstruation: Results of a questionnaire survey. *Annals of Nutrition & Metabolism.* 1999;43(2):69–79. https://doi.org/10.1159/000012770

Kumar S and Kaur G. Intermittent fasting dietary restriction regimen negatively influences reproduction in young rats: a study of hypothalamo-hypophysial-gonadal axis. *PLOS ONE.* 2013;8(1):e52416. https://doi.org/10.1371/journal.pone.0052416

Mueller NT, Jacobs DR, MacLehose RF, et al. Consumption of caffeinated and artificially sweetened soft drinks is associated with risk of early menarche. *American Journal of Clinical Nutrition.* 2015;102(3):648–54. https://doi.org/10.3945/ajcn.114.100958

Mumford SL, Chavarro JE, Zhang C, et al. Dietary fat intake and reproductive hormone concentrations and ovulation in regularly menstruating women. *American Journal of Clinical Nutrition.* 2016;103(3):868–77. https://doi.org/10.3945/ajcn.115.119321

Oertelt-Prigione S. Immunology and the menstrual cycle. *Autoimmunity Reviews.* 2012;11(6):A486–92. https://doi.org/10.1016/j.autrev.2011.11.023

Rostenberg A. "Treating COMT and MAO: The Hormonal Cause of Stress and Anxiety." Beyond MTHFR. Aug. 27, 2015. http://www.beyondmthfr.com/treating-comt-and -mao-the-hormonal-cause-of-stress-and-anxiety/

Sarris J, Logan AC, Akbaraly TN, et al. Nutritional medicine as mainstream in psychiatry. *Lancet Psychiatry.* 2015 Mar;2(3):271–74. https://doi.org/10.1016 /S2215-0366(14)00051-0

Sisson M. *The Keto Reset Diet: Reboot Your Metabolism in 21 Days and Burn Fat Forever.* New York, Harmony, 2017.

Thys-Jacobs S, Starkey P, Bernstein D, et al. Calcium carbonate and the premenstrual syndrome: Effects on premenstrual and menstrual symptoms. *American Journal of Obstetrics and Gynecology.* 1998;179(2):444–52. https://www.ncbi.nlm.nih.gov /pubmed/9731851

Ullrich IH, Peter PJ, and Albrink MJ. Effect of low-carbohydrate diets high in either fat or protein on thyroid function, plasma insulin, glucose, and triglycerides in healthy young adults. *Journal of the American College of Nutrition.* 1985;4(4):451–59. https:// www.ncbi.nlm.nih.gov/pubmed/3900181

Ulrich-Lai YM, Figueiriedo HF, Ostrander MM, et al. Chronic stress induces adrenal hyperplasia and hypertrophy in a subregion-specific manner. *American Journal of Physiology.* 2006; 291(5):E965–73. https://doi.org/10.1152/ajpendo.00070.2006

Wolfrom D and Welsch CW. Caffeine and the development of normal, benign and carcinomatous human breast tissues: a relationship? *Journal of Medicine.* 1990;21(5):225–50. https://www.ncbi.nlm.nih.gov/pubmed/2079614

Wurtman J and Fruzstajer NJ. *The Serotonin Power Diet.* New York: Rodale, 2009.

Wurtman RJ and Wurtman JJ. Brain serotonin, carbohydrate-craving, obesity and depression. *Obesity Research.* 1995;3(suppl 4):477S–80S. https://www.ncbi.nlm.nih .gov/pubmed/8697046

Chapter 5: Work Out Less, Get More Fit

Bruinvels G, Burden RJ, McGregor AJ, et al. Sport, exercise and the menstrual cycle: Where is the research? *British Journal of Sports Medicine.* 2017;51:487–88. https://doi .org/10.1136/bjsports-2016-096279

Clennell B. *The Woman's Yoga Book: Asana and Pranayama for All Phases of the Menstrual Cycle.* Boulder, CO: Shambhala Publications, 2007.

Curtis V, Henry CJK, Birch E, et al. Intraindividual variation in the basal metabolic rate of women: Effect of the menstrual cycle. *American Journal of Human Biology.* 1996;8(5):631–39. https://doi.org/10.1002/(SICI)1520-6300(1996)8:5<631::AID -AJHB8>3.0.CO;2-Y

Janse de Jonge XA. Effects of the menstrual cycle on exercise performance. *Sports Medicine.* 2003;33(11):833–51. https://www.ncbi.nlm.nih.gov/pubmed/12959622

Jarlenski MP, Bennett WL, Bleich SN, et al. Effects of breastfeeding on postpartum weight loss among U.S. women. *Preventive Medicine.* 2014;69:146–50. https://doi.org/10.1016 /j.ypmed.2014.09.018

Johnson KA. *The Fourth Trimester: A Postpartum Guide to Healing Your Body, Balancing Your Emotions, and Restoring Your Vitality.* Boulder, CO: Shambhala Publications, 2017.

Julian R, Hecksteden A, Fullagar HHK, et al. The effects of menstrual cycle phase on physical performance in female soccer players. *PLOS ONE.* 2017;12(3): e0173951. https://doi.org/10.1371/journal.pone.0173951

Landsverk G. "The World Cup-Winning US Women's Soccer Team Tracked Their Periods for Peak Performance, and Evidence Shows Everyday Athletes Can Benefit from Doing the Same." *Insider.* July 23, 2019. https://www.insider.com/world-cup-winning-uswnt -period-tracking-how-to-improve-performance-2019-7

Lee CW, Newman MA, and Riechman SE. Oral contraceptive use impairs muscle gains in young women. *The FASEB Journal.* 2009;23(1-suppl). https://www.fasebj.org/doi/abs/10.1096/fasebj.23.1_supplement.955.25

Ou H. *The First Forty Days: The Essential Art of Nourishing the New Mother.* New York: Abrams, 2016.

Sims ST. *Roar: How to Match Your Food and Fitness to Your Female Physiology for Optimum Performance, Great Health, and a Strong, Lean Body for Life.* New York: Rodale, 2016.

Sung E, Han A, Hinrichs T, et al. Effects of follicular versus luteal phase-based strength training in young women. *SpringerPlus.* 2014;3:668. https://doi.org/10.1186/2193-1801-3-668

Chapter 6: Your Blueprint to Do More with Less Stress

Ansell AB, Rando K, Tuit K, et al. Cumulative adversity and smaller gray matter volume in medial prefrontal, anterior cingulate, and insula regions. *Biological Psychiatry.* 2012;72(1):57–64. https://doi.org/10.1016/j.biopsych.2011.11.022

Chetty A, Friedman AR, Taravosh-Lahn K, et al. Stress and glucocorticoids promote oligodendrogenesis in the adult hippocampus. *Molecular Psychiatry.* 2014;19:1275–83. https://www.nature.com/articles/mp2013190

Forsythe P, Sudo N, Dinan T, et al. Mood and gut feelings. *Brain Behavior, and Immunity.* 2010;24(1):9–16. https://doi.org/ 10.1016/j.bbi.2009.05.058

Mathur MB, Epel E, Kind S, et al. Perceived stress and telomere length: A systematic review, meta-analysis, and methodologic considerations for advancing the field. *Brain, Behavior, and Immunity.* 2016;54:158–69. https://doi.org/10.1016/j.bbi.2016.02.002

Northrup C. *Women's Bodies, Women's Wisdom.* New York: Bantam Books, 2010.

Panda S. *The Circadian Code: Lose Weight, Supercharge Your Energy, and Transform Your Health from Morning to Midnight.* New York: Rodale Books, 2018.

Biohacking Tool Kit

Behre HM, Zitzmann M, Anderson RA, et al. Efficacy and safety of an injectable combination hormonal contraceptive for men. *The Journal of Clinical Endocrinology & Metabolism.* 2016;101(12):4779–88. https://doi.org/10.1210/jc.2016-2141

Berenson AB and Rahman M. Changes in weight, total fat, percent body fat, and central-to-peripheral fat ratio associated with injectable and oral contraceptive use. *American Journal of Obstetrics & Gynecology.* 2009;200(3):329.e1–8. https://doi.org/10.1016/j.ajog.2008.12.052

Ebrahimi E, Khayati Motlagh S, Nemati S, et al. Effects of magnesium and vitamin B6 on the severity of premenstrual syndrome symptoms. *Journal of Caring Sciences.* 2012;1(4):183–89. https://doi.org/10.5681/jcs.2012.026

Faryal U, Rashid S, Hajra B, et al. Effect of hormonal contraceptives on serum serotonin in females of reproductive age group. *Journal of Ayub Medical College Abbottabad.* 2016;28(1):56–58.

Fisher MM, Eugster EA. What is in our environment that effects puberty? *Reproductive Toxicology (Elmsford, NY).* 2014;44:7–14. https://doi.org/10.1016/j.reprotox.2013.03.012

Grosso G, Galvano F, Marventano S, et al. Omega-3 fatty acids and depression: Scientific evidence and biological mechanisms. *Oxidative Medicine and Cellular Longevity.* 2014;2014:313570. https://doi.org/10.1155/2014/313570

Hertel J, König J, and Homuth G. Evidence for stress-like alterations in the HPA-axis in women taking oral contraceptives. *Scientific Reports.* 2017;7(1):14111. https://doi.org/10.1038/s41598-017-13927-7

Hill S. *This Is Your Brain on Birth Control.* New York: Avery, 2019.

Islam MS, Akhtar MM, Ciavattini A, et al. Use of dietary phytochemicals to target inflammation, fibrosis, proliferation, and angiogenesis in uterine tissues: promising options for prevention and treatment of uterine fibroids? *Molecular Nutrition & Food Research*. 2014;58(8):1667–84. https://doi.org/10.1002/mnfr.201400134

Ji K, Kho YL, Park Y, et al. Influence of a five-day vegetarian diet on urinary levels of antibiotics and phthalate metabolites: A pilot study with "Temple Stay" participants. *Environmental Research*. 2010;110(4):375–82. https://doi.org/10.1016/j.envres.2010.02.008

Khalili H, Higuchi LM, Ananthakrishnan AN, et al. Oral contraceptives, reproductive factors and risk of inflammatory bowel disease. *Gut*. 2013;62:1153–59. https://doi.org/10.1136/gutjnl-2012-302362

Kiecolt-Glaser JK, Belury MA, Andridge R, et al. Omega-3 supplementation lowers inflammation and anxiety in medical students: A randomized controlled trial. *Brain, Behavior, and Immunity*. 2011; 25(8):1725–34. https://doi.org/10.1016/j.bbi.2011.07.229

King DE, Mainous AG 3rd, Geesey ME, et al. Dietary magnesium and C-reactive protein levels. *Journal of the American College of Nutrition*. 2005;24(3):166–71. https://www.ncbi.nlm.nih.gov/pubmed/15930481

Lee CW, Newman MA, and Riechman SE. Oral contraceptive use impairs muscle gains in young women. *The FASEB Journal*. 2009;23:1(suppl). https://www.fasebj.org/doi/abs/10.1096/fasebj.23.1_supplement.955.25

Lopez LM, Ramesh S, Chen M, et al. Progestin-only contraceptives: Effects on weight. *Cochrane Database of Systematic Reviews*. 2016;(8):CD008815. https://doi.org/10.1002/14651858.CD008815.pub4

Morabia A. *APHA* Voices from the Nurses' Health Study. *American Journal of Public Health*. 2016;106(9):1530–31. https://doi.org/10.2105/AJPH.2016.303370

Mørch LS, Skovlund CW, Hannaford PC, et al. Contemporary hormonal contraception and the risk of breast cancer. *New England Journal of Medicine*. 2017;377:2228–39. https://doi.org/10.1056/NEJMoa1700732

Oates L, Cohen M, Braun L, et al. Reduction in urinary organophosphate pesticide metabolites in adults after a week-long organic diet. *Environmental Research*. 2014; 132:105–11. https://doi.org/10.1016/j.envres.2014.03.021

Pal L, Shu J, Zeitlian G, et al. Vitamin D insufficiency in reproductive years may be contributory to ovulatory infertility and PCOS. *Fertility and Sterility*. 2008;90:S14. https://doi.org/10.1016/j.fertnstert.2008.07.382

Pletzer BA and Kerschbaum HH. 50 years of hormonal contraception—time to find out, what it does to our brain. *Frontiers in Neuroscience*. 2014;8:256. https://doi.org/10.3389/fnins.2014.00256

Roberts SC, Gosling LM, Carter V, et al. MHC-correlated odour preferences in humans and the use of oral contraceptives. *The Proceedings of the Royal Society B*. 2008, 275(1652): 2715–22. https://doi.org/10.1098/rspb.2008.0825

Rodríguez-Morán M and Gerrero-Romero F. Oral magnesium supplementation improves insulin sensitivity and metabolic control in type 2 diabetic subjects. *Diabetes Care*. 2003; 26(4):1147–52. https://doi.org/10.2337/diacare.26.4.1147

Rudick B, Ingles S, Chung K, et al. Characterizing the influence of vitamin D levels on IVF outcomes. *Human Reproduction*. 2012 Nov;27(11):3321–27. https://doi.org/10.1093/humrep/des280

Sartori SB, Whittle N, Hetzenauer A, et al. Magnesium deficiency induces anxiety and HPA axis dysregulation: Modulation by therapeutic drug treatment. *Neuropharmacology*. 2012;62(1):304–12. https://doi.org/10.1016/j.neuropharm.2011.07.027

Seifert B, Wagler P, Dartsch S, et al. Magnesium—A new therapeutic alternative in primary dysmenorrhea. *Zentralblatt fur Gynakologie*. 1989;111(11):755–60. https://www.ncbi.nlm.nih.gov/pubmed/2675496

Skovlund CW, Mørch LS, Kessing LV, et al. Association of hormonal contraception with depression. *JAMA Psychiatry.* 2016;73(11):1154–62. https://doi.org/10.1001/jamapsychiatry.2016.2387

Tijani JO, Fatoba OO, Babajide OO, et al. Pharmaceuticals, endocrine disruptors, personal care products, nanomaterials and perfluorinated pollutants: A review. *Environmental Chemistry Letters.* 2016;14:27. https://doi.org/10.1007/s10311-015-0537-z

United Nations Environment Programme and World Health Organization. "Effects of Human Exposure to Hormone-Disrupting Chemicals Examined in Landmark UN Report." World Health Organization. Feb. 19, 2013. http://www.who.int/mediacentre/news/releases/2013/hormone_disrupting_20130219/en/

Usselman CW, Luchyshyn TA, Gimon TI, et al. Hormone phase dependency of neural responses to chemoreflex-driven sympathoexcitation in young women using hormonal contraceptives. *Journal of Applied Physiology.* 2013;115(10):1415–22. https://doi.org/10.1152/japplphysiol.00681.2013

Wang Q, Würtz P, Auro K, et al. Effects of hormonal contraception on systemic metabolism: Cross-sectional and longitudinal evidence. *International Journal of Epidemiology.* 2016;45(5):1445–57. https://doi.org/10.1093/ije/dyw147

Webb JL. Nutritional effects of oral contraceptive use: A review. *The Journal of Reproductive Medicine.* 1980;25(4):150–56. https://www.ncbi.nlm.nih.gov/pubmed/7001015

Williams WV. Hormonal contraception and the development of autoimmunity: A review of the literature. *The Linacre Quarterly.* 2017;84(3):275–95. https://doi.org/10.1080/00243639.2017.1360065

Zafari M, Behmanesh F, and Agha Mohammadi A. Comparison of the effect of fish oil and ibuprofen on treatment of severe pain in primary dysmenorrhea. *Caspian Journal of Internal Medicine.* 2011;2(3):279–82. https://www.ncbi.nlm.nih.gov/pmc/articles/PMC3770499/

Chapter 7: Sustainable Success at Work

American Academy of Pediatrics. School start times for adolescents. *Pediatrics.* 2014; 134(3). http://pediatrics.aappublications.org/content/134/3/642?ijkey=ebc1dd1839d660bbbf2008739ab9cd8cd2b407f3&keytype2=tf_ipsecsha

Ariga A and Lleras A. Brief and rare mental "breaks" keep you focused: Deactivation and reactivation of task goals preempt vigilance decrements. *Cognition.* 2011;118(3):439–43. https://doi.org/10.1016/j.cognition.2010.12.007

Baddeley B, Sornalingam S, and Cooper M. Sitting is the new smoking: Where do we stand? *The British Journal of General Practice.* 2016;66(646):258. https://doi.org/10.3399/bjgp16X685009

Baicker K, Cutler D, and Song Z. Workplace wellness programs can generate savings. *Health Affairs.* 2010;29(2). https://doi.org/10.1377/hlthaff.2009.0626

Dunn M. "Who Chooses Part-Time Work and Why?" *Monthly Labor Review,* U.S. Bureau of Labor Statistics. March 2018. https://doi.org/10.21916/mlr.2018.8

Gerzema J and D'Antonio M. *The Athena Doctrine: How Women (and the Men Who Think Like Them) Will Rule the Future.* San Francisco: Jossey-Bass, 2013.

Gorman R. "Women Now Control More Than Half of US Personal Wealth, Which 'Will Only Increase in Years to Come.'" *Business Insider.* Apr. 7, 2015. https://www.businessinsider.com/women-now-control-more-than-half-of-us-personal-wealth-2015-4

Green Carmichael S. "The Research Is Clear: Long Hours Backfire for People and for Companies." *Harvard Business Review.* Aug. 19, 2015. https://hbr.org/2015/08/the-research-is-clear-long-hours-backfire-for-people-and-for-companies

Marano HE. "Biorhythms: Get in Step." *Psychology Today.* 2004. https://www.psychologytoday.com/us/articles/200404/biorhythms-get-in-step

Miller J and Adkins A. "Women Lead Men on Key Workplace Engagement Measures." Gallup. Nov. 16, 2016. http://news.gallup.com/businessjournal/197552/women-lead -men-key-workplace-engagement-measures.aspx

Noland M, Moran T, and Kotschwar B. Is gender diversity profitable? Evidence from a global survey. *Peterson Institute for International Economics Working Paper.* 2016;16–3. http://dx.doi.org/10.2139/ssrn.2729348

Robbins T. *Awaken the Giant Within.* New York: Free Press, 1991.

Sundström Poromaa I and Gingnell M. Menstrual cycle influence on cognitive function and emotion processing—from a reproductive perspective. *Frontiers in Neuroscience.* 2014;8:380. https://doi.org/10.3389/fnins.2014.00380

Trougakos JP and Hideg I. Momentary work recovery: The role of within-day work breaks. In Sonnentag S, Perrewé P, and Ganster DC (eds.), *Research in occupational stress and well being: Vol. 7. Current perspectives on job-stress recovery* (pp. 37–84). Bingley, UK: JAI Press /Emerald Group Publishing. http://psycnet.apa.org/record/2010-12072-002

Watson NF, Martin JL, Wise MS, et al. Delaying middle school and high school start times promotes student health and performance: An American Academy of Sleep Medicine position statement. *Journal of Clinical Sleep Medicine.* 2017;13(4):623–25. https://doi.org /10.5664/jcsm.6558

Woolley CS, Wenzel HJ, and Schwartzkroin PA. Estradiol increases the frequency of multiple synapse boutons in the hippocampal CA1 region of the adult female rat. *The Journal of Comparative Neurology.* 1996;373(1):108–17. https://www.ncbi.nlm.nih.gov /pubmed/8876466

Chapter 8: Get More of What You Want in Sex and Relationships

Barth C, Villringer A, and Sacher J. Sex hormones affect neurotransmitters and shape the adult female brain during hormonal transition periods. *Frontiers in Neuroscience.* 2015;9:37. https://doi.org/10.3389/fnins.2015.00037

Battaglia C, Nappi RE, Mancini F, et al. Menstrual cycle–related morphometric and vascular modifications of the clitoris. *The Journal of Sexual Medicine.* 2008;5(12): 2853–61. https://doi.org/10.1111/j.1743–6109.2008.00972.x

Bly R and Woodman M. *The Maiden King: The Reunion of Masculine and Feminine.* New York: Holt, 1991.

Brilla LR and Conte V. Effects of a novel zinc-magnesium formulation on hormones and strength. *Journal of Exercise Physiology Online.* 2000(3)4:26–36. https://www.research gate.net/publication/288406212_Effects_of_a_novel_zinc-magnesium_formulation _on_hormones_and_strength

Brody S. Slimness is associated with greater intercourse and lesser masturbation frequency. *Journal of Sex & Marital Therapy.* 2004;30(4):251–61. https://doi.org/10.1080 /00926230490422368

Bullivant SB, Sellergren SA, Stern K, et al. Women's sexual experience during the menstrual cycle: Identification of the sexual phase by noninvasive measurement of luteinizing hormone. *The Journal of Sexual Research.* 2004;41(1):82–93. https://doi.org /10.1080/00224490409552216

Charnetski CJ and Brennan FX. Sexual frequency and salivary immunoglobulin A (IgA). *Psychological Reports.* 2004;94(3 Pt 1):839–44. https://doi.org/10.2466/pr0 .94.3.839-844

Cutler WB, Garcia CR, and Kreiger A. Sexual behavior frequency and menstrual cycle length in mature premenopausal women. *Psychoneuroendocrinology.* 1979;4(4):297–309. https://doi.org/10.1016/0306-4530(79)90014-3

Cutler WB, Preti G, Huggins GR, et al. Sexual behavior frequency and biphasic ovulatory type menstrual cycles. *Physiology & Behavior.* 1985;34(5):805–10. https://www.ncbi .nlm.nih.gov/pubmed/4041055

Ellison CR. *Women's Sexualities*. Oakland, CA: New Harbinger Publications, 2000.

Excoffon L, Guillaume YC, Woronoff-Lemsi MC, et al. Magnesium effect on testosterone–SHBG association studied by a novel molecular chromatography approach. *Journal of Pharmaceutical and Biomedical Analysis*. 2009;49(2):175–80. https://doi.org/10.1016/j.jpba.2008.10.041

Fisher H. *Why We Love: The Nature and Chemistry of Romantic Love*. New York: Henry Holt, 2004.

Frederick DA, St. John HK, Garcia JR, et al. Differences in orgasm frequency among gay, lesbian, bisexual, and heterosexual men and women in a U.S. national sample. *Archives of Sexual Behavior*. 2018;47(1):273–88. https://doi.org/10.1007/s10508-017-0939-z

Hambach A, Ever S, Summ O, et al. The impact of sexual activity on idiopathic headaches: An observational study. *Cephalalgia*. 2013;33(6):384–89. https://doi.org/10.1177/0333102413476374

Jung CG. *The Basic Writings of C.G. Jung*. New York: Random House, 1993.

Lê MG, Bachelot A, and Hill C. Characteristics of reproductive life and risk of breast cancer in a case-control study of young nulliparous women. *Journal of Clinical Epidemiology*. 1989;42(12):1227–33. https://www.ncbi.nlm.nih.gov/pubmed/2585013

Legros JJ. Inhibitory effect of oxytocin on corticotrope function in humans: Are vasopressin and oxytocin ying-yang neurohormones? *Psychoneuroendocrinology*. 2001;26(7):649–55. https://www.ncbi.nlm.nih.gov/pubmed/11500247

Leuner B, Glasper ER, and Gould E. Sexual experience promotes adult neurogenesis in the hippocampus despite an initial elevation in stress hormones. *PLOS ONE*. 2010;5(7): e11597. https://doi.org/10.1371/journal.pone.0011597

Lorenz TK, Demas GE, and Heiman JR. Interaction of menstrual cycle phase and sexual activity predicts mucosal and systemic humoral immunity in healthy women. *Physiology & Behavior*. 2015;152(Pt A):92–98. https://doi.org/10.1016/j.physbeh.2015.09.018

Lorenz TK, Heiman JR, and Demas GE. Sexual activity modulates shifts in TH1/TH2 cytokine profile across the menstrual cycle: An observational study. *Fertility and Sterility*. 2015;104(6)1513–21. https://doi.org/10.1016/j.fertnstert.2015.09.001

Martins MA, Moss MB, Mendes IK, et al. Role of dietary fish oil on nitric oxide synthase activity and oxidative status in mice red blood cells. *Food & Function*. 2014;5(12): 3208–15. https://doi.org/10.1039/c4fo00055b

Meston CM. Sympathetic nervous system activity and female sexual arousal. *The American Journal of Cardiology*. 2000;86(2A):30F–34F. https://www.ncbi.nlm.nih.gov/pubmed/10899275

Murrell TG. The potential for oxytocin (OT) to prevent breast cancer: A hypothesis. *Breast Cancer Research and Treatment*. 1995;35(2):225–29. https://www.ncbi.nlm.nih.gov/pubmed/7647345

Om AS and Chung KW. Dietary zinc deficiency alters 5 alpha-reduction and aromatization of testosterone and androgen and estrogen receptors in rat liver. *The Journal of Nutrition*. 1996;126(4):842–48. https://doi.org/10.1093/jn/126.4.842

Panzer C, Wise S, Fantini G, et al. Impact of oral contraceptives on sex hormone-binding globulin and androgen levels: A retrospective study in women with sexual dysfunction. *The Journal of Sexual Medicine*. 2006;3(1):104–13. https://doi.org/10.1111/j.1743-6109.2005.00198.x

Paul KN, Turek FW, and Kryger MH. Influence of sex on sleep regulatory mechanisms. *Journal of Women's Health*. 2008;17(7):1201–8. https://doi.org/10.1089/jwh.2008.0841

Twenge JM, Sherman RA, and Wells BE. Declines in sexual frequency among American adults, 1989–2014. *Archives of Sexual Behavior*. 2017;46(8):2389–401. https://doi.org/10.1007/s10508-017-0953-1

Verhaeghe J, Gheysen R, and Enzlin P. Pheromones and their effect on women's mood and sexuality. *Facts, Views & Vision in ObGyn*. 2013;5(3):189–95. https://www.ncbi.nlm.nih.gov/pmc/articles/PMC3987372/

Wallwiener CW, Wallwiener L-M, Seeger H, et al. Prevalence of sexual dysfunction and impact of contraception in female German medical students. *The Journal of Sexual Medicine.* 2010;7(6):2139–48. https://doi.org/10.1111/j.1743-6109.2010.01742.x

Weeks D. *Secrets of the Superyoung.* New York: Penguin Group, 1998.

Chapter 9: Making Motherhood Easier

Apter D and Hermanson E. Update on female pubertal development. *Current Opinion in Obstetrics & Gynecology.* 2002;14:475–81. https://www.ncbi.nlm.nih.gov/pubmed/12401974

Brown B. *The Gifts of Imperfection: Let Go of Who You Think You're Supposed to Be and Embrace Who You Are.* Center City, MN: Hazelden Publishing, 2010.

Buttke DE, Sircar K, and Martin C. Exposures to endocrine-disrupting chemicals and age of menarche in adolescent girls in NHANES (2003–2008). *Environmental Health Perspectives.* 2012;120(11):1613–18. https://doi.org/10.1289/ehp.1104748

Campbell BC. Adrenarche and middle childhood. *Human Nature.* 2011;22:327. https://doi.org/10.1007/s12110-011-9120-x

Dass R. *Be Here Now.* San Cristobal, New Mexico: Lama Foundation, 1971.

Doss BD and Rhoades GK. The transition to parenthood: Impact on couples' romantic relationships. *Current Opinion in Psychology.* 2017;13:25–28. https://doi.org/10.1016/j.copsyc.2016.04.003

Dunneram Y, Greenwood DC, Burley VJ, et al. Dietary intake and age at natural menopause: Results from the UK Women's Cohort Study. *Journal of Epidemiology & Community Health.* 2018;72:733–40. http://dx.doi.org/10.1136/jech-2017-209887

Friedan B. *The Feminine Mystique* (50th Anniversary Edition). New York: W.W. Norton, 2013.

Galea LA, Wide JK, and Barr AM. Estradiol alleviates depressive-like symptoms in a novel animal model of post-partum depression. *Behavioural Brain Research.* 2001; 122(1):1–9. https://www.ncbi.nlm.nih.gov/pubmed/11287071

Garbes A. *Like a Mother: A Feminist Journey Through Science and Culture of Pregnancy.* New York: Harper Wave, 2018.

Hewlett SA and Buck Luce C. "Off-Ramps and On-Ramps: Keeping Talented Women on the Road to Success." *Harvard Business Review.* Mar. 2005. https://hbr.org/2005/03/off-ramps-and-on-ramps-keeping-talented-women-on-the-road-to-success

Hickey M, Balen A. Menstrual disorders in adolescence: Investigation and management. *Human Reproduction Update.* 2003;9:493–504. https://www.ncbi.nlm.nih.gov/pubmed/14640381

Hoekzema E, Barba-Muller E, Pozzobon C, et al. Pregnancy leads to long-lasting changes in human brain structure. *Nature Neuroscience.* 2017;20(2):287–300. https://doi.org/10.1038/nn.4458

"How Do I Know If My Menstrual Cycle Is Normal?" Planned Parenthood. Accessed Nov. 11, 2019. https://www.plannedparenthood.org/learn/health-and-wellness/menstruation/how-do-i-know-if-my-menstrual-cycle-normal

Kim P, Strathearn L, and Swain JE. The maternal brain and its plasticity in humans. *Hormones and Behavior.* 2016;77:113–23. https://doi.org/10.1016/j.yhbeh.2015.08.001

Koebele SV, et al. Hysterectomy uniquely impacts spatial memory in a rat model: A role for the nonpregnant uterus in cognitive processes. *Endocrinology.* 2019;160(1):1–19. https://www.ncbi.nlm.nih.gov/pubmed/30535329

Lawrence E, Cobb RJ, Rothman AD, et al. Marital satisfaction across the transition to parenthood. *Journal of Family Psychology: JFP: Journal of the Division of Family Psychology of the American Psychological Association (Division 43).* 2008;22(1):41–50. https://doi.org/10.1037/0893-3200.22.1.41

Liedloff, J. *The Continuum Concept: In Search of Happiness Lost.* Cambridge, MA: Perseus Books, 1986.

Mayo Clinic staff. "Menstrual Cycle: What's Normal, What's Not." Mayo Clinic. June 13, 2019. https://www.mayoclinic.org/healthy-lifestyle/womens-health/in-depth /menstrual-cycle/art-20047186

Nazarov I, Lee JW, Soupene E, et al. Multipotent stromal stem cells from human placenta demonstrate high therapeutic potential. *Stem Cells Translational Medicine.* 2012;1(5):359–72. https://doi.org/10.5966/sctm.2011-0021

Northrup C. "The Wisdom of Menopause." DrNorthrop.com. https://www.drnorthrup .com/wisdom-of-menopause/

Northrup C. *Women's Bodies, Women's Wisdom.* New York: Bantam Doubleday, 1997.

Chapter 10: Dynamic, Wise, and Free

Alexander E. *Proof of Heaven: A Neurosurgeon's Journey Into Life After Death.* New York: Simon & Schuster, 2012.

Chen Zeng T, Aw AJ, and Feldman MW. Cultural hitchhiking and competition between patrilineal kin groups explain the post-Neolithic Y-chromosome bottleneck. *Nature Communications.* 2018;9:2077. https://doi.org/10.1038/s41467-018-04375-6

D'Ambra Fagella L. "Women in Artificial Intelligence—A Visual Study of Leadership Across Industries." Sept.14, 2017. https://www.techemergence.com/women-in -artificial-intelligence-visual-study-leaderships-across-industries/

Datta A, Tschantz MC, and Datta A. Automated experiments on ad privacy settings: A tale of opacity, choice, and discrimination. *Proceedings on Privacy Enhancing Technologies.* 2015;(1):92–112. https://www.andrew.cmu.edu/user/danupam /dtd-pets15.pdf

Eller C. *The Myth of Matriarchal Prehistory: Why an Invented Past Won't Give Women a Future.* Boston, MA: Beacon Press, 2001.

Gimbutas, M. *The Civilization of the Goddess.* New York: HarperCollins, 1991.

Graf N, Brown A, and Patten E. "The Narrowing, but Persistent, Gender Gap in Pay." Pew Research Center. Apr. 9, 2018. http://www.pewresearch.org/fact-tank/2018/04/09 /gender-pay-gap-facts/

Gray M. *The Optimized Woman: Using Your Menstrual Cycle to Achieve Success and Fulfillment.* Hants, UK: O Books, 2009.

Johnson PA, Fitzgerald T, Salganicoff A, et al. *Sex-Specific Medical Research: Why Women's Health Can't Wait. A Report of the Mary Hogan Connors Center for Women's Health & Gender Biology at Brigham and Women's Hospital.* 2014. https://www.brighamandwomens .org/assets/BWH/womens-health/pdfs/ConnorsReportFINAL.pdf

Karmin M, Saag L, Vicente M, et al. A recent bottleneck of Y chromosome diversity coincides with a global change in culture. *Genome Research.* 2015;25(4):459–66. https:// doi.org/10.1101/gr.186684.114

Liu KA and Dipietro Mager NA. Women's involvement in clinical trials: Historical perspective and future implications. *Pharmacy Practice.* 2016;14(1):708. https://doi.org /10.18549/PharmPract.2016.01.708

Lorde A. *I Am Your Sister: Collected and Unpublished Writings of Audre Lorde.* Oxford: Oxford University Press, 2009. http://www.pages.drexel.edu/~jc3962/COR/Hierarchy.pdf

Myss C. *Why People Don't Heal and How They Can.* New York: Three Rivers Press, 1997.

Pinkola Estés C. *Women Who Run With the Wolves: Myths and Stories of the Wild Woman Archetype.* New York: Ballantine Books, 1992.

Pope A and Wurlitzer SH. *Wild Power: Discover the Magic of Your Menstrual Cycle and Awaken the Feminine Path to Power.* Carlsbad, CA: Hay House, 2017.

Rose S. *The Path of the Priestess: A Guidebook for Awakening the Divine Feminine.* Rochester, VT: Inner Traditions, 2003.

"The Women's Kingdom." *PBS Frontline.* July 19, 2005. http://www.pbs.org/frontlineworld /rough/2005/07/introduction_to.html

INDEX